Musculoskeletal Research: Biomechanics and Biomaterials for the Treatment of Orthopedic Diseases

Musculoskeletal Research: Biomechanics and Biomaterials for the Treatment of Orthopedic Diseases

Editors

Frank Seehaus
Bastian Welke

MDPI • Basel • Beijing • Wuhan • Barcelona • Belgrade • Manchester • Tokyo • Cluj • Tianjin

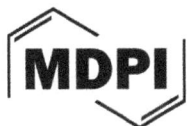

Editors
Frank Seehaus
Friedrich-Alexander
University of
Erlangen-Nürnberg
Erlangen
Germany

Bastian Welke
Hannover Medical School
Hannover
Germany

Editorial Office
MDPI
St. Alban-Anlage 66
4052 Basel, Switzerland

This is a reprint of articles from the Special Issue published online in the open access journal *Applied Sciences* (ISSN 2076-3417) (available at: https://www.mdpi.com/journal/applsci/special_issues/Orthopaedic_Biomaterials_Biomechanics).

For citation purposes, cite each article independently as indicated on the article page online and as indicated below:

LastName, A.A.; LastName, B.B.; LastName, C.C. Article Title. *Journal Name* **Year**, *Volume Number*, Page Range.

ISBN 978-3-0365-6844-7 (Hbk)
ISBN 978-3-0365-6845-4 (PDF)

© 2023 by the authors. Articles in this book are Open Access and distributed under the Creative Commons Attribution (CC BY) license, which allows users to download, copy and build upon published articles, as long as the author and publisher are properly credited, which ensures maximum dissemination and a wider impact of our publications.

The book as a whole is distributed by MDPI under the terms and conditions of the Creative Commons license CC BY-NC-ND.

Contents

Bastian Welke and Frank Seehaus
Special Issue on Musculoskeletal Research: Biomechanics and Biomaterials for the Treatment of Orthopedic Diseases
Reprinted from: *Appl. Sci.* **2022**, *12*, 8968, doi:10.3390/app12188968 1

Junzhe Wu, Dominic Taylor, Raimund Forst and Frank Seehaus
Does Pelvic Orientation Influence Wear Measurement of the Acetabular Cup in Total Hip Arthroplasty—An Experimental Study
Reprinted from: *Appl. Sci.* **2021**, *11*, 10014, doi:10.3390/app112110014 3

Kevin Knappe, Christian Stadler, Moritz Innmann, Mareike Schonhoff, Tobias Gotterbarm, Tobias Renkawitz and Sebastian Jaeger
Does Pressurized Carbon Dioxide Lavage Improve Bone Cleaning in Cemented Arthroplasty?
Reprinted from: *Appl. Sci.* **2021**, *11*, 6103, doi:10.3390/app11136103 17

Eike Franken, Thilo Floerkemeier, Eike Jakubowitz, Alexander Derksen, Stefan Budde, Henning Windhagen and Nils Wirries
What Is the Impact of a CAM Impingement on the Gait Cycle in Patients with Progressive Osteoarthritis of the Hip?
Reprinted from: *Appl. Sci.* **2021**, *11*, 6024, doi:10.3390/app11136024 27

Johanna K. Buschatzky, Michael Schwarze, Nils Wirries, Gabriela von Lewinski, Henning Windhagen, Thilo Floerkemeier and Stefan Budde
The Rate of Correctly Planned Size of Digital Templating in Two Planes—A Comparative Study of a Short-Stem Total Hip Implant with Primary Metaphyseal Fixation and a Conventional Stem
Reprinted from: *Appl. Sci.* **2021**, *11*, 3965, doi:10.3390/app11093965 39

Witit Pothong, Phichayut Phinyo, Yuddhasert Sirirungruangsarn, Kriengkrai Nabudda, Nattamon Wongba, Chatchawarl Sarntipiphat and Dumnoensun Pruksakorn
Biomechanical Analysis of Sagittal Plane Pin Placement Configurations for Pediatric Supracondylar Humerus Fractures
Reprinted from: *Appl. Sci.* **2021**, *11*, 3447, doi:10.3390/app11083447 51

Leandra Bauer, Manuel Kistler, Arnd Steinbrück, Katrin Ingr, Peter E. Müller, Volkmar Jansson, Christian Schröder, et al.
Different ISO Standards' Wear Kinematic Profiles Change the TKA Inlay Load
Reprinted from: *Appl. Sci.* **2021**, *11*, 3161, doi:10.3390/app11073161 61

Maeruan Kebbach, Christian Schulze, Christian Meyenburg, Daniel Kluess, Mevluet Sungu, Albrecht Hartmann, Klaus-Peter Günther, et al.
An MRI-Based Patient-Specific Computational Framework for the Calculation of Range of Motion of Total Hip Replacements
Reprinted from: *Appl. Sci.* **2021**, *11*, 2852, doi:10.3390/app11062852 73

Mareike Schonhoff, Therese Bormann, Kevin Knappe, Tobias Reiner, Linda Stange and Sebastian Jaeger
The Effect of Cement Aging on the Stability of a Cement-in-Cement Revision Construct
Reprinted from: *Appl. Sci.* **2021**, *11*, 2814, doi:10.3390/app11062814 93

Jessica Hembus, Felix Ambellan, Stefan Zachow and Rainer Bader
Establishment of a Rolling-Sliding Test Bench to Analyze Abrasive Wear Propagation of Different Bearing Materials for Knee Implants
Reprinted from: *Appl. Sci.* **2021**, *11*, 1886, doi:10.3390/app11041886 103

Fon-Yih Tsuang, Chia-Hsien Chen, Lien-Chen Wu, Yi-Jie Kuo, Yueh-Ying Hsieh and Chang-Jung Chiang
Partial Threading of Pedicle Screws in a Standard Construct Increases Fatigue Life: A Biomechanical Analysis
Reprinted from: *Appl. Sci.* **2021**, *11*, 1503, doi:10.3390/app11041503 119

Johannes Pordzik, Anke Bernstein, Julius Watrinet, Hermann O. Mayr, Sergio H. Latorre, Hagen Schmal and Michael Seidenstuecker
Correlation of Biomechanical Alterations under Gonarthritis between Overlying Menisci and Articular Cartilage
Reprinted from: *Appl. Sci.* **2020**, *10*, 8673, doi:10.3390/app10238673 129

Jing Xu, Han Cao, Stefan Sesselmann, Dominic Taylor, Raimund Forst and Frank Seehaus
Model-Based Roentgen Stereophotogrammetric Analysis Using Elementary Geometrical Shape Models: Reliability of Migration Measurements for an Anatomically Shaped Femoral Stem Component
Reprinted from: *Appl. Sci.* **2020**, *10*, 8507, doi:10.3390/app10238507 141

Stefan van Drongelen, Hanna Kaldowski, Benjamin Fey, Timur Tarhan, Ayman Assi, Felix Stief and Andrea Meurer
Determination of Leg Alignment in Hip Osteoarthritis Patients with the EOS® System and the Effect on External Joint Moments during Gait
Reprinted from: *Appl. Sci.* **2020**, *10*, 7777, doi:10.3390/app10217777 155

Soo-Bin Lee, Hwan-Mo Lee, Tae-Hyun Park, Sung Jae Lee, Young-Woo Kwon, Seong-Hwan Moon and Byung Ho Lee
Biomechanical Comparison of Posterior Fixation Combinations with an Allograft Spacer between the Lateral Mass and Pedicle Screws
Reprinted from: *Appl. Sci.* **2020**, *10*, 7291, doi:10.3390/app10207291 169

Ilka Schneider, Stephan Zierz, Stephan Schulze, Karl-Stefan Delank, Kevin G. Laudner, Richard Brill and René Schwesig
Characterization of Gait and Postural Regulation in Late-Onset Pompe Disease
Reprinted from: *Appl. Sci.* **2020**, *10*, 7001, doi:10.3390/app10197001 181

Kay Brehme, Thomas Bartels, Martin Pyschik, Manuel Jenz, Karl-Stefan Delank, Kevin G. Laudner and René Schwesig
Postural Stability and Regulation before and after High Tibial Osteotomy and Rehabilitation
Reprinted from: *Appl. Sci.* **2020**, *10*, 6517, doi:10.3390/app10186517 197

Ji-Won Kwon, Hwan-Mo Lee, Tae-Hyun Park, Sung Jae Lee, Young-Woo Kwon, Seong-Hwan Moon and Byung Ho Lee
Biomechanical Analysis of Allograft Spacer Failure as a Function of Cortical-Cancellous Ratio in Anterior Cervical Discectomy/Fusion: Allograft Spacer Alone Model
Reprinted from: *Appl. Sci.* **2020**, *10*, 6413, doi:10.3390/app10186413 217

Kerstin Radtke, Fabian Goede, Michael Schwarze, Peter Paes, Max Ettinger and Bastian Welke
Fixation Stability and Stiffness of Two Implant Systems for Proximal Femoral Varization Osteotomy
Reprinted from: *Appl. Sci.* **2020**, *10*, 5867, doi:10.3390/app10175867 229

René Schwesig, Regina Wegener, Christof Hurschler, Kevin Laudner and Frank Seehaus
Intra- and Interobserver Reliability Comparison of Clinical Gait Analysis Data between Two Gait Laboratories
Reprinted from: *Appl. Sci.* **2020**, *10*, 5068, doi:10.3390/app10155068 237

Editorial

Special Issue on Musculoskeletal Research: Biomechanics and Biomaterials for the Treatment of Orthopedic Diseases

Bastian Welke [1] and Frank Seehaus [2,3,*]

[1] Laboratory for Biomechanics and Biomaterials, Department of Orthopaedic Surgery, Hannover Medical School, 30625 Hannover, Germany
[2] Department of Orthopaedic Surgery, Friedrich Alexander University of Erlangen-Nürnberg, 91054 Erlangen, Germany
[3] Department of Trauma and Orthopedic Surgery, University Hospital Erlangen, Friedrich-Alexander University Erlangen-Nürnberg, 91054 Erlangen, Germany
* Correspondence: frank.seehaus@fau.de

Musculoskeletal research deals with the effects of the orthopedic treatment of pathologies on the biomechanics of the affected areas and on the musculoskeletal system. Biomechanical measurement methods enable the quantitative determination of these influences and the assessment of their extent and size in the patient (in vivo).

The range of examination methods is particularly wide in this field of musculoskeletal research. On one hand, in vitro examinations under laboratory conditions on simplified models, such as artificial bones or specimens from donors, are implemented. With the help of these models, for example, new biomaterials or implants for the treatment of fractures are often examined for their primary stability or to determine the influence of a joint replacement on their kinematics. In contrast to experimental in vitro studies, numerical methods are increasingly applied to analyze a large number of implant configurations and loading scenarios. Using the method of clinical motion analysis, a comprehensive in vivo investigation of the musculoskeletal system is performed directly on the patient. An example of its advantages is that it allows the monitoring and control of therapeutic interventions.

However, it is of great importance to know the limits and possibilities of the applied methodology in its preclinical and clinical applications. In order to reliably answer clinical questions on orthopedic interventions, established and extensively validated methods and measurement protocols are the only choice.

This Special Issue intends to provide the reader with an exciting overview of current research in the field of biomechanical investigations for the treatment of musculoskeletal diseases according topics such as tissue biomechanics [1], in vivo diagnostics [2], numerical simulation [3,4], tribology [4,5], experimental biomechanics [6–12], joint kinematics [3], motion/gait analysis [3,13–17], and implant fixation [18,19]. These accepted manuscripts are just a few examples from the field of musculoskeletal research and its methods. They all have the common goal of increasing patient safety.

Funding: This research received no external funding.

Acknowledgments: We thank all the authors and peer reviewers for their valuable contributions to this Special Issue 'Musculoskeletal Research: Biomechanics and Biomaterials for the Treatment of Orthopedic Diseases'. In particular, we would like to thank the research network Muskuloskelettale Biomechanik (MSB-Net) der Sektion Grundlagengforschung der Deutschen Gesellschaft für Orthopädie und Unfallchirurgie (DGOU) for the numerous contributions submitted. We would also like to express our gratitude to all the staff and people involved in this Special Issue. Finally, we offer special thanks to Karen Yang.

Conflicts of Interest: The authors declare no conflict of interest.

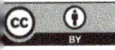

References

1. Pordzik, J.; Bernstein, A.; Watrinet, J.; Mayr, H.O.; Latorre, S.H.; Schmal, H.; Seidenstuecker, M. Correlation of Biomechanical Alterations under Gonarthritis between Overlying Menisci and Articular Cartilage. *Appl. Sci.* **2020**, *10*, 8673. [CrossRef]
2. Buschatzky, J.K.; Schwarze, M.; Wirries, N.; von Lewinski, G.; Windhagen, H.; Floerkemeier, T.; Budde, S. The Rate of Correctly Planned Size of Digital Templating in Two Planes—A Comparative Study of a Short-Stem Total Hip Implant with Primary Metaphyseal Fixation and a Conventional Stem. *Appl. Sci.* **2021**, *11*, 3965. [CrossRef]
3. Kebbach, M.; Schulze, C.; Meyenburg, C.; Kluess, D.; Sungu, M.; Hartmann, A.; Günther, K.P.; Bader, R. An MRI-Based Patient-Specific Computational Framework for the Calculation of Range of Motion of Total Hip Replacements. *Appl. Sci.* **2021**, *11*, 2852. [CrossRef]
4. Bauer, L.; Kistler, M.; Steinbrück, A.; Ingr, K.; Müller, P.E.; Jansson, V.; Schröder, C.; Woiczinski, M. Different ISO Standards' Wear Kinematic Profiles Change the TKA Inlay Load. *Appl. Sci.* **2021**, *11*, 3161. [CrossRef]
5. Hembus, J.; Ambellan, F.; Zachow, S.; Bader, R. Establishment of a Rolling-Sliding Test Bench to Analyze Abrasive Wear Propagation of Different Bearing Materials for Knee Implants. *Appl. Sci.* **2021**, *11*, 1886. [CrossRef]
6. Radtke, K.; Goede, F.; Schwarze, M.; Paes, P.; Ettinger, M.; Welke, B. Fixation Stability and Stiffness of Two Implant Systems for Proximal Femoral Varization Osteotomy. *Appl. Sci.* **2020**, *10*, 5867. [CrossRef]
7. Kwon, J.W.; Lee, H.M.; Park, T.H.; Lee, S.J.; Kwon, J.W.; Moon, S.W.; Lee, B.H. Biomechanical Analysis of Allograft Spacer Failure as a Function of Cortical-Cancellous Ratio in Anterior Cervical Discectomy/Fusion: Allograft Spacer Alone Model. *Appl. Sci.* **2020**, *10*, 6413. [CrossRef]
8. Lee, S.B.; Lee, H.M.; Park, T.H.; Lee, S.J.; Kwon, Y.W.; Moon, S.H.; Lee, B.H. Biomechanical Comparison of Posterior Fixation Combinations with an Allograft Spacer between the Lateral Mass and Pedicle Screws. *Appl. Sci.* **2020**, *10*, 7291. [CrossRef]
9. Tsuang, F.Y.; Chen, C.H.; Wu, L.H.; Kuo, Y.J.; Hsieh, Y.Y.; Chiang, C.J. Partial Threading of Pedicle Screws in a Standard Construct Increases Fatigue Life: A Biomechanical Analysis. *Appl. Sci.* **2021**, *11*, 1503. [CrossRef]
10. Pothong, W.; Phinyo, P.; Sirirungruangsarn, Y.; Nabudda, K.; Wongba, N.; Sarntipiphat, C.; Pruksakorn, D. Biomechanical Analysis of Sagittal Plane Pin Placement Configurations for Pediatric Supracondylar Humerus Fractures. *Appl. Sci.* **2021**, *11*, 3447. [CrossRef]
11. Knappe, K.; Stadler, C.; Innmann, M.; Schonhoff, M.; Gotterbarm, T.; Renkawitz, T.; Jaeger, S. Does Pressurized Carbon Dioxide Lavage Improve Bone Cleaning in Cemented Arthroplasty? *Appl. Sci.* **2021**, *11*, 6103. [CrossRef]
12. Wu, J.; Taylor, D.; Forst, R.; Seehaus, F. Does Pelvic Orientation Influence Wear Measurement of the Acetabular Cup in Total Hip Arthroplasty—An Experimental Study. *Appl. Sci.* **2021**, *11*, 10014. [CrossRef]
13. Schwesig, R.; Wegener, R.; Hurschler, C.; Laudner, K.G.; Seehaus, F. Intra- and Interobserver Reliability Comparison of Clinical Gait Analysis Data between Two Gait Laboratories. *Appl. Sci.* **2020**, *10*, 5068. [CrossRef]
14. Brehme, K.; Bartels, T.; Pyschik, M.; Jenz, M.; Delank, K.S.; Laudner, K.G.; Schwesig, R. Postural Stability and Regulation before and after High Tibial Osteotomy and Rehabilitation. *Appl. Sci.* **2020**, *10*, 6517. [CrossRef]
15. Schneider, I.; Zierz, S.; Schulze, S.; Delank, K.S.; Laudner, K.G.; Brill, R.; Schwesig, R. Characterization of Gait and Postural Regulation in Late-Onset Pompe Disease. *Appl. Sci.* **2020**, *10*, 7001. [CrossRef]
16. van Drongelen, S.; Kaldowski, H.; Fey, B.; Tarhan, T.; Assi, A.; Stief, F.; Meurer, A. Determination of Leg Alignment in Hip Osteoarthritis Patients with the EOS®System and the Effect on External Joint Moments during Gait. *Appl. Sci.* **2020**, *10*, 7777. [CrossRef]
17. Franken, E.; Floerkemeier, T.; Jakubowitz, E.; Derksen, A.; Budde, S.; Windhagen, H.; Wirries, N. What Is the Impact of a CAM Impingement on the Gait Cycle in Patients with Progressive Osteoarthritis of the Hip? *Appl. Sci.* **2021**, *11*, 6024. [CrossRef]
18. Xu, J.; Cao, H.; Sesselmann, S.; Taylor, D.; Forst, R.; Seehaus, F. Model-Based Roentgen Stereophotogrammetric Analysis Using Elementary Geometrical Shape Models: Reliability of Migration Measurements for an Anatomically Shaped Femoral Stem Component. *Appl. Sci.* **2020**, *10*, 8507. [CrossRef]
19. Schonhoff, M.; Bormann, T.; Knappe, K.; Reiner, T.; Stange, L.; Jaeger, S. The Effect of Cement Aging on the Stability of a Cement-in-Cement Revision Construct. *Appl. Sci.* **2021**, *11*, 2814. [CrossRef]

Article

Does Pelvic Orientation Influence Wear Measurement of the Acetabular Cup in Total Hip Arthroplasty—An Experimental Study

Junzhe Wu [1,2], Dominic Taylor [3], Raimund Forst [1] and Frank Seehaus [1,4,*]

[1] Department of Orthopaedic Surgery, Faculty of Medicine, Friedrich-Alexander University Erlangen-Nürnberg (FAU), 91054 Erlangen, Germany; wu.jun.zhe@outlook.com (J.W.); raimund.forst@fau.de (R.F.)
[2] Department of Orthopaedic Surgery, The Second Affiliated Hospital, Fujian Medical University, Quanzhou 362000, China
[3] Department of Orthopaedic and Trauma Surgery, Hospital Coburg, 96450 Coburg, Germany; dominictaylor2000@yahoo.com
[4] Department of Trauma and Orthopaedic Surgery, University Hospital Erlangen, Friedrich-Alexander University Erlangen-Nürnberg (FAU), 91054 Erlangen, Germany
* Correspondence: frank.seehaus@fau.de

Abstract: Roentgen stereophotogrammetric analysis (RSA) is the gold standard to detect in vivo material wear of the bearing couples in hip arthroplasty. Some surgical planning tools offer the opportunity to detect wear by using standard a.p. radiographs ($2D_{wear}$), whilst RSA ($3D_{wear}$) needs a special radiological setup. The aims of this study are to prove the interchangeable applicability of a $2D_{wear}$ approach next to RSA and to assess the influence of different pelvic positions on measurement outcomes. An implant-bone model was used to mimic three different wear scenarios in seven pelvic-femur alignment positions. RSA and a.p. radiographs of the reference and a follow-up (simulated wear) pose were acquired. Accuracy and precision were worse for the $2D_{wear}$ approach (0.206 mm; 0.159 mm) in comparison to the $3D_{wear}$ approach (0.043 mm; 0.017 mm). Changing the pelvic position significantly influenced the $2D_{wear}$ results (4 of 7, $p < 0.05$), whilst $3D_{wear}$ results showed almost no change. The $3D_{wear}$ is superior to the $2D_{wear}$ approach, as it is less susceptible to changes in pelvic position. However, the results suggest that a $2D_{wear}$ approach may be an alternative method if the wear present is in the range of 100–500 µm and a.p. radiographs are available with the pelvis projected in a neutral position.

Keywords: polyethylene wear; roentgen stereophotogrammetric analysis; total hip arthroplasty; precision; accuracy; pelvic orientation

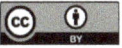

1. Introduction

The success of total hip arthroplasty (THA) depends on good interaction between three factors: (i) the surgeon/surgical technique; (ii) the implant and (iii) the patient [1]. THA replaces the bio-tribological system of the patient's native hip joint. The soft human cartilage of the femoral head and the acetabulum is replaced by some kind of harder material, such as ultra-high molecular weight polyethylene (UHMWPE), cobalt chrome molybdenum alloy or ceramic, which now represents the new "artificial" bearing situation for the patient. The materials used in the THA are subjected to mechanical stress, especially in the area of the bearing couple [2,3]. Each material replacing something within the native human joints is, without exception, susceptible to material wear. Out of a technical perspective, it could be stated that if two materials articulate against each other under enormous stresses, tribological wear results [3]. The applied material, ball head size, or a combination of both within the "artificial" bearing influences the clinical outcome and long-term survival rate [4–6]. However, THA failure is a multifactorial problem. Registries identify aseptic loosening as one of the five main reasons for revision surgery of primary THA [6,7]. Aseptic loosening also has a multifactorial etiology, and its mechanism is not explained by a single theory [8]. One cause of implant loosening is the combination of tribological and biological processes [9]. A major factor leading to aseptic implant loosening is the destruction of the periprosthetic bone. Wear particles are incorporated by macrophages, stimulating osteoclasts and degrading periprosthetic bone. The relative movements of two materials against each other under high compressive forces always lead to tribological abrasion. The material properties of the sliding partners, as well as their quality, determine the degree of wear and the shape of the wear products (so-called particles), which, in each case, determine the concrete biological behaviour in type and extent [3].

Wear detection of artificial joints can be performed within an experimental in vitro or a clinical in vivo setting. Tribological testing of THA bearing couples is essential for the evaluation of wear properties and the resulting debris. This is an important part of the preclinical approval of new medical materials or devices. However, experimental testing is associated with limitations, while the "real world" for the biological behaviour within the human body is not one-to-one exchangeable onto a testing bench. To validate tribological material behaviour under "real world" conditions, an in vivo detection of wear is necessary and required. There is a high priority and relevance for clinical acetabular cup wear measurements to assess common or new types of polymers that implant manufacturers introduce [10].

To detect in vivo wear of THA, several radiographic techniques are available [11], including conventional standard a.p. radiographs of the hip joint, special radiographs using the Roentgen stereophotogrammetric analysis (RSA) method [12], computer tomography [13], and magnetic resonance imaging [14]. These mentioned imaging techniques can be divided into two-dimensional wear detection methods, including standard a.p. radiographs ($2D_{wear}$), and three-dimensional methods ($3D_{wear}$), including multi-plane radiographs (RSA) within a specialized radiological setup or a multilayer stack of radiographs (CT, MRI) of the artificial hip. However, modern $2D_{wear}$ methods are developed and used to detect standard UHMWPE cups with a wear rate between 0.1 mm and 0.2 mm/year [10]. Teeter et al. [15] reported 13 year results and found a wear rate of 0.08 ± 0.03 mm/year for a conventional polyethylene and of 0.04 ± 0.02 mm/year for a crosslinked polyethylene. Wear was measured using RSA as a $3D_{wear}$ method. Within a 7-year follow-up clinical trial, the in vivo total wear data for vitamin E-diffused highly crosslinked polyethylene was reported to be 0.03 mm (SD 0.25), which was lower in comparison to a moderately crosslinked polyethylene of 0.04 mm (SD 0.29) [12]. Consequently, this means that the radiological methods mentioned above must have a sufficiently high resolution to measure beyond these values. With regard to the aforementioned dimensions of PE wear to be determined, it becomes clear in which resolution range the applied measuring methods must be able to work. It should be mentioned that the biological reaction to wear particle size and their quantity with different PE configurations is not the subject of this paper.

$2D_{wear}$ measurements based on conventional a.p. radiographs of the hip prosthesis are common in clinical routines since these radiographs are available at any hospital without the need for additional specialized equipment. However, these approaches yield only a 2D characterisation of the present wear and demonstrate less sensitivity to radiographic projection differences [16]. According to the sensitivity and the resulting radiographic projection differences, Collier et al. [17] reported that the accuracy of wear results varied with acetabular component angulations. It could be stated, thus, that the greater the change of acetabular component angulations within the images, the larger the magnitude of wear measured. A general problem and limitation within a $2D_{wear}$ approach is the detection of wear which occurs out of the image plane of the a.p. radiographs [18].

Ilchman et al. [19] compared clinical hip wear data in 13 patients with THA 3 years after surgery using 4 different radiological methods: (i) RSA, (ii) the Scheier–Sandel method, (iii) the Charnley–Duo method and (iv) "Ein-Bild-Roentgenanalyse (EBRA)". Mean (SD) measurement error for EBRA was, in the worst case, 0.11 mm (±0.12 mm). After excluding radiographs with the presence of a pelvic tilt (rotation around the horizontal axis), the error decreased to 0.08 mm (±0.11 mm). In comparison to RSA, the mean difference of the Scheier–Sandel method was reported in a worst case to be 0.17 mm (SD 0.21 mm) and a best case to be 0.14 mm (SD 0.25 mm). For the Charnley–Duo method, the mean difference was 0.27 mm (SD 0.27 mm). The EBRA method was found to be the most accurate compared to the gold standard RSA, and the Scheier–Sandel method was not recommended for wear analysis. However, Ilchman et al. [19] recommended the Charnley–Duo method, because this method demonstrated good correlation in relation to the RSA approach as the gold standard. Within a related paper, Ilchman [20] identified a pelvic tilt as the main error influencing measured wear results.

Langlois et al. [21] validated the computerized semiautomatic edge detection method for cemented PE components (Hip Analysis Suite, version 8.0.1.4.3; UCTech the University of Chicago) within an experimental setting. Accuracy and precision were reported to be 0.060 ± 0.021 mm (mean ± SD) and 0.207 ± 0.099 mm, respectively. In comparison to validation values of the RSA approach [22], the accuracy was comparable to, and precision was inferior to, RSA.

Derbyshire and Barkatali [10] reported achieving a similar accuracy to RSA by using a customized $2D_{wear}$ measurement tool. Bias, defined as the mean (SD) error of the simulated head penetration measurements, was about −0.002 mm (±0.028 mm), and precision was 0.055 mm for this 2D approach.

RSA is a $3D_{wear}$ approach which presents an accurate measurement tool for the in vivo assessment of polyethylene wear in THA [13] and is regarded as the gold standard [16,23]. An associated disadvantage of the RSA approach is its complexity in the acquisition of RSA image pairs. In addition, a second X-ray source, as well as a calibration box, is required during image acquisition. Furthermore, special analysis software must be purchased. However, besides the mentioned additional roentgen equipment, additional X-ray images are also required, as the standard a.p. radiographs cannot be used for wear detection using the RSA approach. These additional X-ray images mean an additional radiation exposure for the patient, which is challenging in the context of radiation hygiene for the patient.

Von Schewelov et al. [24] reported that it was difficult to determine small amounts of wear in vivo if the RSA method was not used. The accuracy of RSA, irrespective of the prosthetic component studied or the direction of wear, was reported to be about 0.4; mean error was reported to be 0.010 mm. These were compared to two 2D approaches, which demonstrated an accuracy of 1.3 for each and a mean error of 0.19 mm (Charnley–Duo method) and 0.13 mm (Imagika). However, the authors reported the effect of image quality as well and applied RSA technology. The results indicated that a digital RSA analysis decreased the mean measurement error from 0.011 to 0.004 mm. The authors therefore hypothesized that using a digital RSA measurement setup would probably culminate in better results [24].

Preoperative planning software enables, in addition to the preoperative planning of total joint arthroplasty, the measurement of THA wear using standard a.p. radiographs of the pelvic region. Wear measurement using these kinds of radiographs is conducted for two reasons. Firstly, wear along the x-axis and y-axis on the coronal plane is extensively considered to be the site of occurrence of the most wear [25]. Secondly, lateral radiographs are of low quality and do not meet the requirements for wear measurement [26].

The main question, therefore, is whether a simple measurement method, such as the mentioned $2D_{wear}$ method used in the manuscript, which is integrated within commercially available preoperative planning software can determine the in vivo wear of THA bearing couples in a manner that is equivalent to the gold standard. The current gold standard measurement method could be associated with some challenges; likewise, its complexity in the acquisition of RSA image pairs has been mentioned above. Therefore, if a clinic has an in vivo wear measuring tool available, e.g., already integrated in a software solution for preoperative planning, the assessment of its accuracy is essential before its clinical application. To the authors' knowledge, to date, there have not been many studies comparing $2D_{wear}$ with $3D_{wear}$ methods to detect acetabular cup insert wear. There is no data available within literature which validates the investigated $2D_{wear}$ approach. Testing the interchangeability of a $2D_{wear}$ method next to the gold standard RSA is rarely described in the literature; the potential influence of the pelvic orientation onto wear measurement outcomes is also rarely described in the literature. Therefore, pelvic positioning could be added as an influencing factor within this investigation.

The aims of this experimental study are:

(1) to evaluate the interchangeability of $2D_{wear}$ next to the gold standard $3D_{wear}$ method by comparing the accuracy and reproducibility of both methods;
(2) to determine further the extent to which the two different methods are influenced by changing pelvic orientation.

The authors hypothesize that the $3D_{wear}$ detection method would show higher precision and accuracy than the $2D_{wear}$ detection method and be insensitive to pelvic misalignment.

2. Materials and Methods

The measurement protocol required a measurement setup that was capable of imaging an implant-bone model with two radiographic wear detection methods in parallel. The same implant-bone model setting was presented within the resulting radiographs. Out of these RSA and a.p. radiographs, the linear wear was detected by both methods.

2.1. Measurement Setup

A classical radiological setup using ceiling-fixed roentgen tubes (Multix RD 82477-01 Vertix ACS, Siemens, Berlin, Germany) to acquire standard a.p. pelvic radiographs was used (Figure 1a). While changing the classical radiological setup to a uniplanar RSA setup, the implant-bone model positions on the roentgen table were unchanged (Figure 1b). The uniplanar RSA setup consisted of a ceiling-fixed (Multix RD 82477-01 Vertix ACS, Siemens, Berlin, Germany) and a mobile roentgen tube (Mobilett Plus, Siemens, Berlin, Germany), which were arranged relative to a calibration box (Umea Cage 43, RSA BioMedical Developments AB, Umea, Sweden). The implant-bone model was located within the intersection of the two X-ray beams. The two X-ray tubes were triggered manually for simultaneous generation of RSA radiographs (Figure 1c).

2.2. Implant-Bone Model

The implant-bone model should make it possible to simulate a sequential linear penetration of the femoral ball head into the acetabular cup insert. This penetration is used to simulate polyethylene (PE) wear.

A synthetic femoral and pelvic model (Sawbone Foam Cortical Shell, Pacific Research Laboratories Inc., Vashon, WA, USA) presented the basic elements of the implant-bone-model (Figure 2). Within the synthetic femoral bone model, an uncemented stem component (VECTOR-TITAN, Peter Brehm, Weisendorf, Germany) was inserted according to all rules of a surgical THA procedure. Onto the taper of the femoral stem component, a 32 mm cobalt-chromium ball head was connected. The ball head was positioned as the reference position in the center of an uncemented, 58 mm titanium acetabular cup without PE insert (PHÖNIX-TITAN, Peter Brehm, Weisendorf, Germany), which was implanted into the acetabulum of the synthetic pelvic bone. The femoral bone model was rigidly fixed to 3D micrometer screw equipment (Mitutoyo, Kanagawa, Japan), which enabled a movement of the femoral stem-head junction around three degrees of freedom along medio-lateral, cranio-caudal, and anterior-posterior axes relative to the global coordinate system cup. This free mobility was possible because only the metallic cup component was used without a PE insert inside.

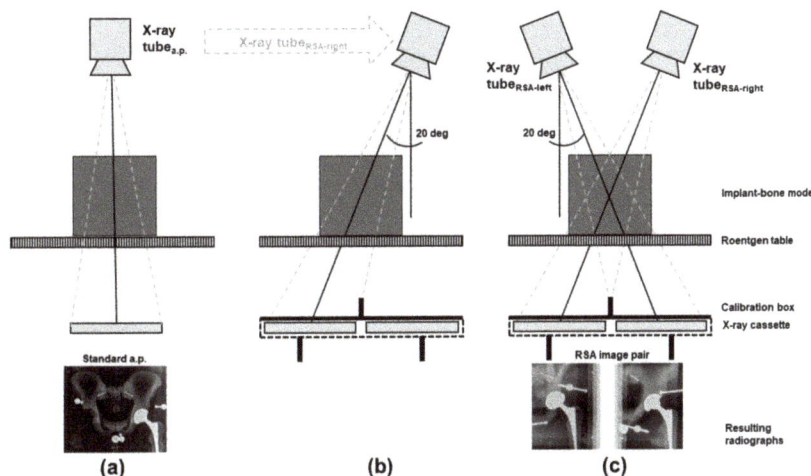

Figure 1. Radiological setup. (**a**) Classical set up to generate an a.p. radiograph of the pelvis. The implant-bone model is located in the middle of the central X-ray beam. (**b**) When X-ray tube$_{a.p.}$ shifts to the X-ray tube$_{RSA-right}$ position, the classical radiological setup is converted to (**c**) a uniplanar RSA setup. Both roentgen tubes are arranged at an angle of 20 deg to the vertical above the calibration box. The implant-bone model is located at the intersection of both X-ray beams.

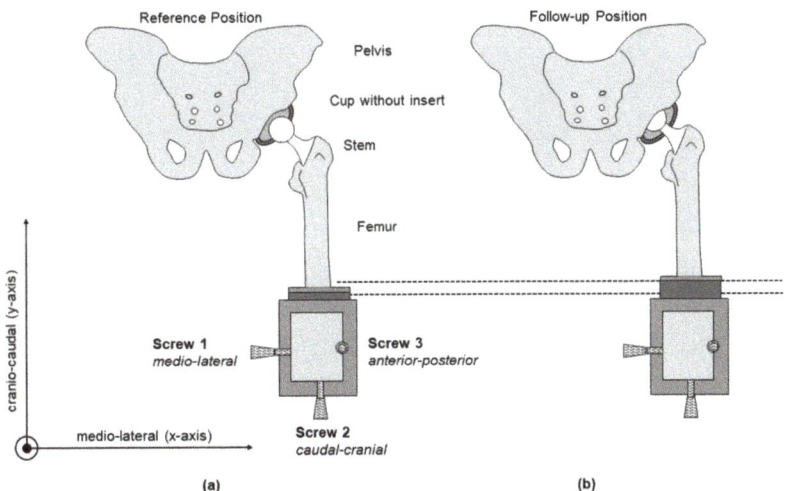

Figure 2. A schematic drawing of the implant-bone model with a femoral and pelvic element in (**a**) the reference position and (**b**) the follow-up position. The femoral part of the implant-bone model was moved according to the measurement protocol by the three screws (see Section 2.3). The alignment of the implant-bone model, as well as the wear simulation and pelvic positions, were performed according to the global coordinate system: medio-lateral axis (x-axis), cranio-caudal axis (y-axis), and anterior-posterior axis (z-axis).

Additionally, the pelvic element of the implant-bone-model could be relatively aligned to the femoral stem-ball head junction. In summary, the pelvis could be positioned in seven different positions.

2.3. Measurement Protocol

In accordance with the study protocol of Stilling et al. [27], 3 different wear settings were predefined, all of which could be mimicked by the implant-bone-model: low wear (0.01 to 0.05 mm), medium wear (0.1 to 0.5 mm), and high wear (1 to 5 mm). For each individual wear setting, a 3D wear vector could be simulated, which was defined as a set point value, representing the calculated true vector length by use of Pythagoras' theorem.

According to the wear setting (low, medium, high), the micrometer screws increased sequentially along medio-lateral, cranio-caudal, and anterior-posterior axes of 0.01 mm, 0.1 mm, and 1 mm, respectively.

In addition to a neutral pelvic position (Figure 3a), the pelvic model element could be aligned in six other positions: pelvic tilt (Figure 3b), pelvic obliquity (Figure 3c), and pelvic rotation (Figure 3d). A reference and follow-up radiographs—the RSA image pair and classical a.p.—were taken before (as reference) and after (follow up) the performed measurement protocol. All the iterative simulations for the wear and pelvic position protocol were repeated five times.

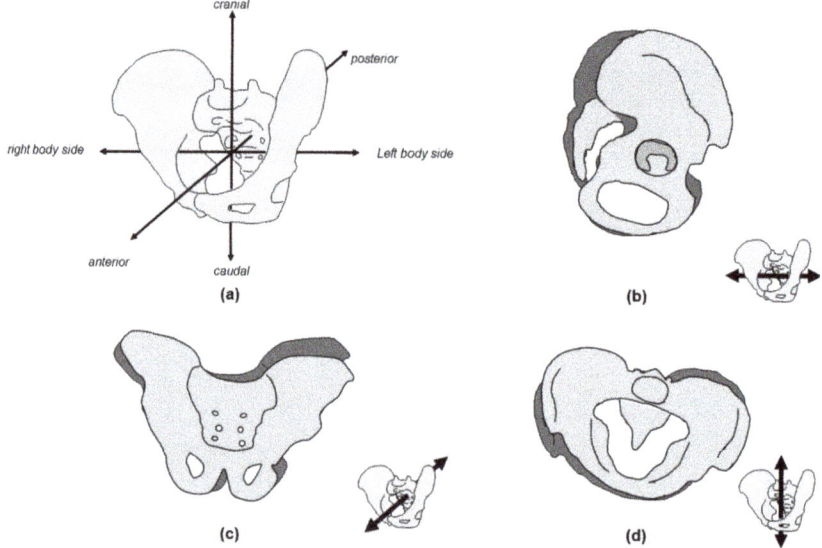

Figure 3. Pelvic model element and its alignment options. (**a**) Local coordinate system based on an anatomical axis of the pelvic model element. (**b**) Anterior/posterior inclination up to ±5 deg of so-called pelvic tilt, presenting a motion within the sagittal plane, representing rotation around the medio-lateral axis. (**c**) Lateral inclination up to ±5 deg of so-called pelvic obliquity, presenting a motion within the frontal plane and rotation around the anterior-posterior axis. (**d**) Pelvic rotation up to ±5 deg, presenting a motion within the transverse plane and rotation around the cranio-caudal axis.

2.4. Data Analysis

The resulting radiographs of the implant-bone model setting from the three wear simulation protocols and seven pelvic orientations were analysed by $2D_{wear}$ and $3D_{wear}$ approaches.

For the $2D_{wear}$ method, wear analysis was performed using plain radiographs and the wear analysis tool of a standard digital surgical planning software (mediCAD Classic, version 5.1, mediCAD Hectec GmbH, Landshut, Germany). Wear detection could be performed with two or more follow-up radiographic images. According to the instructions for use provided by the manufacturer, the wear procedure was only applicable for acetabular cups with a spherical outer contour and a bearing couple PE inlay with a ceramic or metal ball head. Radiographs required the presence of a calibration sphere within the radiographs (original mediCAD calibration sphere, diameter: 25 mm; tolerance: ±0.1 mm). To enable THA wear detection within two scaled X-ray images, a correctly drawn reference line, detected ball head centres, and acetabular cup centres were required. The reference line was located and defined by the Köhler's "tear drop" or by the tangent of the os ischii. The centre of the femoral ball head was defined by the centre point of a circle over three detected points on the circumference of the femoral ball head. This procedure was done manually by the clinician or technician performing the analysis. The same procedure was carried out for the acetabular cup component: with three points on the cup rim, the resulting centre point of the circle was created by the software.

For the $3D_{wear}$ method, wear analysis was performed using RSA image pairs and a model-based RSA approach using elementary geometrical shape (EGS) models to calculate wear (MBRSA v.4.1, RSAcore, LMUC, Leiden, The Netherlands). EGS model spheres and hemispheres were used to represent the femoral ball head and the acetabular cup component. Scaling of these EGS models was performed according to the known diameter of both components. Counter-detection for the ball head and cup was performed at the region of interest within the left and right RSA image pair. Pose estimation algorithms matched the detected contour within the RSA image pair (actual contour) to the virtual contour of the EGS models, until the three-dimensional pose and orientation of the models within the RSA image pair were matched. Relative wear, presenting the displacement of the centre of the ball head model with respect to the cup model, was calculated in consecutive examinations relative to the reference (baseline) examination.

The wear results obtained from $2D_{wear}$ and $3D_{wear}$ approaches were compared to set-point wear values.

2.5. Statistics

The statistical analysis was performed using the statistical software package SPSS for Windows (Version 23, SPSS Inc., Chicago, IL, USA). In order to compare the two methods, precision and accuracy were evaluated. Precision was indicated as the standard deviation (SD) of the repeated measurements. Accuracy was defined as the bias, which was described as the average difference between the measured and true values. Box plots to visualize data distribution or outliers were plotted, as well as Bland–Altman plots [28] to assess the interchangeable applicability of the $2D_{wear}$ next to the golden standard $3D_{wear}$ method. Within these scatter plots, the calculated differences for detected wear by both methods were plotted against their average value. The limit of agreement (LoA) was set to mean ± 1.96 standard deviations of the measured differences, representing approximately 95% of all measured values. The influence of pelvic position was statistically proven using a paired t-test or Wilcoxon matched-pair signed-rank test, which was applied between each paired wear position depending on whether the difference between the two positions conformed to a normal distribution. The level of significance was adjusted to $p < 0.05$.

3. Results

Precision and accuracy values of the $3D_{wear}$ approach were all within the range of a hundredth of a millimeter. Values were below 0.054 mm (precision) and 0.025 mm (accuracy), respectively, for the three wear protocols. In comparison to $2D_{wear}$ methodology, these values were all within the range of a tenth of a millimeter, below 0.304 mm and 0.263 mm, respectively.

Overall precision was 0.206 mm for the $2D_{wear}$ and 0.043 mm for the $3D_{wear}$ approach (Table 1). For overall accuracy, an identical trend was observable. With an accuracy value of 0.159 mm, the $2D_{wear}$ approach was worse in comparison with the $3D_{wear}$ methodology, with an accuracy value of 0.017 mm (Table 2). Only within the medium wear group, the accuracy of the $2D_{wear}$ approach was 0.069 mm below 0.1 mm, and for detectable wear in this range, close to the $3D_{wear}$ value of 0.011 mm.

Table 1. Precision (SD) of overall and individual wear groups in $2D_{wear}$ and $3D_{wear}$.

	$2D_{wear}$ [mm]	$3D_{wear}$ [mm]
In total	0.206	0.043
Low	0.107	0.033
Medium	0.154	0.038
High	0.304	0.054

Remark: SD = standard deviation.

Table 2. Accuracy (bias) of overall and individual wear groups in $2D_{wear}$ and $3D_{wear}$.

	$2D_{wear}$ [mm]	$3D_{wear}$ [mm]
In total	0.159	0.017
Low	0.146	0.025
Medium	0.069	0.011
High	0.263	0.016

The wear results of the $3D_{wear}$ approach did not change significantly with a change in pelvic position (Figure 4). Significant changes in wear results could be identified only for the pelvic lateral tilted left 5 deg position relative to the pelvic neutral position ($p < 0.05$). The $2D_{wear}$ p values illustrated a contrary picture to the findings for $3D_{wear}$. With the exception of the pelvic lateral tilted left 5 deg position and the pelvic rotated left 5 deg position, the remaining four pelvic positions showed significantly different wear results ($p < 0.05$) relative to the pelvic neutral position.

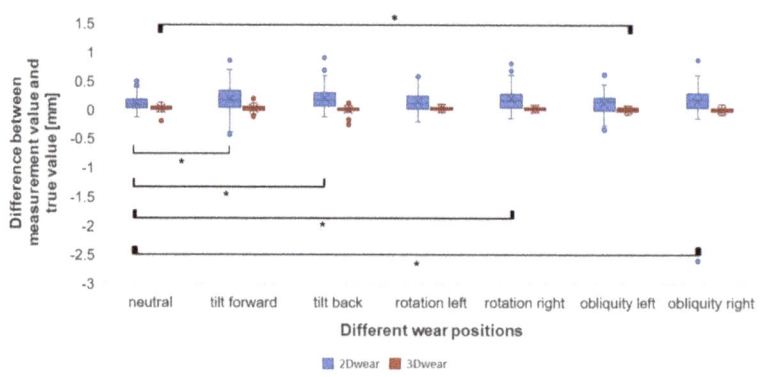

Figure 4. Box plot between $2D_{wear}$ and $3D_{wear}$ (the x-axis reveals different wear positions, and the y-axis reveals the difference between the measurement value and true value. The blue and brown boxes illustrate $2D_{wear}$ and $3D_{wear}$, respectively. Stars (*): $p < 0.05$).

The assessment for interchangeable applicability of the $2D_{wear}$ next to the $3D_{wear}$ wear approach within the neutral pelvic position scenario indicated the largest range of the LoA for high wear group. LoA ranged from a minimum of −0.16 up to 0.49 mm (mean difference: 0.16 mm), as well as from a minimum of −0.06 up to 0.20 mm (mean difference: 0.07 mm) for the low wear group, respectively (Figure 5). For different pelvic orientations, the largest LoA was observed in the high wear group, with values ranging from −1.06 to 1.36 mm (mean difference: 0.15 mm) within the pelvic lateral tilted right 5 deg position (Table 3). The lowest LoA existed in the medium wear group and was from −0.24 to 0.25 mm (mean difference: 0.00 mm) within the pelvic rotated left 5 deg position. In general, LoAs were increased for changed pelvic positions relative to the neutral position within all the wear groups.

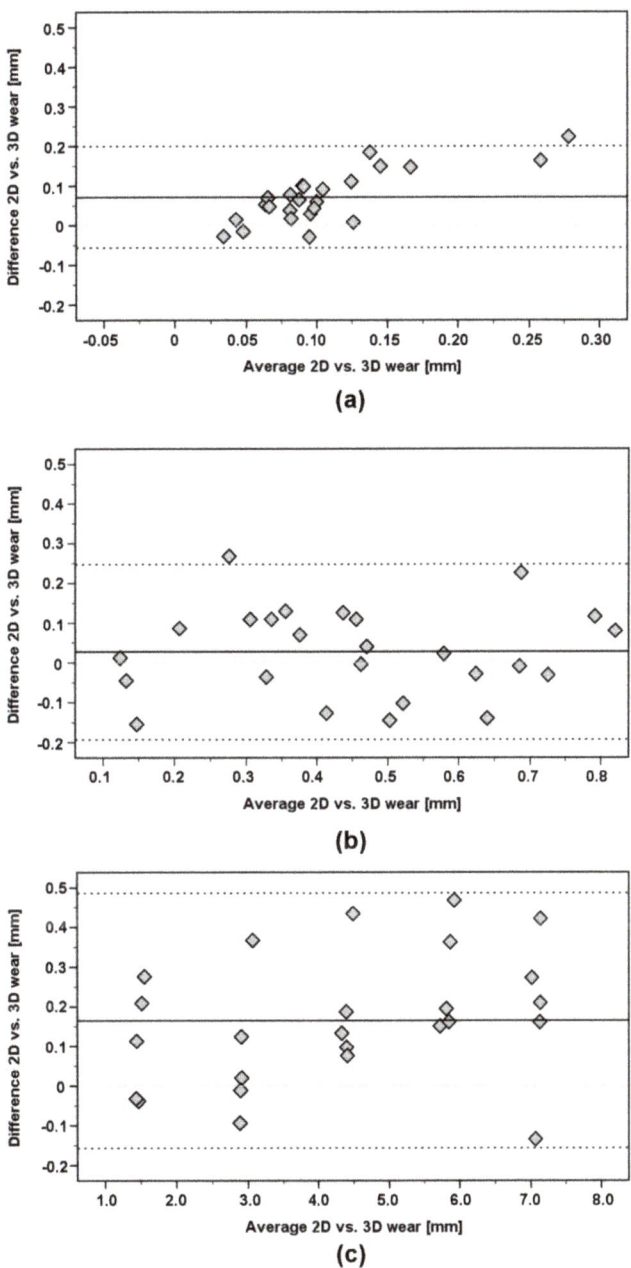

Figure 5. Bland–Altman [28] scatter plots in the pelvic neutral position between $2D_{wear}$ and $3D_{wear}$ for (**a**) the low wear group (**b**) the medium wear group and (**c**) the high wear group. Each data point of the plots presents the computed differences between the $2D_{wear}$ and $3D_{wear}$ approach (ordinate), which is plotted versus the mean difference (abscissa) of both methods, respectively. LoA is visualized by the horizontal lines, representing the mean value of calculated differences, and the two dashed lines (mean ± 1.96 SD) represent bounding criteria.

Table 3. Mean value with upper and lower LoA for six changed pelvic positions.

Protocol		Tilt Forward	Tilt Back	Rotation Left	Rotation Right	Lateral Tilted Left	Lateral Tilted Right
Low wear	LoA (↑)	0.29	0.37	0.29	0.27	0.38	0.42
	mean	0.07	0.15	0.11	0.12	0.14	0.18
	LoA (↓)	−0.15	−0.07	−0.07	−0.02	−0.10	−0.06
Medium wear	LoA (↑)	0.54	0.41	**0.25**	0.32	0.34	0.39
	mean	0.07	0.10	0.00	0.07	0.03	0.11
	LoA (↓)	−0.40	−0.21	**−0.24**	−0.17	−0.28	−0.17
High wear	LoA (↑)	0.76	0.75	0.61	0.82	0.52	**1.36**
	mean	0.37	0.32	0.23	0.33	0.17	0.15
	LoA (↓)	−0.03	−0.11	−0.16	−0.17	−0.18	**−1.06**

Remark: Bold values indicate LoA with the highest and lowest ranges.

4. Discussion

In vivo wear of THA could be detected by 2D and 3D measurement techniques. Within this experimental study, a $2D_{wear}$ approach was compared to the gold standard $3D_{wear}$ methodology, the RSA method. The results indicated superior accuracy (0.017 mm) and precision (0.043 mm) of the $3D_{wear}$ method in comparison to the $2D_{wear}$ approach (Tables 1 and 2). No significant effect of mal-aligned pelvic positions on the $3D_{wear}$ measurement outcome existed. These results of the 2D and 3D measurement techniques could be confirmed already by Ilchman et al. [20] and the results of Stilling et al. [27].

Ilchman et al. [20] detected in vivo wear by four different methods: (i) RSA, (ii) the Scheier–Sandel method, (iii) the Charnley–Duo method, and (iv) EBRA. The 2D EBRA approach was observed to be the most accurate $2D_{wear}$ approach in comparison to the gold standard (RSA). After excluding radiographs with the presence of a pelvic tilt (rotation around the horizontal axis), the measurement error was 0.08 ± 0.11 mm (mean ± SD), which was superior to the investigated $2D_{wear}$ approach of this study, but inferior to the RSA result.

Stilling et al. [27] reported precision for RSA and a 2D method (Poly Wear 3D Pro 5.10, Draftware Developers Inc., Vevay, Indiana) as 2D wear measurements of 0.078 mm and 0.076 mm and for 3D wear measures of 0.189 mm and 0.244 mm, respectively. In comparison to the outcome of this study, the $3D_{wear}$ (as the RSA method using EGS models) was within 0.043 mm of the prior results of Stilling et al. [27], but the 2D approach (Poly-Wear) performed better than the applied $2D_{wear}$ method (mediCAD) in this study, with 0.206 mm (Table 1). However, for reported accuracy, the results of Stilling et al. [27] for 2D measures of 0.055 mm (RSA) and 0.335 mm (Poly-Wear) and 3D measures of 0.2 mm and 0.3 mm respectively, were worse in comparison to the investigated $3D_{wear}$ and $2D_{wear}$ approach of this study, with 0.017 mm and 0.159 mm, respectively (Table 2).

In contrast, clinical validation of 12 patients undergoing total hip replacement surgery by the same wear measurement tools showed similar repeatability of PolyWare and RSA with a LoA of ± 0.22 mm and ± 0.23 mm, respectively, and good concurrent validity between them with limits of agreement of ± 0.55 mm [29]. LoA of this experimental study range in a worst case (high wear protocol) from −0.16 up to 0.49 mm (mean difference: 0.16 mm) to a best case (low wear protocol) from −0.06 up to 0.20 mm (mean difference: 0.07 SD) (Figure 5). There seemed to be a discrepancy in accuracy between clinical and experimental images.

Based on the results of this investigation and the available literature, the $2D_{wear}$ detection technique could be used to some degree as a substitute for the 3D technique to investigate in vivo wear. Langlois et al. [21] reported for Martell's Hip Analysis Suite software (version 8.0.1.4.3; UCTech the University of Chicago) accuracy and precision as mean ± SD to be 0.060 ± 0.021 mm and 0.207 ± 0.099 mm, respectively. A mean bias of 0.089 mm and reproducibility of 0.106 mm existed for this 2D approach. The bias of this investigation is a quarter less of the value for the 3D$_{wear}$ approach. 2D$_{wear}$ bias is, for the medium wear protocol, approximate to the results of Langlois et al. [21] for high and low wear protocols of inferior accuracy.

Derbyshire & Barkatali [10] reported for their customized software (programmed in C++ language) a mean error of −0.002 mm. The precision was 0.055 mm and the performed comparison tests with the RSA method showed similar accuracy. Hui et al. [30] investigated the outcome of two in vivo methods (PolyWare and Martell Hip Analysis Suite) with the direct wear measurement of the articulating surface of the retrieved polyethylene liners. Wear was detected by a coordinate measuring machine. Results suggested that both 2D methods accounted for the majority of 3D ex vivo results. Martell et al. [18] analysed radiographs of 140 patients using both 3D and 2D techniques and showed that 3D analysis detected 10% more wear, but its repeatability was four times worse than 2D. The decrease in repeatability was explained by the authors by poor quality of the lateral radiographs.

Taking into account that 2D$_{wear}$ methods were used originally to measure wear rates less than 0.2 mm/year for UHMWPE cup inserts [10] and that a decreased rate with vitamin E-diffused or crosslinked polyethylene to 0.04 mm or less [12,15] is possible, the gold standard RSA is certainly to be given preference in the clinical measurement of wear in vivo.

In clinical practice, anteroposterior pelvic radiographs are standard to monitor the performance of THA. This radiological image material has the advantage that it can be widely applied at any follow-up point in place of RSA. However, the pelvis is often not in a neutral position at the time of X-ray generation due to patient or radiology technician factors. Patient factors are usually due to lumbar spine disease or hip pain. The technician factor is usually a lack of compliance with standard specifications or quality control for radiographs. This affects the projection of the implant component within the X-ray, resulting in errors in wear measurements for the applied 2D$_{wear}$ technique. It must be taken into account that wear measurements of the investigated 2Dwear or 3Dwear approach could be influenced by subjective error by the clinician or technician performing the analysis. A possible error source could be point detection defining the centre point of the ball head via a circle over three detected points within the 2Dwear approach. Similarly, within the 3D$_{wear}$ method, a user interaction is also necessary and may result in a subjective error. However, many of the points needed to be defined and produced by the application of edge detection algorithms, for which thresholds are determined by the user. In the context of point detection in the 2D$_{wear}$ approach, the detection of the points is manual in nature. Accordingly, a user interaction is also present here, which can cause higher subjective errors. The difference compared to the gold standard RSA method is that within the 2Dwear, no points are specified by image processing algorithms. However, intra- and interrater reliability was not investigated within this study.

Please take into account that the investigated approaches are only applicable for hard-soft bearings. According to standard analysis protocols for both technologies, the contours of the ball head, which are within the X-ray located inside the acetabular insert, must be detectable. For hard-hard bearings, this yields poor image quality, which makes it difficult to detect the exact outline of the ball head. However, this visibility problem represents a problem for the RSA method as well [27,31]. In summary, these facts limit the application of the investigated 2D$_{wear}$ method to a fraction of the existing THA systems and bearing couples in the "real world".

5. Conclusions

Based on the results of this investigation, it can be concluded that a 3D$_{wear}$ method presents the best methodological approach to detect linear wear of THA in vivo. The accuracy and precision of the 3D$_{wear}$ method are superior to the 2D$_{wear}$ approach. When using a 3D$_{wear}$ approach, pelvic positioning will not affect the measurement outcome. Associated disadvantages of such specialized 3D$_{wear}$ methods, such as RSA, are as follows:

- The acquisition of additional RSA radiographs compared to standard a.p. X-rays is required, resulting in additional radiation exposure for patients;
- Additional necessary equipment is required for RSA, such as a calibration box or a second X-ray tube;
- No wear for hard-hard bearings is detectable.

However, the investigated $2D_{wear}$ method can be an alternative approach if several conditions are met. Especially in the medium wear group (simulated wear between 0.1 mm to 0.5 mm), this approach presents an alternative to $3D_{wear}$. Due to the influence of pelvic position factors, $2D_{wear}$ is more susceptible to poorly aligned positions of the pelvis. Therefore, the pelvis should be kept in a standard neutral position during image capturing so that $2D_{wear}$ can obtain accurate results. A significant advantage is that this approach enables wear detection using standard a.p. radiographs of the treated hip joint, meaning no additional radiation exposure for patients.

Author Contributions: Conceptualization, J.W., R.F. and F.S.; formal analysis, J.W.; investigation, J.W.; resources, R.F.; data curation, J.W.; writing—original draft preparation, J.W., D.T., R.F. and F.S.; writing—review and editing, J.W., D.T., R.F. and F.S.; visualization, J.W. and F.S.; supervision, R.F. and F.S.; project administration, F.S. All authors have read and agreed to the published version of the manuscript.

Funding: A fellowship (J.W.) was supported by China Scholarship Council.

Institutional Review Board Statement: Not applicable.

Informed Consent Statement: Not applicable.

Data Availability Statement: Not applicable.

Acknowledgments: This work was supported by a fellowship (J.W.) from the China Scholarship Council.

Conflicts of Interest: The authors declare no conflict of interest.

References

1. Karachalios, T.; Komnos, G.; Koutalos, A. Total hip arthroplasty: Survival and modes of failure. *EFORT Open Rev.* **2018**, *3*, 232–239. [CrossRef]
2. Bleß, H.H.; Kip, M. *White Paper On Joint Replacement—Status of Hip and Knee Arthroplasty Care in Germany*; Springer Nature: Heidelberg, Germany, 2018. [CrossRef]
3. Kretzer, J.P.; Uhler, M.; Jager, S.; Bormann, T.; Sonntag, R.; Schonhoff, M.; Schroder, S. Tribology in hip arthroplasty: Benefits of different materials. *Orthopade* **2021**, *50*, 259–269. [CrossRef]
4. Zagra, L.; Gallazzi, E. Bearing surfaces in primary total hip arthroplasty. *EFORT Open Rev.* **2018**, *3*, 217–224. [CrossRef] [PubMed]
5. Tsikandylakis, G.; Mohaddes, M.; Cnudde, P.; Eskelinen, A.; Karrholm, J.; Rolfson, O. Head size in primary total hip arthroplasty. *EFORT Open Rev.* **2018**, *3*, 225–231. [CrossRef]
6. (AOAJR), A.N.J.R. 2019 Annual Report—Hip, Knee & Shoulder Arthroplasty. 2019.
7. Kärrholm, J.; Rogmark, C.; Nauclèr, E.; Vinblad, J.; Mohaddes, M.; Rolfson, O. Swedish Hip Arthroplasty Register—Annual Report 2018. 2019.
8. Sundfeldt, M.; Carlsson, L.V.; Johansson, C.B.; Thomsen, P.; Gretzer, C. Aseptic loosening, not only a question of wear: A review of different theories. *Acta Orthop.* **2006**, *77*, 177–197. [CrossRef]
9. Evans, J.T.; Evans, J.P.; Walker, R.W.; Blom, A.W.; Whitehouse, M.R.; Sayers, A. How long does a hip replacement last? A systematic review and meta-analysis of case series and national registry reports with more than 15 years of follow-up. *Lancet* **2019**, *393*, 647–654. [CrossRef]
10. Derbyshire, B.; Barkatali, B. Validation of a new 2-D technique for radiographic wear measurement of cemented, highly cross-linked polyethylene acetabular cups. *Med. Eng. Phys.* **2017**, *47*, 159–166. [CrossRef] [PubMed]
11. Rahman, L.; Cobb, J.; Muirhead-Allwood, S. Radiographic methods of wear analysis in total hip arthroplasty. *J. Am. Acad. Orthop. Surg.* **2012**, *20*, 735–743. [CrossRef] [PubMed]
12. Galea, V.P.; Rojanasopondist, P.; Laursen, M.; Muratoglu, O.K.; Malchau, H.; Bragdon, C. Evaluation of vitamin E-diffused highly crosslinked polyethylene wear and porous titanium-coated shell stability: A seven-year randomized control trial using radiostereometric analysis. *Bone Jt. J.* **2019**, *101-B*, 760–767. [CrossRef]
13. Goldvasser, D.; Hansen, V.J.; Noz, M.E.; Maguire, G.Q., Jr.; Zeleznik, M.P.; Olivecrona, H.; Bragdon, C.R.; Weidenhielm, L.; Malchau, H. In vivo and ex vivo measurement of polyethylene wear in total hip arthroplasty: Comparison of measurements using a CT algorithm, a coordinate-measuring machine, and a micrometer. *Acta Orthop.* **2014**, *85*, 271–275. [CrossRef]

14. Koff, M.F.; Esposito, C.; Shah, P.; Miranda, M.; Baral, E.; Fields, K.; Bauer, T.; Padgett, D.E.; Wright, T.; Potter, H.G. MRI of THA Correlates With Implant Wear and Tissue Reactions: A Cross-sectional Study. *Clin. Orthop. Relat. Res.* **2019**, *477*, 159–174. [CrossRef]
15. Teeter, M.G.; Yuan, X.; Somerville, L.E.; MacDonald, S.J.; McCalden, R.W.; Naudie, D.D. Thirteen-year wear rate comparison of highly crosslinked and conventional polyethylene in total hip arthroplasty: Long-term follow-up of a prospective randomized controlled trial. *Can. J. Surg.* **2017**, *60*, 212–216. [CrossRef]
16. Stilling, M.; Soballe, K.; Andersen, N.T.; Larsen, K.; Rahbek, O. Analysis of polyethylene wear in plain radiographs. *Acta Orthop.* **2009**, *80*, 675–682. [CrossRef] [PubMed]
17. Collier, M.B.; Kraay, M.J.; Rimnac, C.M.; Goldberg, V.M. Evaluation of Contemporary Software Methods Used to Quantify Polyethylene Wear After Total Hip Arthroplasty. *J. Bone Jt. Surg. Am.* **2003**, *85*, 2410–2418. [CrossRef] [PubMed]
18. Martell, J.M.; Berkson, E.; Berger, R.A.; Jacobs, J. Comparison of two and three-dimensional computerized polyethylene wear analysis after total hip arthroplasty. *J. Bone Jt. Surg. Am.* **2003**, *85*, 1111–1117. [CrossRef]
19. Ilchmann, T.; Mjöberg, B.; Wingstrand, H. Measurement accuracy in acetabular cup wear. *J. Arthroplast.* **1995**, *10*, 636–642. [CrossRef]
20. Ilchmann, T. Radiographic assessment of cup migration and wear after hip replacement. *Acta Orthop. Scand.* **1997**, *68*, i-26. [CrossRef] [PubMed]
21. Langlois, J.; Zaoui, A.; Scemama, C.; Martell, J.; Bragdon, C.; Hamadouche, M. Validation of a computer-assisted method for measurement of radiographic wear in total hip arthroplasty using all polyethylene cemented acetabular components. *J. Orthop. Res.* **2015**, *33*, 417–420. [CrossRef] [PubMed]
22. Bragdon, C.R.; Malchau, H.; Yuan, X.; Perinchief, R.; Kärrholm, J.; Börlin, N.; Estok, D.M.; Harris, W.H. Experimental assessment of precision and accuracy of radiostereometric analysis for the determination of polyethylene wear in a total hip replacement model. *J. Orthop. Res.* **2002**, *20*, 688–695. [CrossRef]
23. Uddin, M.S.; Mak, C.Y.E.; Callary, S.A. Evaluating hip implant wear measurements by CMM technique. *Wear* **2016**, *364–365*, 193–200. [CrossRef]
24. Von Schewelov, T.; Sanzen, L.; Borlin, N.; Markusson, P.; Onsten, I. Accuracy of radiographic and radiostereometric wear measurement of different hip prostheses: An experimental study. *Acta Orthop. Scand.* **2004**, *75*, 691–700. [CrossRef]
25. McCalden, R.W.; Naudie, D.D.; Yuan, X.; Bourne, R.B. Radiographic methods for the assessment of polyethylene wear after total hip arthroplasty. *J. Bone Jt. Surg. Am.* **2005**, *87*, 2323–2334. [CrossRef]
26. Sychterz, C.J.; Young, A.M.; Engh, C.A. Effect of Radiographic Quality on Computer-Assisted Head Penetration Measurements. *Clin. Orthop. Rel. Res.* **2001**, *386*, 150–158. [CrossRef]
27. Stilling, M.; Kold, S.; de Raedt, S.; Andersen, N.T.; Rahbek, O.; Soballe, K. Superior accuracy of model-based radiostereometric analysis for measurement of polyethylene wear: A phantom study. *Bone Jt. Res.* **2012**, *1*, 180–191. [CrossRef] [PubMed]
28. Bland, J.M.; Altman, D.G. Statistical methods for assessing agreement between two methods of clinical measurement. *Lancet* **1986**, *327*, 307–310. [CrossRef]
29. Stilling, M.; Larsen, K.; Andersen, N.T.; Soballe, K.; Kold, S.; Rahbek, O. The final follow-up plain radiograph is sufficient for clinical evaluation of polyethylene wear in total hip arthroplasty. A study of validity and reliability. *Acta Orthop.* **2010**, *81*, 570–578. [CrossRef] [PubMed]
30. Hui, A.J.; McCalden, R.W.; Martell, J.M.; MacDonald, S.J.; Bourne, R.B.; Rorbaeck, C.H. Validation of Two and Three-Dimensional Radiographic Techniques for Measuring Polyethylene Wear After Total Hip Arthroplasty. *J. Bone Jt. Surg. Am.* **2003**, *95*, 505–511. [CrossRef] [PubMed]
31. Borlin, N.; Rohrl, S.M.; Bragdon, C.R. RSA wear measurements with or without markers in total hip arthroplasty. *J. Biomech.* **2006**, *39*, 1641–1650. [CrossRef]

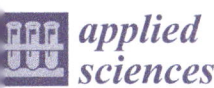

Article

Does Pressurized Carbon Dioxide Lavage Improve Bone Cleaning in Cemented Arthroplasty?

Kevin Knappe [1,2,*], Christian Stadler [3], Moritz Innmann [1,2], Mareike Schonhoff [2], Tobias Gotterbarm [3], Tobias Renkawitz [1] and Sebastian Jaeger [2]

1. Clinic for Orthopedic and Trauma Surgery, Heidelberg University Hospital, Schlierbacher Landstrasse 200a, 69118 Heidelberg, Germany; moritz.innmann@med.uni-heidelberg.de (M.I.); tobias.renkawitz@med.uni-heidelberg.de (T.R.)
2. Laboratory of Biomechanics and Implant Research, Clinic for Orthopedics and Trauma Surgery, Heidelberg University Hospital, 69118 Heidelberg, Germany; mareike.schonhoff@med.uni-heidelberg.de (M.S.); sebastian.jaeger@med.uni-heidelberg.de (S.J.)
3. Clinic for Orthopedics and Trauma Surgery, Kepler University Hospital, 4020 Linz, Austria; christian.stadler@kepleruniklinikum.at (C.S.); tobias.gotterbarm@kepleruniklinikum.at (T.G.)
* Correspondence: kevin.knappe@med.uni-heidelberg.de

Abstract: Cemented implant fixation in total joint arthroplasty has been proven to be safe and reliable with good long-term results. However, aseptic loosening is one of the main reasons for revision, potentially caused by poor cementation with low penetration depth in the cancellous bone. Aim of this prospective laboratory study was, to compare impact pressure and cleaning effects of pulsatile saline lavage to novel carbon dioxide lavage in a standardized carbon foam setup, to determine whether or not additional use of carbon dioxide lavage has any impact on cleaning volume or cleaning depth in cancellous bone. Carbon specimens simulating human cancellous bone were filled with industrial grease and then underwent a standardized cleaning procedure. Specimens underwent computed tomography pre- and post-cleaning. Regarding the impact pressure, isolated carbon dioxide lavage showed significant lower pressure compared to pulsatile saline lavage. Even though the combination of carbon dioxide lavage and pulsatile saline lavage had a positive cleaning effect compared to the isolated use of pulsatile saline lavage or carbon dioxide lavage, this was not significant in terms of cleaning volume or cleaning depth.

Keywords: carbon dioxide lavage; pulsatile lavage; joint arthroplasty; bone preparation; cement; total knee arthroplasty; total hip arthroplasty

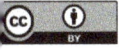

1. Introduction

Cemented implant fixation in total joint arthroplasty has demonstrated to be a reliable and safe procedure with excellent long-term results [1–4]. However, there are many regional differences if cemented or non-cemented fixation is performed. Regarding cemented fixation in total hip arthroplasty, those differences vary from 76% (Sweden) to 29% (Denmark) [5]. National registries demonstrate slight differences in the technique for total knee arthroplasty as well. In Germany, the Netherlands and New Zealand, 95% and more of total knee arthroplasties are performed using the cemented technique [6–8], whereas in Sweden it was only 92% in 2019 [9].

Despite regional differences in the choice of technique, the procedure for cemented arthroplasty is standardized. In total knee arthroplasty this includes to use high-pressure pulsatile saline lavage irrigation, drilling holes into the tibia, drying the bone and applying vacuum-mixed-cement to both, implant and bone [10]. In total hip arthroplasty third generation cementing technique is performed. This includes preparing bone bed properly by aggressive rasping, using high-pressure pulsatile saline lavage irrigation, using a distal cement restrictor, applying vacuum-mixed-cement in retrograde technique into the femur via cement gun, pressurizing the cement and inserting the stem with a distal centralizer [11]. Despite improved technique of cementing, aseptic loosening is still the main reason for revision after cemented total knee and hip arthroplasty [6,12,13].

Implant stability can be increased by adequate cleaning of the bone bed prior to cement application. In addition, pulsatile lavage can have a protective effect on implant stability in case of reduced bone density [14]. This preparation requires removal of bone marrow containing residual bone material, blood and fat. Even the presence of blood between bone and cement can reduce integrity of bone-cement interface [15]. Bone cement interface and penetration depth of cement are directly related to prior cleaning. For stable anchorage, desired cement thickness is described as 2–5 mm [16,17]. With this cement penetration depth, implant failure rates are significantly lower compared to cement thickness below 2 mm [18]. In addition, harmful thermal effects of polymerizing cement are not observed, which are described for a cement thickness of more than 5 mm [19,20].

A reliable method for this crucial cleaning procedure of cancellous bone is using saline high-pressure pulsatile lavage and subsequent drying of bone bed with abdominal cloth and suction. However, after this procedure liquid and fatty material often remains and may prevent cement from penetrating in the desired depth into the cancellous bone. Many studies have shown, that cleaning cancellous bone using pulsatile lavage is more efficient than manual rinse cleaning by bladder syringe alone [21–25]. For the application of pulsatile lavage, different rinsing pressures are recommended in the literature depending on the area of application or tissue type, since pulsatile lavage is used to clean contaminated wounds as well. When comparing pressures of these procedures, it is important to distinguish whether the pressure specifications are "output pressure" or "impact pressure". The US Department of Health and Human Services recommends an impact pressure between 0.03 N/mm^2 (4 PSI) and 0.10 N/mm^2 (15 PSI) for cleaning wounds [26]. This recommendation is based on a number of studies that have shown a pressure of less than 0.03 N/mm^2 being inefficient in removing surface pathogens. Also, pressure of more than 0.10 N/mm^2 can potentially facilitate bacterial contamination in deeper tissue layers or cause traumatic soft tissue damage. Regarding the topic of this study, much higher pressures for cleaning cancellous bone have been reported in the literature. They reach from 0.48 N/mm^2 (70 PSI) to 0.59 N/mm^2 (85 PSI) [27,28].

A novel type of high-pressure carbon dioxide lavage, which is recommended for usage after standard saline lavage, is designed to advance cleaning and simultaneous drying of the bone [29]. A cadaveric study demonstrated that a combination of pressurized carbon dioxide and common pulsatile saline lavage produced a significantly deeper bone cement penetration than saline lavage alone [30]. Another study from 2019 showed that by using sterile compressed CO_2 in addition to the established pulsatile lavage, a significantly deeper cement penetration in three of seven defined zones (Knee Society Radiographic Evaluation System) could be achieved in 303 total knee endoprosthesis [31]. In addition bone cement interface was stronger in an experimental study using human radii [32]. However, cases of embolic events using carbon dioxide lavage in intramedullary cleaning during cemented hip arthroplasty have been reported [33,34].

Aim of this prospective laboratory study was to compare impact pressure and cleaning effects of pulsatile saline lavage to novel carbon dioxide lavage in a standardized carbon foam setup and to determine whether or not additional use of carbon dioxide lavage has any impact on cleaning volume or cleaning depth in cancellous bone.

2. Materials and Methods

First, we investigated impact pressure to the surface of two different devices. This was followed by measurements of cleaning volume and cleaning depth of the two devices and their combination in a standardized laboratory setting.

2.1. Devices and Investigated Carbon Specimens

2.1.1. Lavage and Cleaning Systems

In an in vitro study, we investigated the bone cleaning effect of carbon dioxide lavage compared to pulsatile lavage and in addition to pulsatile bone cleaning. We used the InterPulse (Stryker, Kalamazoo, MI, USA) for conventional bone cleaning with saline solution and the CarboJet (Kinamed, Camarillo, CA, USA) for carbon dioxide cleaning (Figure 1). The bone cleaning tip (REF 0210-010-00) for the InterPulse and the supplied Wide-Angle-Knee-Nozzle of the CarboJet were used for the experiments (Figure 1). To investigate the impaction pressure, the cleaning systems were divided into the InterPulse and CarboJet group. For the analysis of the cleaning effect, the two systems were investigated separately and in combination. This resulted in the groups InterPulse (A), CarboJet (B) and InterPulse + CarboJet (C).

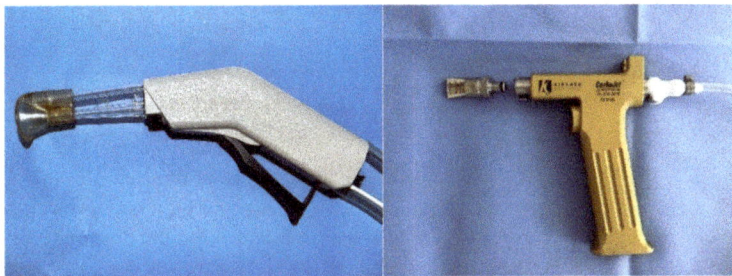

Figure 1. (**left**) Handpiece of InterPulse by Stryker. (**right**) Handpiece of CO_2 lavage CarboJet by KINAMED.

2.1.2. Determination Impact Pressure

The impact pressure of both investigated lavage systems was determined under standardized condition. Therefore, we used a custom-made setup with mounting platform for the lavage systems and a target with integrated force measuring plate (Figure 2). Each lavage system was firmly fixed on the movable mounting platform. This was necessary to place the tip with splash shield for the InterPulse and the nozzle for the CarboJet at a defined distance of 2 mm in front of the force measuring plate (Figure 2). A distance of 2 mm was maintained to avoid interference between the force plate and the tip due to the flushing liquid or carbon dioxide. The flushing medium was applied centrally onto the force plate. The distance of the tip of the saline lavage device to the force measuring plate was specified by the splash shield (Figure 1, left). For the InterPulse this was 17 mm (15 + 2 mm) and in case of the CarboJet, the distance was 2 mm because there was no splash shield.

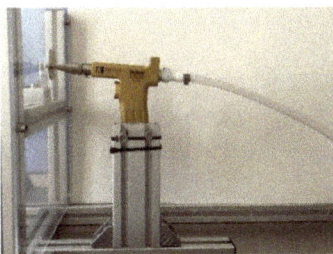

Figure 2. Force measuring plate with 2 mm distance to the CO_2 nozzle.

The impact pressure was calculated by dividing the force and the area of the nozzle orifice (Figure 3). The nozzle openings of the two lavage systems investigated were measured using a calibrated digital microscope (Digital Microscope VHX-500 by Keyence, Osaka, Japan). Both lavage systems were tested four times within the first minute of powering up. The force values were recorded at a sampling rate of 1000 Hz and the mean values were calculated.

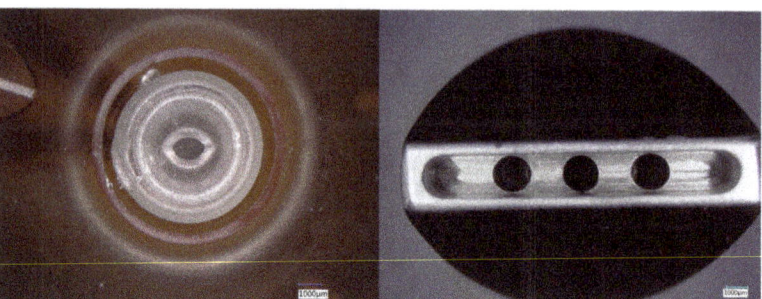

Figure 3. Top view of: (**left**) Stryker- InterPuls bone cleaning tip, (**right**) KINAMED—CarboJet Wide-Angle Knee—Nozzle.

2.1.3. Determination of the Cleaning Effect

The two lavage systems were divided into group InterPulse (A), CarboJet (B) and InterPulse + CarboJet (C) as described. A sample size of 10 specimens per group (30 in total) were used. In case of the InterPulse a saline irrigation volume of one liter per specimen was used. The cleaning distance was determined by the splash shield. Following the manufacturer's specifications, a cleaning duration of 30 s was used for the CarboJet.

The determination of the cleaning effect of the investigated lavage systems were performed using validated and standardized carbon foam specimens (RVC foam; ERG Materials and Aerospace, Oakland, CA, USA) as substitutes for human cancellous bone [35]. The carbon specimens showed a porosity of 30 PPI (pores per inch), which corresponds to 1.2 PPM (pores per millimeter). During the manufacturing process, the specimens were compressed twice, resulting in similar trabecular bone structure (Figure 4, right). The carbon foam specimens were filled with standardized technical fat (Bechem Rhus FA 37; Carl Bechem GmbH, Hagen, Germany), to simulate human bone marrow [36]. One ingredient of the fat was an aluminum-complex soap which we used as contrast medium for the radiological analysis. The fat-filled carbon specimens were coated with a shrink-on tube simulating the cortex (Figure 4, left).

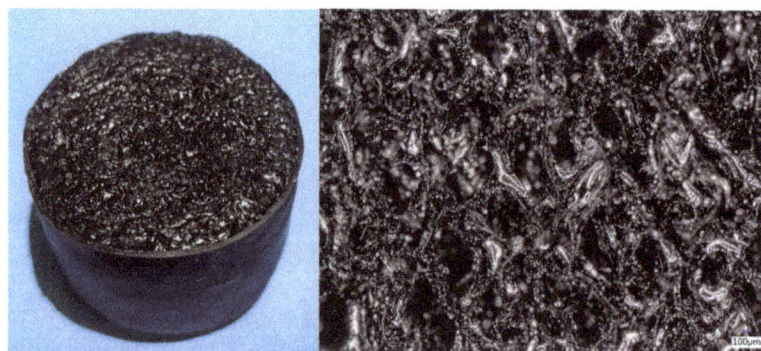

Figure 4. (**Left**) Fat filled carbon specimen with shrink tube, (**right**) close up of Carbon foam.

The evaluation of cleaning effects was determined by using computer tomography scans (SOMATOM Emotion, Siemens Healthcare GmbH, Erlangen, Germany). For this purpose, the fat-filled specimens were scanned before and after cleaning with a slice thickness of 0.75 mm. For volume determination, a reference volume was recorded for each scan. The segmentation and calculation of the cleaning volume was performed with the software itk-Snap [37]. The mean flushing depth was calculated using the volume and the geometric parameters. Exclusion criteria were air inclusions or if specimens would not have been fully filled with fat. One specimen in Group A had to be excluded due to air inclusions that would have biased the cleaning effect. Therefore, only 9 out of 10 samples could be analyzed for Group A. Beyond that, no other specimens had to be excluded.

2.2. Statistics

Using SPSS V.25 (IBM Corp. Released 2017. IBM SPSS Statistics for Windows, Version 25.0. Armonk, NY: IBM Corp., Armonk, NY, USA) a descriptively data analysis was performed. A Shapiro- Wilk test was used to test for normal distribution. A t-test was done to detect significances in impact pressure. Analysis of variance (ANOVA) was used to determine if there are significant differences regarding cleaning effects. $p < 0.05$ was set to be the significance level.

3. Results

3.1. Impact Pressure

The t-test revealed a statistically significant difference for the impact pressure between the InterPulse 0.76 ± 0.02 N/mm^2 and CarboJet 0.12 ± 0.01 N/mm^2 group, t(3.4) = 59.0, $p < 0.001$, (95% CI [0.61–0.68]). Whereas this was a mean difference increase of 0.64 N/mm^2 for the InterPulse system (Figure 5).

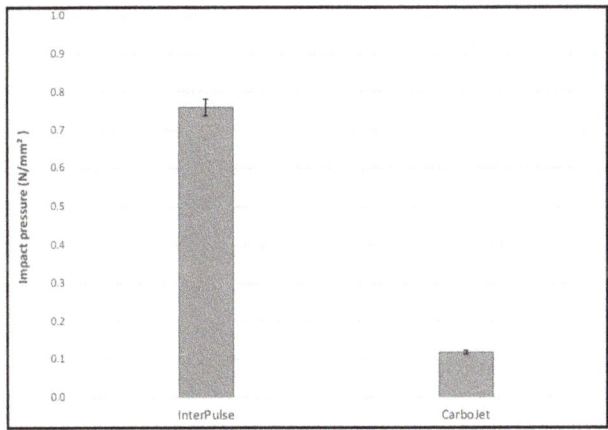

Figure 5. Impact pressure in N/mm^2.

3.2. Cleaning Effect

The ANOVA-test comparing cleaning volumes showed no statistically significant difference between the InterPulse, CarboJet and the combination of both, F(2,26) = 1.14, $p = 0.334$ (Table 1, Figure 6). Cleaning depth showed also no significant differences between the investigated groups, F(2,26) = 1.07, $p = 0.259$ (Table 1, Figure 7).

Table 1. Mean cleaning volume and cleaning depth in carbon foam specimens.

	Mean Cleaning Volume	Mean Cleaning Depth
InterPulse	2832.1 ± 1236.6 mm^3	2.1 ± 0.9 mm
CarboJet	2755.4 ± 906.3 mm^3	2.1 ± 0.7 mm
InterPulse + CarboJet	3428.4 ± 1100.0 mm^3	2.6 ± 0.8 mm

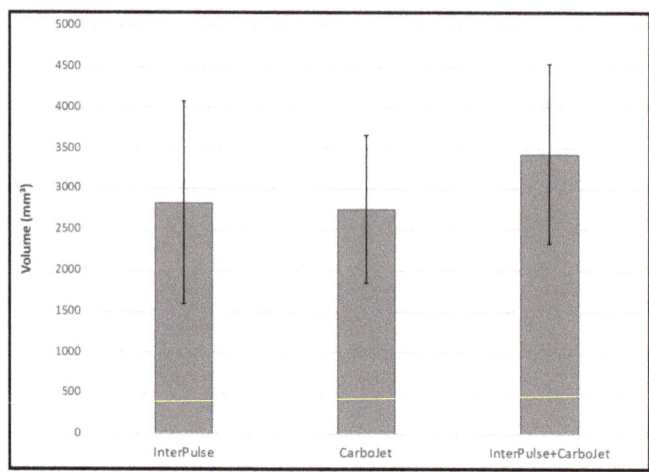

Figure 6. Volume of removed grease in standardized carbon foam specimens.

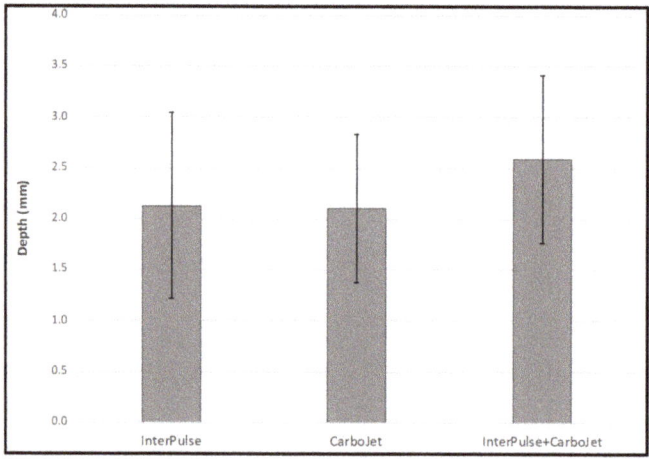

Figure 7. Cleaning depth in mm in standardized carbon foam specimens.

4. Discussion

The use of pulsatile lavage is known to enhance the fixation of cemented total knee arthroplasty [38]. Highly significant improvements of cement penetration into cancellous bone can be demonstrated in vitro comparing manual rinsing and pulsed saline lavage [25]. In addition, cleaning of cancellous bone leads to improved cement penetration and therefore to a stronger bone cement interface, which reduces the probability of aseptic loosening [18,39]. However, aseptic loosening is the main reason for revision in cemented total knee and hip arthroplasty [12,13]. Modern cementing technique requires pulsed saline lavage, drying bone by abdominal cloth and suction, drilling holes in the tibia and applying vacuum-mixed-cement either on both, metal and bone in total knee arthroplasty, or filling the femur in retrograde technique using a cement gun in total hip arthroplasty. Considering this, many factors besides the cancellous bone cleaning result can affect cementation. Bone density or sclerotic bone also can cause reasonable differences [40]. Cement storage temperature, humidity, cement viscosity or timing of cement application are other aspects that have to be considered [41,42].

In our experimental in vitro study, we compared a standard high-pressure pulsatile saline lavage to a novel lavage system using compressed carbon dioxide to enhance cleaning efficiency of cancellous bone under standardized conditions. Cancellous bone was simulated by standardized fat-filled carbon foam. In this experimental setup, impact pressure was applied to a force-measuring-plate. We detected significantly higher pressures in pulsatile saline lavage (InterPulse) than in pressurized carbon dioxide lavage (CarboJet). Although we showed higher cleaning volume and deeper penetration in carbon foam, when using carbon dioxide lavage additionally to high-pressure pulsatile saline lavage (Group C) these differences were not significant. Similar results were obtained for the single use of carbon dioxide lavage (Group B) in comparison to the single use of pulsatile saline lavage (Group A) (Figures 6 and 7).

So far, there is only limited data available about carbon dioxide lavage. A cadaveric study in 10 knees in 2016 demonstrated that a combination of pressurized carbon dioxide and common pulsatile saline lavage produced a significantly deeper bone cement penetration than saline lavage alone [30]. In addition, another study demonstrated that bone cement interface was stronger [32]. In 2019, Gapinski et al. revealed that using sterile compressed carbon dioxide in addition to the established pulsatile jet lavage, resulted in a deeper cement penetration in six of seven defined zones (Knee Society Radiographic Evaluation System) in 303 total knee endoprostheses. This difference was significant in three out of seven zones [31].

In this standardized laboratory setup, which was established in earlier studies [35,36], no significant difference between the three experimental groups was detected although higher cleaning volumes and cleaning depth using additional carbon dioxide lavage (Group C) was discovered. In this study the aspect of preparing bone bed prior to cementation was investigated. Other aspects such as pressure during cementing, viscosity of cement, remaining blood or fat in the interface or the timing of cement-application were excluded from the investigations. With this test setup, the ability of carbon dioxide lavage to clean cancellous bone was examined closely. Whether or not the slightly enhanced cleaning ability will result in deeper cement penetration remains uncertain. The use of additional carbon dioxide lavage needs extra devices, sterilization and carbon dioxide gas cylinders, which need adequate storage and the exact following of safety instructions. Moreover, the additional time needed for the procedure extends duration of operation and time of anesthesia. Since we saw similar results for single use carbon dioxide lavage (Group B) compared to single use of pulsatile lavage (Group A) it has to be considered, that using carbon dioxide lavage only, might be faster, less wet and more controlled to saline lavage. Studies showed that using high-pressure lavage to clean contaminated wounds can cause irreversible insult to tissue, resulting in myonecrosis and dystrophic calcification [43,44]. Even bacteria can be propagated into soft tissue or significant damage to the architecture of the bone can occur [45,46]. Therefore, lower impact pressure as shown in our investigation can hold advantages. Despite these potential advantages case reports are published showing gas embolisms occurred during femoral intramedullary usage of carbon dioxide lavage [33,34]. Further investigation focusing on in vivo impact can help revealing, if a specific range of pressure orchestrates all benefits while avoiding complications.

In this experimental in vitro study where we compared high-pressure saline lavage to carbon dioxide lavage and its combination, we detected significant lower impact pressure and a deeper cleaning effect with carbon dioxide lavage used additionally to high-pressure pulsatile saline lavage in standardized carbon foam specimens representing cancellous bone. However, these effects were statistically not significant. We found no evidence that using carbon dioxide lavage reduces the effect of saline lavage. Using carbon dioxide lavage only had similar outcomes compared to high-pressure pulsatile lavage. Since aseptic loosening still is the main reason for implant failure due to poor cementing, better cleaning of cancellous bone prior to cementing will have a positive effect on implant durability.

In conclusion, using a combination of high-pressure saline lavage followed by carbon dioxide lavage showed a clear tendency of resulting in improved cleaning effects prior to cementing and therefore seems to have a positive effect on stability of endoprosthesis. Further investigation in human bone and larger clinical trials will determine, if using additional carbon dioxide lavage will confirm its positive effect on bone cement interface and therefore on success of endoprosthesis implantation itself.

Author Contributions: Conceptualization, K.K. and S.J.; Data curation, K.K., M.S., C.S. and S.J.; Formal analysis, K.K., S.J. and C.S.; Methodology, K.K. and S.J.; Project administration, K.K., S.J. and M.I.; Writing—original draft, K.K. and S.J.; Writing—review & editing, K.K., C.S., M.I., M.S., T.G., T.R. and S.J. All authors have read and agreed to the published version of the manuscript.

Funding: This research received no external funding.

Institutional Review Board Statement: Not applicable.

Informed Consent Statement: Not applicable.

Data Availability Statement: Not applicable.

Conflicts of Interest: The authors declare no pertinent conflict of interest. S.J. reports grants from B Braun Aesculap, Johnson & Johnson Depuy Synthes, Heraeus Medical, Waldemar Link, Peter Brehm and Zimmer Biomet that are not related to the current study. T.G. reports personal fees paid to T.G. during the conduct of the study from Zimmer Biomet, Europe and from Depuy Synthes Orthopädie GmbH, Peter Brehm GmbH, ImplanTec GmbH outside the submitted work. Research grants paid to the institution during the conduct of the study from Zimmer Biomet, Europe, Mathys AG Switzerland, Anika Therapeutics outside the submitted work that are not related to the current study. TR reports research funding/travel expenses and/or paid speaking engagements by the German Federal Ministry of Education and Research (BMBF), The German Federal Ministry for Economic Cooperation and Development (BMZ), Otto Bock Foundation, Stiftung Oskar-Helene-Heim Berlin, DePuy Int, Zimmer, Aesculap/B. Braun, the Vielberth Foundation, German Society of Orthopaedics and Traumatology (DGOU) and the German Association of Orthopaedics and Orthopaedic Surgery (DGOOC). TR is associate editor of "Der Orthopäde" and "Der Unfallchirurg" (Springer Heidelberg, Berlin, New York) and member of the International Advisory Board of the Journal of the American Academy of Orthopaedic Surgeons (AAOS).

References

1. Dalury, D.F. Cementless total knee arthroplasty: Current concepts review. *Bone Jt. J.* **2016**, *98*, 867–873. [CrossRef]
2. Ritter, M.A.; Keating, E.M.; Sueyoshi, T.; Davis, K.E.; Barrington, J.W.; Emerson, R.H. Twenty-Five-Years and Greater, Results After Nonmodular Cemented Total Knee Arthroplasty. *J. Arthroplast.* **2016**, *31*, 2199–2202. [CrossRef]
3. Herberts, P.; Malchau, H. Long-term registration has improved the quality of hip replacement: A review of the Swedish THR Register comparing 160,000 cases. *Acta Orthop. Scand.* **2000**, *71*, 111–121. [CrossRef]
4. Malchau, H.; Herberts, P.; Eisler, T.; Garellick, G.; Soderman, P. The Swedish Total Hip Replacement Register. *J. Bone Jt. Surg. Am.* **2002**, *84* (Suppl. 2), 2–20. [CrossRef] [PubMed]
5. Bunyoz, K.I.; Malchau, E.; Malchau, H.; Troelsen, A. Has the Use of Fixation Techniques in THA Changed in This Decade? The Uncemented Paradox Revisited. *Clin. Orthop. Relat. Res.* **2020**, *478*, 697–704. [CrossRef] [PubMed]
6. Grimberg, A.; Jansson, V.; Melsheimer, O.; Steinbrück, A. German Arthroplasty Registry (EPRD)—2019 Annual Report. 2019. Available online: https://www.eprd.de/fileadmin/user_upload/Dateien/Publikationen/Berichte/EPRD_Jahresbericht_2019_EN_doppelseitig_F_Web-Stand-251120.pdf (accessed on 30 June 2021).
7. *The New Zealand Joint Registry—Fifteen Year Report January 1999 to December 2013*; NZOA: Christchurch, New Zealand, 2014; Volume 15, Available online: https://nzoa.org.nz/sites/default/files/NZJR2014Report.pdf (accessed on 30 June 2021).
8. Gademan, M.G.J.; van Steenbergen, L.N.; Cannegieter, S.C.; Nelissen, R.; Marang-Van De Mheen, P.J. Population-based 10-year cumulative revision risks after hip and knee arthroplasty for osteoarthritis to inform patients in clinical practice: A competing risk analysis from the Dutch Arthroplasty Register. *Acta Orthop.* **2021**, *92*, 1–5. [CrossRef] [PubMed]
9. Robertsson, O. (Ed.) *The Swedish Knee Arthroplasty Register—Anual Report 2020*; Skånes University Hospital: Lund, Sweden, 2020.
10. Refsum, A.M.; Nguyen, U.V.; Gjertsen, J.E.; Espehaug, B.; Fenstad, A.M.; Lein, R.K.; Ellison, P.; Høl, P.J.; Furnes, O. Cementing technique for primary knee arthroplasty: A scoping review. *Acta Orthop.* **2019**, *90*, 582–589. [CrossRef]
11. Niculescu, M.; Solomon, B.L.; Viscopoleanu, G.; Antoniac, I.V.; Viscopoleanu, G.; Antoniac, I.V. Evolution of Cementation Techniques and Bone Cements in Hip Arthroplasty. In *Handbook of Bioceramics and Biocomposites*; Springer International Publishing: Cham, Switzerland, 2016; pp. 859–899.
12. Khan, M.; Osman, K.; Green, G.; Haddad, F.S. The epidemiology of failure in total knee arthroplasty: Avoiding your next revision. *Bone Jt. J.* **2016**, *98* (Suppl. 1), 105–112. [CrossRef]

3. Kochbati, R.; Rbai, H.; Jlailia, M.; Makhlouf, H.; Bouguira, A.; Daghfous, M.S. Predictive factors of aseptic loosening of cemented total hip prostheses. *Pan. Afr. Med. J.* **2016**, *24*, 260.
4. Jaeger, S.; Rieger, J.S.; Bruckner, T.; Kretzer, J.P.; Clarius, M.; Bitsch, R.G. The protective effect of pulsed lavage against implant subsidence and micromotion for cemented tibial unicompartmental knee components: An experimental cadaver study. *J. Arthroplast.* **2014**, *29*, 727–732. [CrossRef]
5. Benjamin, J.B.; Gie, G.A.; Lee, A.J.; Ling, R.S.; Volz, R.G. Cementing technique and the effects of bleeding. *J. Bone Jt. Surg. Br.* **1987**, *69*, 620–624. [CrossRef]
6. Wetzels, T.; van Erp, J.; Brouwer, R.W.; Bulstra, S.K.; van Raay, J. Comparing Cementing Techniques in Total Knee Arthroplasty: An In Vitro Study. *J. Knee Surg.* **2019**, *32*, 886–890. [CrossRef]
7. Huiskes, R. Some fundamental aspects of human joint replacement. Analyses of stresses and heat conduction in bone-prosthesis structures. *Acta Orthop. Scand. Suppl.* **1980**, *185*, 1–208. [CrossRef] [PubMed]
8. Hampton, C.B.; Berliner, Z.P.; Nguyen, J.T.; Mendez, L.; Smith, S.S.; Joseph, A.D.; Padgett, D.E.; Rodriguez, J.A. Aseptic Loosening at the Tibia in Total Knee Arthroplasty: A Function of Cement Mantle Quality? *J. Arthroplast.* **2020**, *35*, S190–S196. [CrossRef] [PubMed]
9. Cawley, D.T.; Kelly, N.; McGarry, J.P.; Shannon, F.J. Cementing techniques for the tibial component in primary total knee replacement. *Bone Jt. J.* **2013**, *95*, 295–300. [CrossRef] [PubMed]
10. Sih, G.C.; Connelly, G.M.; Berman, A.T. The effect of thickness and pressure on the curing of PMMA bone cement for the total hip joint replacement. *J. Biomech.* **1980**, *13*, 347–352. [CrossRef]
11. Clarius, M.; Hauck, C.; Seeger, J.B.; James, A.; Murray, D.W.; Aldinger, P.R. Pulsed lavage reduces the incidence of radiolucent lines under the tibial tray of Oxford unicompartmental knee arthroplasty: Pulsed lavage versus syringe lavage. *Int. Orthop.* **2009**, *33*, 1585–1590. [CrossRef] [PubMed]
12. Breusch, S.J.; Norman, T.L.; Schneider, U.; Reitzel, T.; Blaha, J.D.; Lukoschek, M. Lavage technique in total hip arthroplasty: Jet lavage produces better cement penetration than syringe lavage in the proximal femur. *J. Arthroplast.* **2000**, *15*, 921–927. [CrossRef]
13. Seeger, J.B.; Jaeger, S.; Bitsch, R.G.; Mohr, G.; Rohner, E.; Clarius, M. The effect of bone lavage on femoral cement penetration and interface temperature during Oxford unicompartmental knee arthroplasty with cement. *J. Bone Jt. Surg. Am.* **2013**, *95*, 48–53. [CrossRef]
14. Helwig, P.; Konstantinidis, L.; Hirschmuller, A.; Miltenberger, V.; Kuminack, K.; Sudkamp, N.P.; Hauschild, O. Tibial cleaning method for cemented total knee arthroplasty: An experimental study. *Indian J. Orthop.* **2013**, *47*, 18–22. [CrossRef]
15. Kalteis, T.; Pforringer, D.; Herold, T.; Handel, M.; Renkawitz, T.; Plitz, W. An experimental comparison of different devices for pulsatile high-pressure lavage and their relevance to cement intrusion into cancellous bone. *Arch. Orthop. Trauma Surg.* **2007**, *127*, 873–877. [CrossRef]
16. Granick, M.S.; Tenenhaus, M.; Knox, K.R.; Ulm, J.P. Comparison of wound irrigation and tangential hydrodissection in bacterial clearance of contaminated wounds: Results of a randomized, controlled clinical study. *Ostomy Wound Manag.* **2007**, *53*, 64–66, 68–70, 72.
17. Sobel, J.W.; Goldberg, V.M. Pulsatile irrigation in orthopedics. *Orthopedics* **1985**, *8*, 1019–1022. [CrossRef]
18. Morgan, J.; Holder, G.; Desoutter, G. The measurement and comparison of jet characteristics of surgical pulse lavage devices. *J. Arthroplast.* **2003**, *18*, 45–50. [CrossRef]
19. Goldstein, W.M.; Gordon, A.; Goldstein, J.M.; Berland, K.; Branson, J.; Sarin, V.K. Improfement of Cement mantle thickness with pressurized carbon dioxide lavage. In Proceedings of the 20th Annual Meeting of the International Society for Technology in Arthroplasty 2007, Paris, France, 28 July 2007.
20. Boontanapibul, K.; Ruangsomboon, P.; Charoencholvanich, K.; Pornrattanamaneewong, C. Effectiveness Testing of Combined Innovative Pressurized Carbon Dioxide Lavage and Pulsatile Normal Saline Irrigation to Enhance Bone Cement Penetration in Total Knee Replacement: A Cadaveric Study. *J. Med. Assoc. Thai.* **2016**, *99*, 1198–1202.
21. Gapinski, Z.A.; Yee, E.J.; Kraus, K.R.; Deckard, E.R.; Meneghini, R.M. The Effect of Tourniquet Use and Sterile Carbon Dioxide Gas Bone Preparation on Cement Penetration in Primary Total Knee Arthroplasty. *J. Arthroplast.* **2019**, *34*, 1634–1639. [CrossRef]
22. Ravenscroft, M.J.; Charalambous, C.P.; Mills, S.P.; Woodruff, M.J.; Stanley, J.K. Bone-cement interface strength in distal radii using two medullary canal preparation techniques: Carbon dioxide jet cleaning versus syringed saline. *Hand Surg.* **2010**, *15*, 95–98. [CrossRef] [PubMed]
23. Lax-Prez, R.; Ferrero-Manzanal, F.; Marin-Penia, O.; Murcia-Asensio, A. Gas embolism after the use of the CarboJet lavage system during hip hemiarthroplasty. Clinical case and literature review. *Acta Ortop. Mex.* **2014**, *28*, 45–48. [PubMed]
24. Garcia Martinez, M.R.; Ruiz, G.M.V.; Perez, J.M.R.; Perez, R.L. Air embolism after cleaning the intramedullary canal with a high pressure CO_2 wash in hip fracture. *Rev. Esp. Anestesiol. Reanim* **2013**, *60*, 353–354. [PubMed]
25. Jaeger, S.; Rieger, J.S.; Obermeyer, B.; Klotz, M.C.; Kretzer, J.P.; Bitsch, R.G. Cement applicator use for hip resurfacing arthroplasty. *Med. Eng. Phys.* **2015**, *37*, 447–452. [CrossRef]
26. Bitsch, R.G.; Loidolt, T.; Heisel, C.; Schmalzried, T.P. Cementing techniques for hip resurfacing arthroplasty: Development of a laboratory model. *J. Bone Jt. Surg. Am.* **2008**, *90* (Suppl. 3), 102–110. [CrossRef]
27. Yushkevich, P.A.; Piven, J.; Hazlett, H.C.; Smith, R.G.; Ho, S.; Gee, J.C.; Gerig, G. User-guided 3D active contour segmentation of anatomical structures: Significantly improved efficiency and reliability. *Neuroimage* **2006**, *31*, 1116–1128. [CrossRef]

38. Schlegel, U.J.; Siewe, J.; Delank, K.S.; Eysel, P.; Puschel, K.; Morlock, M.M.; de Uhlenbrock, A.B. Pulsed lavage improves fixation strength of cemented tibial components. *Int. Orthop.* **2011**, *35*, 1165–1169. [CrossRef] [PubMed]
39. Miller, M.A.; Terbush, M.J.; Goodheart, J.R.; Izant, T.H.; Mann, K.A. Increased initial cement-bone interlock correlates with reduced total knee arthroplasty micro-motion following in vivo service. *J. Biomech.* **2014**, *47*, 2460–2466. [CrossRef] [PubMed]
40. Bitsch, R.G.; Jager, S.; Lurssen, M.; Loidolt, T.; Schmalzried, T.P.; Clarius, M. Influence of bone density on the cement fixation of femoral hip resurfacing components. *J. Orthop. Res.* **2010**, *28*, 986–991. [CrossRef]
41. Buller, L.T.; Rao, V.; Chiu, Y.F.; Nam, D.; McLawhorn, A.S. Primary Total Knee Arthroplasty Performed Using High-Viscosity Cement is Associated With Higher Odds of Revision for Aseptic Loosening. *J. Arthroplast.* **2020**, *35* (Suppl. 6), S182–S189. [CrossRef] [PubMed]
42. Koh, B.T.; Tan, J.H.; Ramruttun, A.K.; Wang, W. Effect of storage temperature and equilibration time on polymethyl methacrylate (PMMA) bone cement polymerization in joint replacement surgery. *J. Orthop. Surg. Res.* **2015**, *10*, 178. [CrossRef] [PubMed]
43. Chiaramonti, A.M.; Robertson, A.D.; Nguyen, T.P.; Jaffe, D.E.; Hanna, E.L.; Holmes, R.; Barfield, W.R.; Fourney, W.L.; Stains, J.P.; Pellegrini, V.D., Jr. Pulsatile Lavage of Musculoskeletal Wounds Causes Muscle Necrosis and Dystrophic Calcification in a Rat Model. *J. Bone Jt. Surg. Am.* **2017**, *99*, 1851–1858. [CrossRef]
44. Boyd, J.I., 3rd; Wongworawat, M.D. High-pressure pulsatile lavage causes soft tissue damage. *Clin. Orthop. Relat. Res.* **2004**, *427*, 13–17. [CrossRef]
45. Bhandari, M.; Adili, A.; Lachowski, R.J. High pressure pulsatile lavage of contaminated human tibiae: An in vitro study. *J. Orthop. Trauma* **1998**, *12*, 479–484. [CrossRef]
46. Hassinger, S.M.; Harding, G.; Wongworawat, M.D. High-pressure pulsatile lavage propagates bacteria into soft tissue. *Clin Orthop. Relat. Res.* **2005**, *439*, 27–31. [CrossRef] [PubMed]

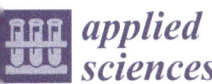

Article

What Is the Impact of a CAM Impingement on the Gait Cycle in Patients with Progressive Osteoarthritis of the Hip?

Eike Franken [1], Thilo Floerkemeier [2], Eike Jakubowitz [3], Alexander Derksen [4], Stefan Budde [4], Henning Windhagen [4] and Nils Wirries [4,*]

1. Department for Orthopaedic Surgery and Traumatology, Hospital Agnes Karll, 30880 Laatzen, Germany; Eike.Franken@krh.eu
2. go:h Gelenkchirurgie Orthopädie: Hannover, 30159 Hannover, Germany; thilo.floerkemeier@g-o-hannover.de
3. Laboratory for Biomechanics and Biomaterials, Hannover Medical School, 30625 Hannover, Germany; Jakubowitz.Eike@mh-hannover.de
4. Department for Orthopaedic Surgery at Diakovere Annastift, Hannover Medical School, 30625 Hannover, Germany; Alexander.Derksen@diakovere.de (A.D.); st-budde@t-online.de (S.B.); Henning.Windhagen@diakovere.de (H.W.)
* Correspondence: Nils.Wirries@diakovere.de; Tel.: +49-(511)-5354-0

Citation: Franken, E.; Floerkemeier, T.; Jakubowitz, E.; Derksen, A.; Budde, S.; Windhagen, H.; Wirries, N. What Is the Impact of a CAM Impingement on the Gait Cycle in Patients with Progressive Osteoarthritis of the Hip? *Appl. Sci.* 2021, *11*, 6024. https://doi.org/10.3390/app11136024

Academic Editor: Hanatsu Nagano

Received: 27 February 2021
Accepted: 27 June 2021
Published: 29 June 2021

Publisher's Note: MDPI stays neutral with regard to jurisdictional claims in published maps and institutional affiliations.

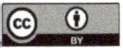

Copyright: © 2021 by the authors. Licensee MDPI, Basel, Switzerland. This article is an open access article distributed under the terms and conditions of the Creative Commons Attribution (CC BY) license (https://creativecommons.org/licenses/by/4.0/).

Abstract: (1) Background: The femoroacetabular impingement (FAI) type cam leads to a conflict between the acetabular rim and a bony thickening of the femoral neck junction. While maximal excursions in flexion, adduction and internal rotation provoke pain, the aim of this study was to analyze if a cam morphology shows an impact on gait pattern. (2) Methods: Fifty-five patients with end-stage hip osteoarthritis performed gait analysis before hip replacement as well as three, six and 12 months postoperatively. Thirty-three (60%) of them presented an FAI type cam. An ANOVA was used to compare the hip angles in sagittal, frontal and transversal planes between patients with a FAI type cam (group "+cam") and without (group "−cam"). (3) Results: Before surgery the patients of the +cam-group showed a tendency towards a reduced flexion and internal rotation at the heel strike ($p > 0.05$). Over time, the differences were adjusted by total hip arthroplasty. (4) Conclusions: We did not find any differences in the gait analysis of patients with a FAI type cam compared to patients without.

Keywords: hip deformity; femoroacetabular impingement (FAI); gait analysis; range of motion; heel strike; toe off

1. Introduction

Osteoarthritis of the hip (OA) is an irreversible degeneration of the cartilage that affects the functionality of the joint due to reduction of the range of motion (ROM). These limitations result multifactorially from bone remodeling with osteophytes and inflammatory processes of muscles, tendons and the joint capsule [1]. The accompanied pain leads to compensatory movements and relieving postures. Previous studies showed that patients with hip OA were characterized with a reduced stride length, gait velocity and maximum joint excursions [2,3]. The surgical treatment of the hip OA with a total hip arthroplasty (THA) is considered to be one of the most successful orthopedic operations [4]. This procedure leads to a higher physical performance in treated patients with severe OA compared to untreated patients, as well as to a very high post operational satisfaction in patients [5]. While older patients usually suffer from an idiopathic joint degeneration, the OA in younger patients commonly occur due to a specific trigger, in most cases dysplasia or a femoro-acetabular impingement (FAI) [6]. FAI is an incongruence between the acetabular rim and the femoral neck. Three different types of an articular FAI were differentiated: FAI type pincer, FAI type cam and a mixed type. While the type pincer represents a local or general over coverage of the femoral head, comparable with osteophytes of the acetabular rim, the type cam affects the femoral neck with anterior-lateral bone thickening [7]. In clinical examination, the conflict between the cam morphology and the acetabular rim could be provoked with a maximal excursion in flexion, adduction and internal rotation (FADIR or anterior impingement test) [8]. This test leads to pain and shows the restrictions in the maximum excursions caused by the bony conflict in the presence of an FAI [9,10]. Some studies showed that the presence of a cam deformity influences the gait pattern and joint moments [11,12]. In spite of joint-preserving surgeries, differences in healthy individuals were notable or with a questionable clinical relevance [13–15]. Due to studies showing differences in the gait pattern of patients with a FAI type cam, the aim of the current study was to analyze if the functionality of the affected joint was comparable after THA, or if there were notable remaining changes. Another goal was to compare the gait pattern of patients with hip OA depend on the presence of an FAI type cam.

2. Materials and Methods

This prospective clinical study was approved by the local IRB (4565) and registered in the German Clinical Trail Register (Trail-ID: DRKS00010421). The primary aim of the project was to compare the gait pattern between patients who received a short-stem total hip replacement (METHA, Fa. Aesculap, Tuttlingen, Germany) and cementless cup (PLASMAFIT, Fa. Aesculap, Tuttlingen, Germany) through a standard lateral approach and a minimal-invasive antero-lateral approach. Power analysis for this yielded a size of 30 patients in each group. The current study question regarding the impact of a FAI type cam represents a secondary aim. Thus, all results only represent assumptions. All patients provided an informed consent. After written informed consent, the patients were consecutively included with respect to the following inclusion and exclusion criteria.

Inclusion criteria:
- end-stage, therapy-resistant osteoarthritis of the hip in patients with ages between 18 and 75 years on the day of surgery;
- no deficiency in the motoric and neurologic function of the lower extremity, documented by the preoperative clinical examination.

Exclusion criteria:
- cardiovascular disease as contraindication for physical exercise, e.g., cardiac insufficiency (NYHA class IV);
- intake of drugs affecting the patient's balance;
- changes in balance and sensitivity affecting the lower extremity due to diseases such as Ménière's disease, complete loss of eyesight, polyneuropathy, multiple sclerosis;
- previous bony surgery on the affected hip;
- arthrodesis or replacement of the knee or ankle joint.

All patients sustained an end-stage hip OA and were planned for THA. Based on the axial radiograph of the hip, the alpha angle described by Nötzli was used to determine the incidence of a CAM impingement in the patient population (alpha angle > 65°) [16]. As patients with primary OA may build osteophytes around the femoral neck junction, we decided to enhance the usually used cut-off value for a FAI type CAM from 55° to 65° to achieve a clearer selection between patients with osteophytes and a bony bump. Furthermore, the offset and the caput-collum-diaphyseal (CCD) angle was measured on the native hip joint of the preoperative anterior-posterior (a.p.) pelvic planning radiograph, standardized in the supine position, to define the hip morphology [17,18]. The measurements were repeated after hip replacement on the control a.p. pelvic at the 12-months follow-up examination according to our clinical routine. Direct postoperative radiographs were not used for evaluation due to possible inaccuracies caused by postoperative pain resulting in limitations of positioning. All radiographs were analyzed with Carestream® (Carestream Solutions, Vue Solutions).

The clinical observations were published [19,20]. However, to compare the preoperative findings with the 12-month follow-up results between patients with or without an FAI type CAM, the Harris Hip Score (HHS) was added.

From the original total study group of 60 patients, five patients (8.3%) were subsequently excluded due to more than two missing follow-up examinations. Two further patients missed two (3.3%) and 19 one (31.6%) follow-up examinations. As a result, 34 patients (56.8%) attended all follow-up points. In the case of participation, all data were attained in total. In accordance with our biometric procedure, the missing values for the 21 patients with one to two follow-ups less could be filled with the results of the previous values of the earlier one to two examination time points.

2.1. Gait Cycle Analysis

The recording of gait cycle was carried out preoperatively as well as three, six and 12 months postoperatively after THA. To trace the joint movement, 16 reflective markers of a Plug-In Gait-Marker set were attached to the subject's skin [21]. These markers were placed bilaterally over specific bony landmarks (spina iliaca anterior superior, spina iliaca posterior superior, lateral thigh, lateral epicondyle, lateral lower leg, lateral malleolus, base of os metatarsale II, posterior calcaneus). To determine the correct orientation of the markers, as well as to compute the position of the joint centers and the individual segments of the lower limb, a static standing trial was recorded subsequently. Eight infrared MX-cameras sampling at 200 Hz were used to track the markers (Vicon Motion Systems Ltd., Oxford, UK) while the ground reaction forces were measured with two in-ground mounted force plates type BP400600 sampling at 1000 Hz (AMTI, Watertown, MA, USA). The captured kinetic and kinematic data were further processed using Nexus software Version 1.8.5 (Vicon Motion Systems Ltd.), as were spatio-temporal parameters (walking speed, cadence, step length). For the dynamic measurements the subjects walked a distance of 10 m barefooted at a self-selected speed. At about 5 m the two in-ground force plates were located. Ten valid trials were recorded. A trial was counted as valid when the subject struck each plate with one foot without stepping over the plate's borderline.

The joint movements of the operated and nonoperated limb in each degree of freedom (hip: flexion/extension, abduction/adduction, external/internal rotation) were described in courses of curves. Events of the gait (toe off/heel strike on the in-ground force plates) were detected automatically. Kinematic and kinetic data were time normalized with respect to the gait cycle (101 parts, 0–100% of the gait cycle; Figure 1), whereas kinetic data were additionally normalized to the body weight. The normalization and averaging were performed with Polygon software Version 3.5.2 (Vicon Motion Systems Ltd.). Single values were picked out from continuous joint kinematics regarding heel strike (0% of gait cycle) and toe-off (~60% of gait cycle) for comparisons (Figure 1).

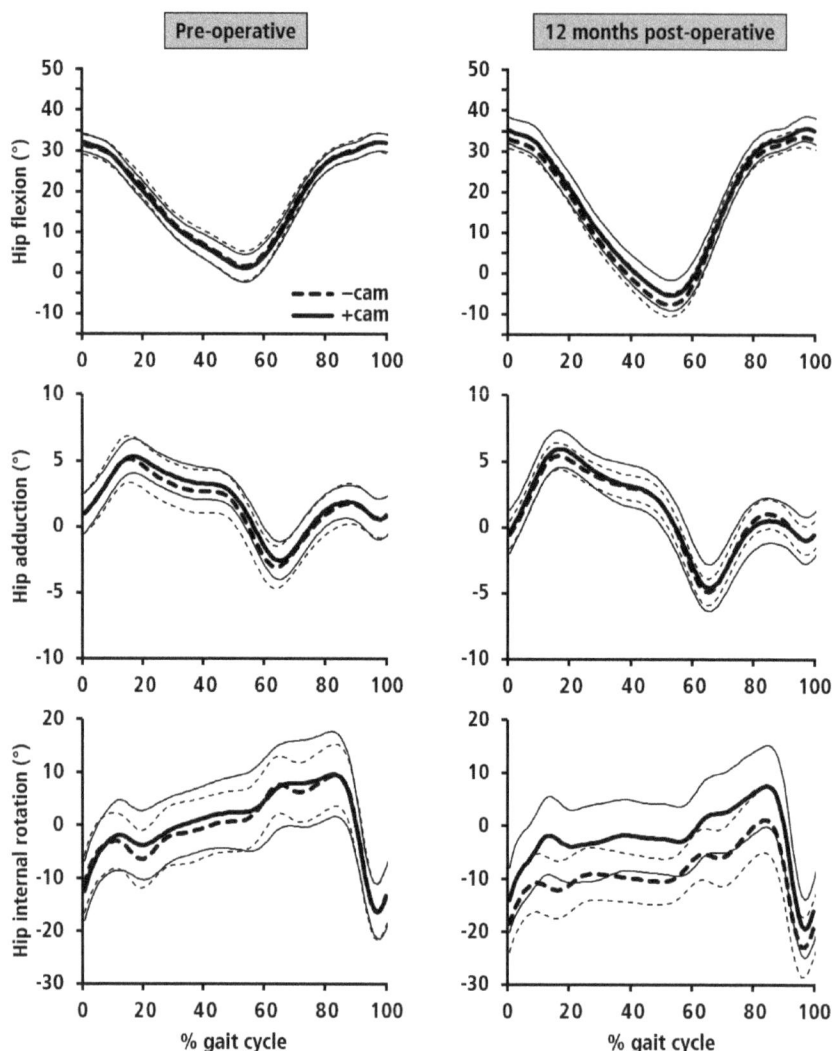

Figure 1. Mean value graphs (bold lines) with standard deviation (fine lines) of the gait cycles (0–100%) for both patient groups with (+cam) or without (−cam) an FAI type cam before surgery and at the last follow-up. The analysis was based on the values at 0% (heel strike) and 60% (toe off).

2.2. Statistics

For statistical analysis SPSS (Version 26, IBM, Armonk, NY, USA) was used. In the describing assay, metric values are given as the means and standard deviations (1.96), ordinal and nominal data as absolute values and percentages. For the demographic analysis and the comparison of the approach data, hip morphology and the clinical results between patients with (+cam group) and without cam (−cam group), unpaired t-tests (metric data) or chi^2 tests (nominal data) were performed. Analysis of the gait cycle was performed on the time at the toe off and the heel strike preoperatively and at the 12-month follow-up, because we expected steady state values at these times with the least influence of the postoperative healing processes. To achieve a more detailed development of the range of motion over the time, the three and six months postoperative follow-ups were used for creating figures. We selected hip angles in the sagittal (flexion/extension), frontal (adduction/abduction) and transversal plane (internal/external rotation) to investigate the impact of the bony cam on the hip movements and gait pattern. The values were measured relative to the pelvic position. First, a linear regression was performed to compare the preoperative and the 12-month follow-up results, and the difference between patients with or without cam. The level of significance of p-value was $<0.05/3 = 0.017$ according to a Bonferroni correction resulting from two previously published paper with the current study group [19,20]. Further, significant parameters were tested using multiple linear regression to identify the potential influence of the patient's age, body-mass index (BMI), gender, the performed approach and the hip morphology (difference of the pre to postoperative offset and CCD angle) as covariants. In addition, a post hoc analysis (CI 95.0%, $p < 0.05$) was used to describe the power of the comparisons.

3. Results

The total study group included 55 patients (33 males/60.0%; 22 females/40.0%) with a mean age of 57.8 years (±8.4; 36.0–71.0) and a mean body mass index (BMI) of 27.3 kg/m^2 (±5.2; 20.6–54.9). The affected side was the left hip in 20 cases (36.4%) and the right hip in 33 cases (63.6%). In 33 cases (60.0%) a cam morphology was present, and in 22 (40.0%) it was not. Both groups, cam + and cam −, were comparable in terms of age, BMI, gender, performed hip approach, the hip morphology (offset/CCD angle) and the clinical results (HHS) ($p > 0.05$) (Table 1).

Table 1. Demographic data, approach data, hip morphology and clinical outcomes between both groups, +cam and −cam. Lat. = standard lateral hip approach, ant.-lat. = minimal-invasive antero-lateral hip approach. Both groups were comparable in terms of age, BMI, gender and approach ($p > 0.05$). The +cam group showed a tendency towards younger patient age (2.8 years) and lower BMI (1.7).

Mean ± SD	−cam (n = 22)	+cam (n = 33)	95% CI
Age	59.5 ± 8.2	56.7 ± 8.5	−1.8; 7.4
BMI	28.3 ± 6.1	26.6 ± 3.1	−1.2; 4.5
Gender (♂/♀)	10/12	21/12	>0.05
Approach (Lat./Ant.-lat.)	8/14	19/14	>0.05
Offset preop.	44.9 ± 10.1	47.7 ± 6.4	−7.2; 1.8
Offset 12M FU	52.6 ± 7.8	54.0 ± 7.5	−5.7; 2.8
difference offset	7.7 ± 6.6	6.2 ± 6.5	−2.1; 5.1
CCD preop.	131.8 ± 9.7	130.7 ± 5.2	−1.0; 7.2
CCD 12M FU	130.9 ± 5.9	130.8 ± 4.6	−2.8; 2.9
Difference CCD	−0.9 ± 6.9	0.09 ± 5.7	−5.5; 1.6
HHS preop.	51.7 ± 11.9	53.7 ± 11.4	−8.4; 4.4
HHS 12M FU	95.7 ± 7.0	94.6 ± 9.9	−3.9; 6.1
Difference HHS	43.6 ± 13.9	42.9 ± 15.8	−7.8; 9.2

3.1. Heel Strike

The comparison between the hip angles of the treated side to the nontreated side showed that a preoperative tendency in the sagittal and transversal plane was balanced up to the last follow-up. In detail, the mean values in the sagittal/transversal planes of the treated leg tended, preoperatively, to be inferior compared to the untreated side, and approximated over the time. However, the results showed no statistical significance ($p > 0.05$). The values of the treated and nontreated sides in the frontal plane were nearly constant over time ($p > 0.05$). In spite of a preoperative trend to an inferior mean flexion, abduction and internal rotation in the presence of a cam deformity compared to patients without a FAI type CAM, the results showed no statistical significance ($p > 0.05$) (Table 2).

Table 2. Mean values and standard deviation at the heel strike of the treated hip before and 12 months after surgery dependent on a cam shaped femoral neck junction. The difference in the frontal plane was statistically significant with a lower reduction to the adduction after treatment in patients with an FAI type cam. The mean differences between the hip angles in presence of a cam deformity and absence ranged between 0.9–2.7°.

Heel Strike	−cam	+cam	Difference −/+cam	95% CI
Hip sag. preop.	32.9 ± 6.2	30.5 ± 5.7	2.4	−0.89; 5.7
Hip sag. 12 M FU	34.6 ± 7.8	33.5 ± 6.2	1.1	−3.0; 5.0
difference preop. − 12 M	1.7 ± 10.7	3.1 ± 7.9	1.4	−6.4; 3.7
Hip front. preop.	1.7 ± 3.0	0.01 ± 4.2	1.69	−0.42; 3.8
Hip front. 12 M FU	−1.1 ± 3.1	−0.05 ± 3.6	1.05	−3.0; 0.8
difference preop. − 12 M	−2.8 ± 4.1	−0.06 ± 3.6	2.74	−4.9; −0.66
Hip trans. preop.	−12.1 ± 16.2	−10.8 ± 11.7	1.3	−8.8; 6.2
Hip trans. 12 M FU	−18.1 ± 17.0	−15.8 ± 11.5	2.3	−9.9; 5.4
difference preop. − 12 M	−5.9 ± 22.2	−5.0 ± 10.6	0.9	−9.9; 8.0

Comparison between the baseline values and the 12-month results in all planes showed a greater increase in the +cam group for the frontal plane, with statistical significance ($p = 0.011$, Cohen's d = −0.73, post-hoc power = 0.72) (Figure 2).

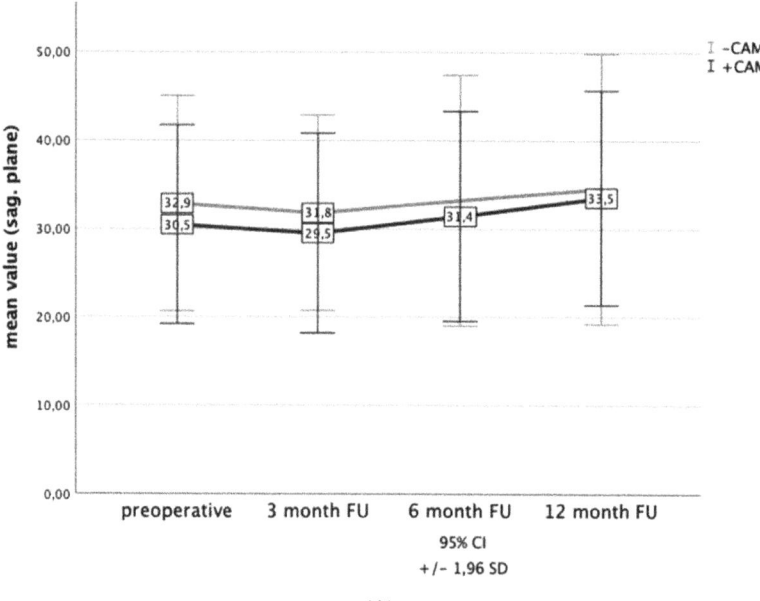

(A)

Figure 2. Cont.

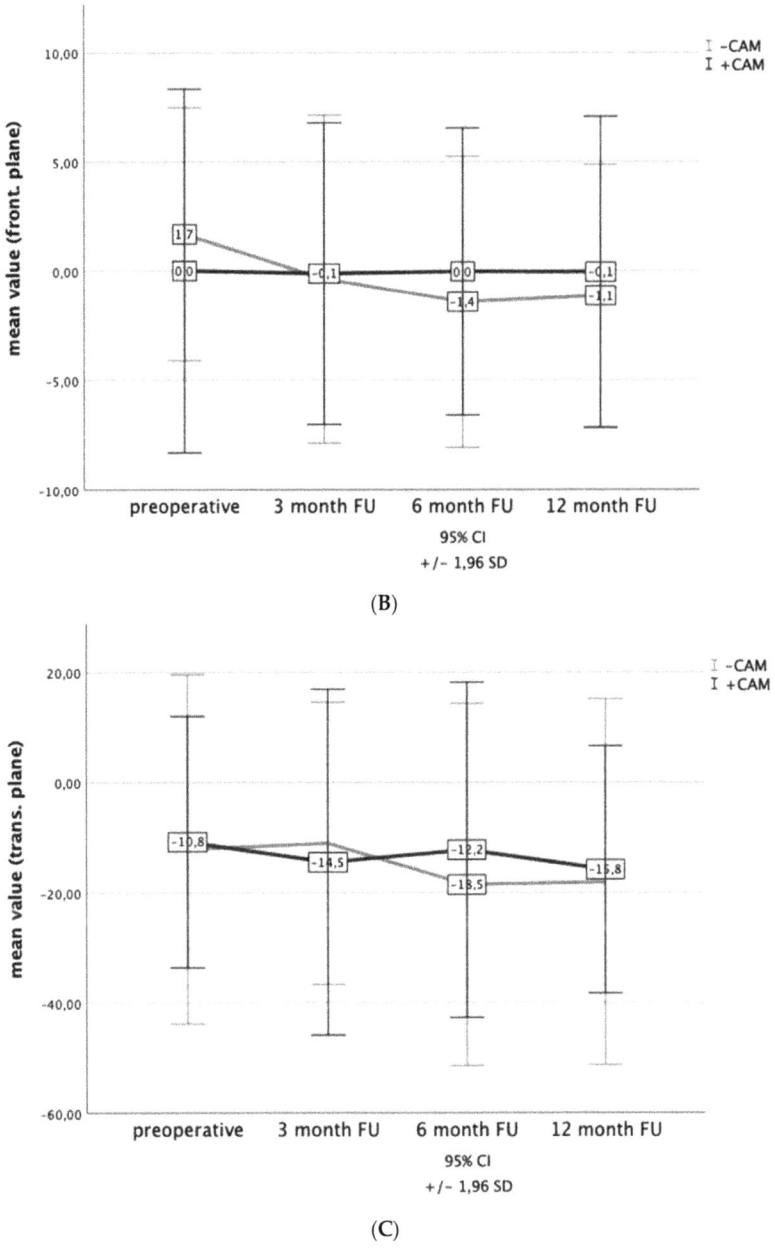

Figure 2. (**A**–**C**) The hip angles at the point of heel strike showed a constant course in the sagittal and frontal plane. Consistent with the results in Table 2, the transversal values decreased from the preoperative status to the last time of follow-up. Overall, no significant differences between patients with or without a cam morphology were observed.

Multiple linear analysis showed that the patient's age ($p = 0.1$), BMI ($p = 0.85$), gender ($p = 0.43$), the performed approach ($p = 0.91$) and the pre to postoperative changes of the offset ($p = 0.59$) and the CCD angle ($p = 0.96$) had no statistically significant impact on the difference values in the frontal plane ($p > 0.05$). The r^2 of the whole model regarding all analyzed cofactors was 0.18, resulting in a power of 0.7.

3.2. Toe off

Before surgery the treated side stood tendentially in flexion at the toe off, while the contralateral side had an extended position. Over time, the treated hip tended to an extension at 12-month follow-up examination. The curves of the frontal plane proceeded nearly in parallel. Here the treated hip showed a mean 0.8° abduction, and the nontreated had about 0.9° adduction. Furthermore, preoperatively the treated side showed on average 2.5° internal rotation, and the nontreated side about a 3.9° external rotation. Over time the curves crossed, so that the treated leg turned towards an external rotation. All these differences showed no statistical significance and were thus interpreted as tendencies ($p > 0.05$). At the toe off, the mean angles at the hip joint were tendentially in all planes inferior in the presence of a CAM ($p > 0.05$) (Table 3).

Table 3. Mean values and standard deviations at the toe off of the treated hip before and 12 months after surgery, as well as the difference between both time points depending on the presence of a cam deformity. No statistically significant differences were found. The mean differences between the hip angles in patients with and without a cam deformity ranged between 0.1–4.2°.

Toe off	−cam	+cam	Difference −/+cam	95% CI
Hip sag. preop.	2.2 ± 7.8	2.1 ± 10.2	0.1	−5.1; 5.2
Hip sag. 12 M FU	−3.2 ± 9.1	−6.3 ± 8.0	3.1	−1.6; 7.7
Difference preop. − 12 M	−5.4 ± 10.3	−8.4 ± 8.8	3.0	−2.2; 8.2
Hip front. preop.	−0.7 ± 2.9	−1.1 ± 4.5	0.4	−1.8; 2.5
Hip front. 12 M FU	−1.2 ± 4.1	−1.1 ± 2.8	0.1	−2.0; 1.7
Difference preop. − 12 M	−0.5 ± 3.8	0.02 ± 4.5	0.51	−2.8; 1.8
Hip trans. preop.	3.0 ± 17.4	2.1 ± 15.7	0.9	−8.2; 9.9
Hip trans. 12 M FU	−4.0 ± 14.7	−8.2 ± 10.7	4.2	−2.8; 11.0
Difference preop. − 12 M	−7.0 ± 18.5	−10.3 ± 18.0	3.3	−6.8; 13.3

The difference between the baseline values and the 12-month follow-up results tended towards a greater decrease in sagittal and transversal, and a greater rise in frontal planes for all hip angles in case of a CAM being present ($p > 0.05$) (Figure 3).

4. Discussion

The incongruence between the femoral neck and the acetabular rim in the case of a FAI is provoked in maximal flexion, adduction and internal rotation by the FADIR test. The purpose of the present study was to analyze the impact of a CAM deformity on the gait cycle of patients with an OA of the hip. A gait analysis was performed in fifty-five patients before THA and were followed up three, six and 12 months postoperatively to determine if preoperative differences existed, and if these adjusted over the time.

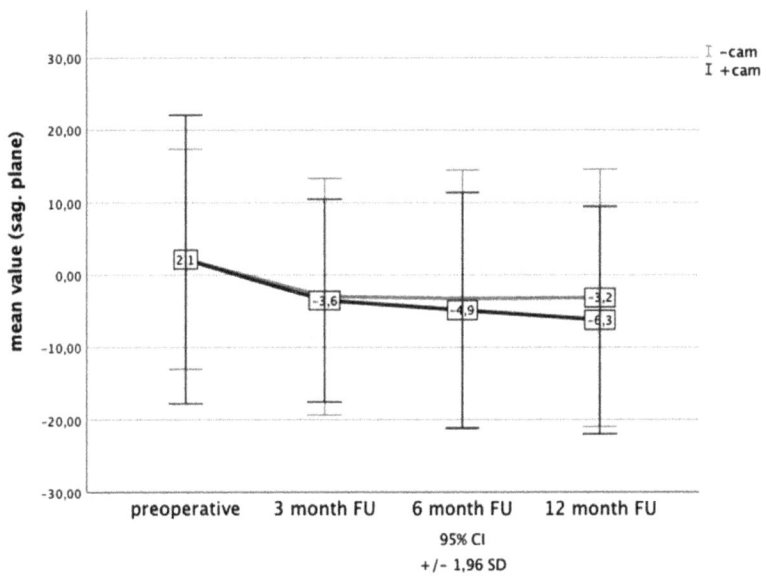

(A)

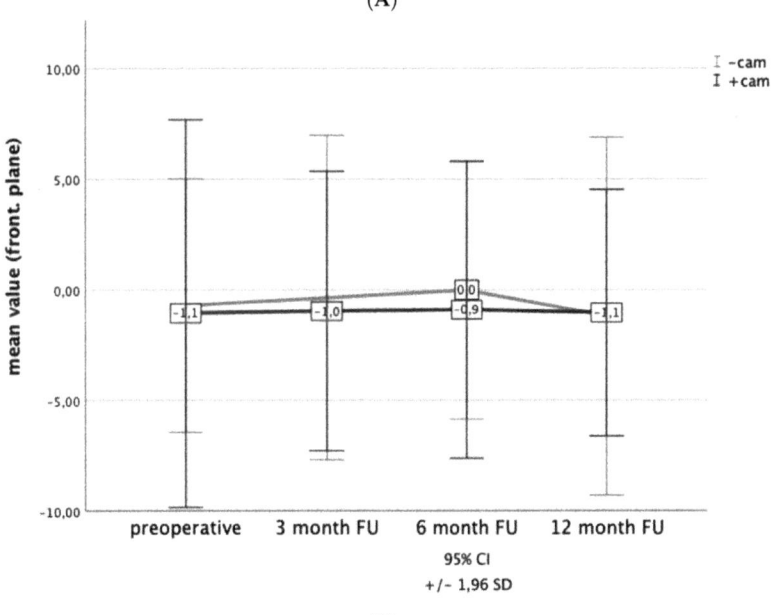

(B)

Figure 3. Cont.

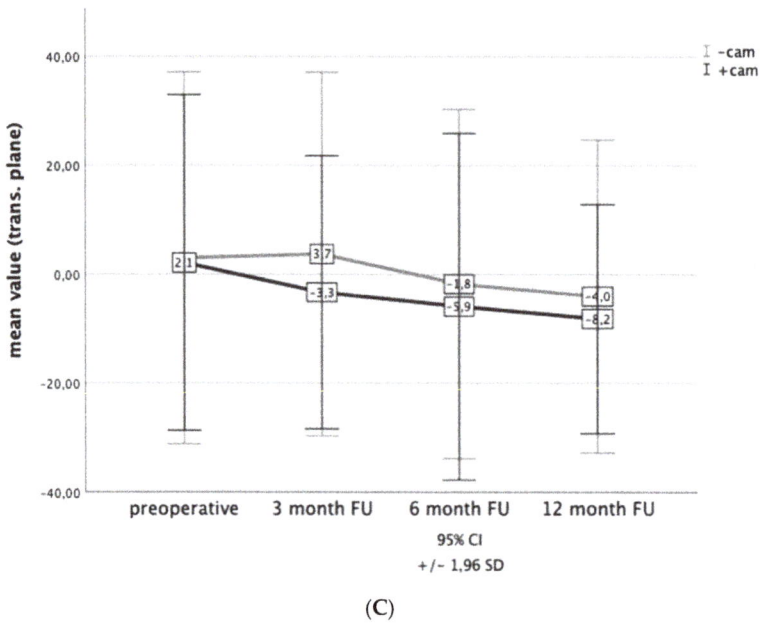

(C)

Figure 3. (A–C) The hip angles at the toe off in both groups were in the frontal plane before surgery and after. All the values in the sagittal and transversal plane had positive angles preoperatively and decreased to negative results at the 12-month examination.

Due to the great volume of collected parameters, the focus was set to the hip position at heel strike and toe off. At the heel strike, the hip position was tendentially in all planes inferior in the +cam group ($p > 0.05$), resulting in a flexion about 30.5°, an internal rotation about 10.8° and a neutral position in frontal plane. At the last examination the hip angles adjusted to 33.5° flexion, 0.5° adduction and 15.8 internal rotation in presence of a CAM. The differences at the toe off between patients with or without an FAI type CAM were not significant for the hip position ($p > 0.05$). Preoperatively, the hips showed a comparable position in sagittal and frontal planes with a tendentially inferior internal rotation in the presence of a CAM deformity ($p > 0.05$). At the examination 12 months after THA, the angles in the frontal plane remained comparable, while the mean values in the sagittal plane tended towards an extension and external rotation in the +cam group ($p > 0.05$). Overall, the results of the hip position while walking with a CAM deformity showed no statistical significance, and the differences were too small to determine relevant clinical consequence. However, the observed tendencies might hint at an impact of an FAI on gait pattern with limited flexion and internal rotation, the trigger movements for the bony conflict of this hip disease. Our results indicate that patients who suffer from an FAI may avoid provoking movements while walking. Comparable findings were presented in previous studies. Rutherford et al. compared 20 asymptomatic patients with 20 patients suffering from FAI. Both groups showed comparable ranges of angles while walking. The authors estimated differences in testing these groups in impingement position and provoking maneuvers [22]. Further, Diamond et al. observed minimal impairments in gait pattern with an unclear impact on the patient's symptoms or the hip function. The authors performed a three-dimensional gait analysis with 15 symptomatic FAI patients before arthroscopic treatment compared to 15 symptoms-free patients [23]. In addition, compared to a healthy group of 18 subjects, the FAI type CAM patients had slower walking speeds as described in a gait analysis study by Ng et al. [24]. However, Kennedy et al. showed a reduced frontal and sagittal range of motion during gait. The authors compared 17 patients with a cam shaped femoral neck with a control group of 14 without, and explained the results by soft tissue restriction and limited mobility at the spino-pelvic joint [25]. The interaction of the spino-pelvic joint was also analyzed by Catelli et al., who found stronger hip extensors in patients with an FAI type cam, allowing a higher degree of posterior pelvic tilt to prevent symptoms [26].

The current study had some limitations. First, all patients suffered from high-grade osteoarthritis of the hip. As a result, their restrictions in movements might not have been caused only by the FAI type cam, but may also have been due to inflammatory and remodeling processes during degeneration. Therefore, the cut off value of the alpha-angle was elevated to 65°. Only results above that were defined as FAI type cam. The second limitation was that maximal joint movements of the hip were not assessed. Although the main aim of the study was to analyze the impact of a FAI type cam on gait pattern, there may have been some differences between the groups in maximal joint excursion. However, the limitations of flexion and internal rotation in FAI patients were known and used for clinical diagnosis (FADIR-test) [8], and might be proved in further studies with a cost-intensive adapted study population. Further, since the data were reanalyzed post hoc with respect to CAM, an analysis of confounders according to the usual procedures is not possible [27]. Therefore, we tried to identify the influencing covariates using a linear regression model. However, none of the included variables showed a significant influence. In spite of that, the current study is one of the first in the literature that observed the gait pattern of patients with coexistence of a hip OA and an FAI type cam before and after THA. Repeated gait assessments postoperatively allowed detection of changes after surgery to determine if preoperative differences adapted over time.

5. Conclusions

We did not find any differences in the gait analysis of patients with a FAI type cam compared to patients without.

Author Contributions: Conceptualization, H.W., T.F., S.B.; methodology, H.W., T.F., E.J.; software, E.F., E.J.; formal analysis, E.F., E.J., N.W.; investigation, E.F., E.J.; data curation, E.F., E.J., N.W.; writing—original draft preparation, E.F., N.W.; writing—review and editing, E.J., N.W.; visualization, A.D., E.J.; supervision, H.W., T.F., S.B., E.F., E.J.; project administration, E.F., T.F., N.W.; All authors have read and agreed to the published version of the manuscript.

Funding: This research received no external funding.

Institutional Review Board Statement: The study was conducted according to the guidelines of the Declaration of Helsinki, and approved by the Institutional Review Board (or Ethics Committee) of the Medical School Hannover (No. 4565).

Informed Consent Statement: Informed consent was obtained from all subjects involved in the study.

Data Availability Statement: The data presented in this study are available on request from the corresponding author. The data are not publicly available due to data protection.

Conflicts of Interest: The authors declare no conflict of interest.

References

1. Bijlsma, J.W.; Berenbaum, F.; Lafeber, F.P. Osteoarthritis: An update with relevance for clinical practice. *Lancet* **2011**, *377*, 2115–2126. [CrossRef]
2. Bennett, D.; Ogonda, L.; Elliott, D.; Humphreys, L.; Beverland, D.E. Comparison of gait kinematics in patients receiving minimally invasive and traditional hip replacement surgery: A prospective blinded study. *Gait Posture* **2006**, *23*, 374–382. [CrossRef] [PubMed]
3. Foucher, K.C.; Schlink, B.R.; Shakoor, N.; Wimmer, M.A. Sagittal plane hip motion reversals during walking are associated with disease severity and poorer function in subjects with hip osteoarthritis. *J. Biomech.* **2012**, *45*, 1360–1365. [CrossRef] [PubMed]
4. Tanaka, R.; Shigematsu, M.; Motooka, T.; Mawatari, M.; Hotokebuchi, T. Factors influencing the improvement of gait ability after total hip arthroplasty. *J. Arthroplasty* **2010**, *25*, 982–985. [CrossRef]
5. Mariconda, M.; Galasso, O.; Costa, G.G.; Recano, P.; Cerbasi, S. Quality of life and functionality after total hip arthroplasty: A long-term follow-up study. *BMC Musculoskelet Disord.* **2011**, *12*, 222. [CrossRef]

6. Ganz, R.; Leunig, M.; Leunig-Ganz, K.; Harris, W.H. The etiology of osteoarthritis of the hip: An integrated mechanical concept. *Clin. Orthop. Relat. Res.* **2008**, *466*, 264–272. [CrossRef]
7. Ganz, R.; Parvizi, J.; Beck, M.; Leunig, M.; Notzli, H.; Siebenrock, K.A. Femoroacetabular impingement: A cause for osteoarthritis of the hip. *Clin. Orthop. Relat. Res.* **2003**, 112–120. [CrossRef]
8. Philippon, M.J.; Maxwell, R.B.; Johnston, T.L.; Schenker, M.; Briggs, K.K. Clinical presentation of femoroacetabular impingement. *Knee Surg. Sports Traumatol. Arthrosc.* **2007**, *15*, 1041–1047. [CrossRef]
9. Byrd, J.W. Femoroacetabular impingement in athletes, part 1: Cause and assessment. *Sports Health* **2010**, *2*, 321–333. [CrossRef]
10. Kapron, A.L.; Anderson, A.E.; Peters, C.L.; Phillips, L.G.; Stoddard, G.J.; Petron, D.J.; Toth, R.; Aoki, S.K. Hip internal rotation is correlated to radiographic findings of cam femoroacetabular impingement in collegiate football players. *Arthroscopy* **2012**, *28*, 1661–1670. [CrossRef] [PubMed]
11. Farkas, G.J.; Cvetanovich, G.L.; Rajan, K.B.; Espinoza Orias, A.A.; Nho, S.J. Impact of Femoroacetabular Impingement Morphology on Gait Assessment in Symptomatic Patients. *Sports Health* **2015**, *7*, 429–436. [CrossRef]
12. Samaan, M.A.; Schwaiger, B.J.; Gallo, M.C.; Sada, K.; Link, T.M.; Zhang, A.L.; Majumdar, S.; Souza, R.B. Joint Loading in the Sagittal Plane During Gait Is Associated With Hip Joint Abnormalities in Patients With Femoroacetabular Impingement. *Am. J. Sports Med.* **2017**, *45*, 810–818. [CrossRef]
13. Catelli, D.S.; Ng, K.C.G.; Kowalski, E.; Beaule, P.E.; Lamontagne, M. Modified gait patterns due to cam FAI syndrome remain unchanged after surgery. *Gait Posture* **2019**, *72*, 135–141. [CrossRef]
14. Alradwan, H.; Khan, M.; Grassby, M.H.; Bedi, A.; Philippon, M.J.; Ayeni, O.R. Gait and lower extremity kinematic analysis as an outcome measure after femoroacetabular impingement surgery. *Arthroscopy* **2015**, *31*, 339–344. [CrossRef]
15. Brisson, N.; Lamontagne, M.; Kennedy, M.J.; Beaule, P.E. The effects of cam femoroacetabular impingement corrective surgery on lower-extremity gait biomechanics. *Gait Posture* **2013**, *37*, 258–263. [CrossRef]
16. Notzli, H.P.; Wyss, T.F.; Stoecklin, C.H.; Schmid, M.R.; Treiber, K.; Hodler, J. The contour of the femoral head-neck junction as a predictor for the risk of anterior impingement. *J. Bone Jt. Surg. Br.* **2002**, *84*, 556–560. [CrossRef]
17. Kutzner, K.P.; Freitag, T.; Donner, S.; Kovacevic, M.P.; Bieger, R. Outcome of extensive varus and valgus stem alignment in short-stem THA: Clinical and radiological analysis using EBRA-FCA. *Arch. Orthop. Trauma Surg.* **2017**, *137*, 431–439. [CrossRef]
18. Kutzner, K.P.; Kovacevic, M.P.; Roeder, C.; Rehbein, P.; Pfeil, J. Reconstruction of femoro-acetabular offsets using a short-stem. *Int. Orthop.* **2015**, *39*, 1269–1275. [CrossRef] [PubMed]
19. Floerkemeier, T.; Budde, S.; Lewinski, G.V.; Windhagen, H.; HurSchler, C.; Schwarze, M. Greater early migration of a short-stem total hip arthroplasty is not associated with an increased risk of osseointegration failure: 5th-year results from a prospective RSA study with 39 patients, a follow-up study. *Acta Orthop.* **2020**, *91*, 266–271. [CrossRef]
20. Schwarze, M.; Budde, S.; von Lewinski, G.; Windhagen, H.; Keller, M.C.; Seehaus, F.; Hurschler, C.; Floerkemeier, T. No effect of conventional vs. minimally invasive surgical approach on clinical outcome and migration of a short stem total hip prosthesis at 2-year follow-up: A randomized controlled study. *Clin. Biomech.* **2018**, *51*, 105–112. [CrossRef] [PubMed]
21. Kadaba, M.P.; Ramakrishnan, H.K.; Wootten, M.E.; Gainey, J.; Gorton, G.; Cochran, G.V. Repeatability of kinematic, kinetic, and electromyographic data in normal adult gait. *J. Orthop. Res.* **1989**, *7*, 849–860. [CrossRef] [PubMed]
22. Rutherford, D.J.; Moreside, J.; Wong, I. Differences in Hip Joint Biomechanics and Muscle Activation in Individuals With Femoroacetabular Impingement Compared With Healthy, Asymptomatic Individuals: Is Level-Ground Gait Analysis Enough? *Orthop. J. Sports Med.* **2018**, *6*. [CrossRef] [PubMed]
23. Diamond, L.E.; Wrigley, T.V.; Bennell, K.L.; Hinman, R.S.; O'Donnell, J.; Hodges, P.W. Hip joint biomechanics during gait in people with and without symptomatic femoroacetabular impingement. *Gait Posture* **2016**, *43*, 198–203. [CrossRef]
24. Ng, K.C.G.; Mantovani, G.; Modenese, L.; Beaule, P.E.; Lamontagne, M. Altered Walking and Muscle Patterns Reduce Hip Contact Forces in Individuals With Symptomatic Cam Femoroacetabular Impingement. *Am. J. Sports Med.* **2018**, *46*, 2615–2623. [CrossRef] [PubMed]
25. Kennedy, M.J.; Lamontagne, M.; Beaule, P.E. Femoroacetabular impingement alters hip and pelvic biomechanics during gait Walking biomechanics of FAI. *Gait Posture* **2009**, *30*, 41–44. [CrossRef]
26. Catelli, D.S.; Kowalski, E.; Beaule, P.E.; Smit, K.; Lamontagne, M. Asymptomatic Participants With a Femoroacetabular Deformity Demonstrate Stronger Hip Extensors and Greater Pelvis Mobility During the Deep Squat Task. *Orthop. J. Sports Med.* **2018**, *6*. [CrossRef]
27. Shrier, I.; Platt, R.W. Reducing bias through directed acyclic graphs. *BMC Med. Res. Methodol.* **2008**, *8*, 70. [CrossRef]

Article

The Rate of Correctly Planned Size of Digital Templating in Two Planes—A Comparative Study of a Short-Stem Total Hip Implant with Primary Metaphyseal Fixation and a Conventional Stem

Johanna K. Buschatzky [1], Michael Schwarze [2], Nils Wirries [1], Gabriela von Lewinski [3], Henning Windhagen [1], Thilo Floerkemeier [4] and Stefan Budde [1,*]

1. Department of Orthopaedic Surgery at Diakovere Annastift, Hannover Medical School, 30625 Hannover, Germany; j.buschatzky@yahoo.de (J.K.B.); Nils.Wirries@diakovere.de (N.W.); Henning.Windhagen@diakovere.de (H.W.)
2. Laboratory for Biomechanics and Biomaterials, Hannover Medical School, 30625 Hannover, Germany; Schwarze.Michael@mhh-hannover.de
3. Department of Orthopaedic Surgery, Göttingen Medical School, 37075 Göttingen, Germany; gabriela.lewinski@med.uni-goettingen.de
4. Go:h Gelenkchirurgie Orthopädie, 30159 Hannover, Germany; thilo.floerkemeier@g-o-hannover.de
* Correspondence: Stefan.Budde@diakovere.de

Abstract: (1) Background: Preoperative templating is mainly conducted on an anteroposterior pelvic overview X-ray. For short stem hip arthroplasty, the choice of the optimal size is especially crucial to avoid complications. Thus, the study aimed to determine if there is an increased rate of correctly planned sizes using two radiological planes. (2) Methods: 50 patients with a conventional stem and 100 with a short stem total hip arthroplasty were analyzed. Without knowing the implanted size, three independent orthopedic surgeons performed digital templating: once using the anteroposterior pelvic overview only and once using the lateral view in addition. (3) Results: The rate of correctly planned sizes (+/−1 size compared to the inserted size) of templating with one plane was 86.3% ± 9.5% in short stem hip arthroplasty and 88.4% ± 6.0% in conventional stem arthroplasty. By adding the lateral view, the rate of correctly planned sizes was 89.9% ± 12.0% for the short stem hip arthroplasty group and 89.4% ± 9.8% for the conventional group ($p > 0.1$). (4) A potential positive effect of preoperative templating using an additional lateral X-ray view for short stem implants may be suggested based on the results of this study, which did, however, not reach statistical significance.

Keywords: digital templating; short-stem; lateral view; femoral torsion

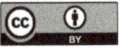

1. Introduction

The implantation of the optimal stem size is important for the implantation of a total hip arthroplasty (THA) in order to reduce complications. Digital templating of a THA is a helpful tool for preoperative planning of surgery regarding implant type, implant size, reconstruction of the center of rotation, offset, and limb lengths [1]. This tool assists in order to receive a good outcome after a THA and to avoid complications due to anatomic variations. It helps to reduce the incidence of undersizing the femoral implant with the associated risk of increased micromotions, subsidence, and early aseptic loosening [2–4] and the incidence of oversizing associated with the risk of femoral fractures. Furthermore, it is helpful to avoid limb length discrepancies, instability, or excessive tension of the periarticular soft tissues by inaccurate reconstruction of the center of rotation of the hip [3,5–10].

Meanwhile, preoperative planning with plastic templates on radiographs or digital templating as a valid method to determine the correct size of the femoral stem and acetabular component belongs to the standard preoperative procedures prior to a THA [5,11,12]. Digital templating of a THA is usually performed on the anteroposterior (a.p.) pelvic overview X-ray [13]. Some software programs allow for digital templating also use the lateral view of the proximal femur for templating the stem. Although efforts have been made to further improve the accuracy of preoperative templating by using CT-based three-dimensional computerized models [14], the simple method using only the pelvic overview X-ray is still the standard procedure in clinical routine due to its high practicability on the one hand and the high radiation exposure when using CT scans on the other. The fixation of short stem THA (STHA) with predominantly metaphyseal anchorage is different from conventional THA (CTHA). While the conventional stem has a metaphyseal-diaphyseal anchorage with an intramedullary fixation within the proximal third of the femur [11], STHA with predominantly metaphyseal anchorage adapts its orientation to the femoral neck and thus to its ante torsion (Figure 1).

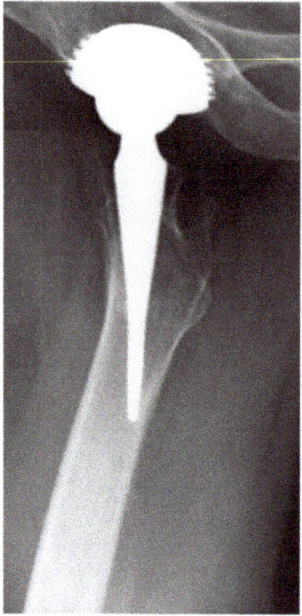

Figure 1. Lateral view of the METHA short stem total hip arthroplasty (STHA), showing the striven positioning parallel to the femoral neck and thus reconstructing the physiological ante torsion of the femoral neck.

This study aimed to determine whether there is a difference in accuracy when templating THA stems using not only the a.p. view of the pelvis but also the lateral view of the proximal femur. Furthermore, we analyzed whether there is a difference in the rate of correctly planned sizes when templating CTHA stems in comparison to STHA implants with a predominantly metaphyseal anchorage.

2. Materials and Methods

One hundred fifty patients with a good radiological outcome after implantation of a THA were selected: 50 after implantation of a THA using a conventional femoral stem (CTHA group) and 100 after implantation of a THA using a short stem with primary metaphyseal fixation (STHA group). A good radiological outcome was judged on the postoperative X-rays by three senior surgeons according to the following criteria: under- or oversizing, early subsidence, and intra- or postoperative fractures.

Undersizing was defined as either a too low fit of the implant that could have been avoided by choosing a bigger size or by the presence of a visible distance between the cortical bone and the implant in a region of bone that is crucial for the anchorage of the implant (calcar region and lateral cortex for CTHA and cortical ring of the resected femoral neck basis as well as lateral cortex for STHA). Oversizing was defined as a too high fit of the implant that could have been avoided by choosing a smaller size, indicated by the shoulder of the implant exceeding the highest point of the greater trochanter for CTHA or the shoulder of the implant exceeding the cortical ring of the femoral neck basis by more than 10 mm for STHA. Early subsidence after full load-bearing, which was allowed for all patients, was defined as an unambiguous (>2 mm) migration of the implant within the surrounding bone in a follow-up X-ray examination 3 months after surgery. The occurrence of intra- or postoperative fractures were retrieved from the surgery reports and patients' charts.

For these patients, who were included consecutively and underwent THA between 2010 and 2011, preoperative and postoperative digital X-rays in pairs were selected from the database of the department of orthopedic surgery of a university hospital. All these patients underwent standardized X-ray examinations, including an a.p. pelvic overview and an lateral view (Lauenstein) of the proximal femur. These X-rays existed for the preoperative and postoperative state and with a follow-up of at least 3 months. All X-rays were taken with a standardized film-focus-distance of 100 cm. An external calibration marker of 25 mm diameter was positioned between the legs of each patient for the preoperative pelvic overview.

Digital templating was performed by three senior surgeons experienced in THA. When conducting digital templating, the examiners were only able to see the preoperative, but not the postoperative X-rays.

The software used for digital templating was OrthoView (OrthoView Orthopaedic Digital Planning Version 6.3, Meridian Technique Limited, Southampton, UK). For this software tool, templates for the conventional BICONTACT stem (CTHA) and the METHA short stem (STHA; both Aesculap B. Braun, Tuttlingen, Germany) were available (Figures 2 and 3).

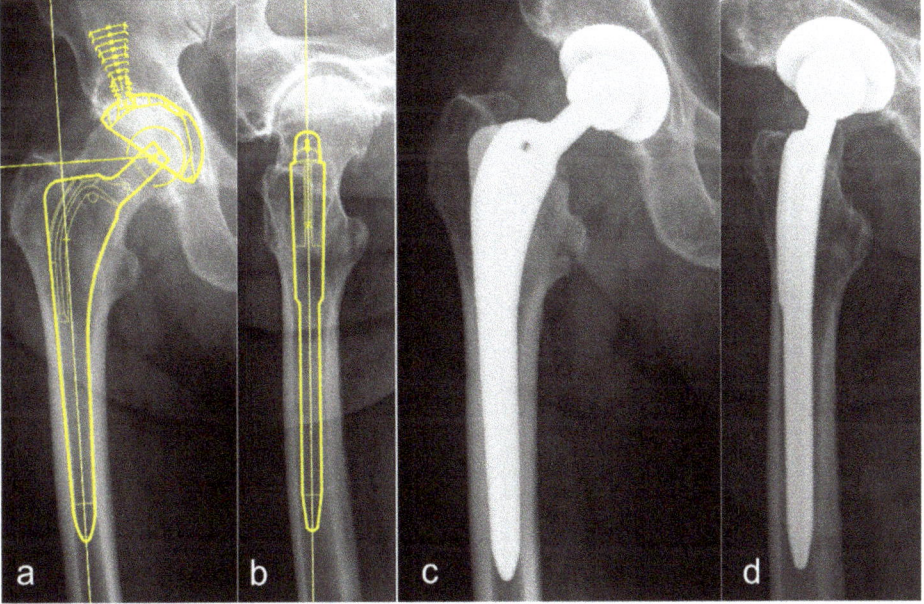

Figure 2. Digital templating of the BICONTACT stem (CTHA) in an anteroposterior (**a**) and lateral (**b**) view with the corresponding postoperative radiographs (**c,d**).

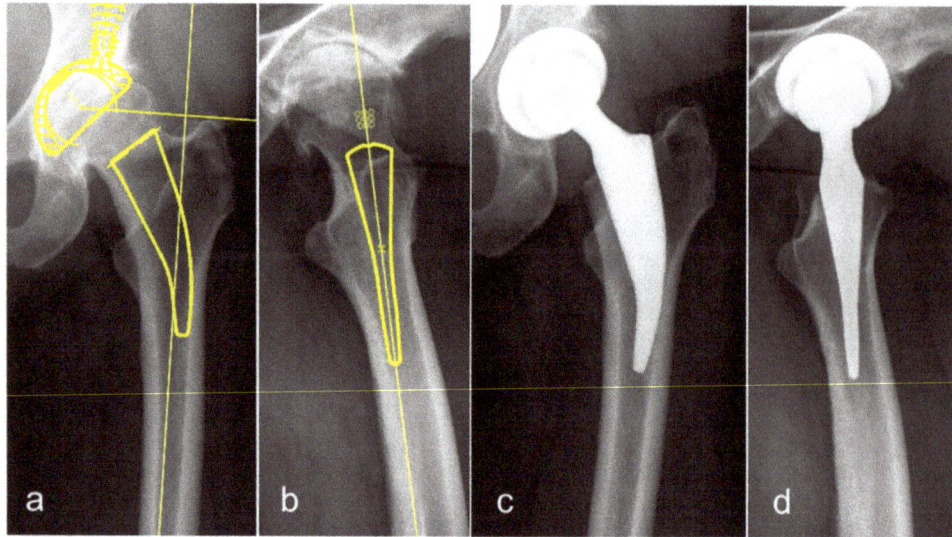

Figure 3. Digital templating of the METHA stem (STHA) in an anteroposterior (**a**) and lateral (**b**) view with the corresponding postoperative radiographs (**c**,**d**).

One hundred patients received a cementless METHA prosthesis with a caput-collum-diaphysis (CCD) angle of 130°, 135°, or 140°. All these stems are available in a size range of 0 to 7. The median stem size of the implanted METHA short stems was 3.

Fifty patients received a cementless conventional BICONTACT stem. These stems are monobloc-types with different offset variations: S for standard, H for High offset, and SD for dysplastic femurs. In our study, we templated and implanted only S and H types. BICONTACT stems are available in stem sizes 10–21. From the 50 truly implanted hip implants, the median stem size was 14.

Statistics

First, the results of all three raters were described with the cumulative rate of consistency between the templated and the implanted stem size. The difference was described as size derivation from the actual stem size. In addition, the planned stem sizes were presented in scatterplots. The intra-class correlation (ICC) 3,1 for consistency and 3,k for conformity for all raters was measured and quantified using Fleiss Kappa and Kendall's coefficient of concordance. For the correlation between the templated stem size and the actual implanted stem size, a Spearman's rank correlation coefficient was determined. Analysis was conducted in R (Version 4.0.3) [15], and figures were produced using the package ggplot2 [16].

3. Results

The study population consisted of 66 males and 84 females. The average age was 60 +/−12.8 years, ranging from 21 to 86 years. The CTHA group included 25 males and 25 females, the STHA group 41 males and 59 females. The CTHA group was significantly older than the STHA group (71 ± 14.3 years vs. 55 ± 11.5 years).

3.1. Conventional Stem Total Hip Arthroplasty (CTHA)—Conventional Templating in One Plane on the a.p. Pelvic Overview

The rate of correctly planned size of preoperative templating in one plane (a.p. view) predicted the exact CTHA stem size in 44.4% ± 6.8% cases. With a difference of +/−1 stem size, the rate of correctly planned size 88.4% ± 6.0% was detected. In 93.8% ± 5.4% of cases, the stem size was predicted within two stem sizes. In the remaining 6.2% of measurements, the templated stem size showed a deviation of +/−3 stem sizes (Table 1). The preoperative templating showed an oversizing in 27.5% and an undersizing in 28.1% of the cases.

Table 1. Cumulative percentages of the three raters for the conventional (CTHA) and short stem total hip arthroplasty (STHA) groups, using one and two planes, separated in accordance with the variation between the real stem size and the measured size while templating.

Difference in Templated Size Compared to the Truly Implanted Prosthesis		0	+/−1	+/−2	+/− > 2
CTHA (Templating a.p.)	Rater 1	52.0%	82.0%	90.0%	100.0%
	2	39.1	89.1	91.3	100.0
	3	42.0	94.0	100.0	100.0
	Mean ± Standard Deviation	44.4 ± 6.8	88.4 ± 6.0	93.8 ± 5.4	100.0 ± 0
CTHA (Templating 2 Planes)	Rater 1	64.0%	96.0%	100.0%	100.0%
	2	26.1	78.2	97.8	100.0
	3	30.0	94.0	100.0	100.0
	Mean ± Standard Deviation	40.0 ± 20.8	89.4 ± 9.8	99.3 ± 1.3	100.0 ± 0
STHA (Templating a.p.)	Rater 1	45.0%	83.0%	99.0%	100.0%
	2	16.7	78.9	100.0	100.0
	3	47.0	97.0	100.0	100.0
	Mean ± Standard Deviation	36.2 ± 16.9	86.3 ± 9.5	99.7 ± 0.6	100.0 ± 0
STHA (Templating 2 Planes)	Rater 1	60.0%	93.0%	100.0%	100.0%
	2	18.9	76.7	94.5	100.0
	3	71.0	100.0	100.0	100.0
	Mean ± Standard Deviation	50.0 ± 27.5	89.9 ± 12.0	98.2 ± 3.2	100.0 ± 0

3.2. CTHA—Templating in Two Planes—a.p. and Lateral View

Preoperative templating in two planes (a.p. view and lateral "Lauenstein" view) of CTHA showed an exact match of the implanted stem size in 40.0% ± 20.8% of cases. In 89.4% ± 9.8% an implanted size within a deviation of +/−1 stem size was found. In 99.3% ± 1.3% of our cases, we could predict the implanted stem size within a range of +/−2 sizes. The remaining 1.7% showed a deviation of +/−3 stem sizes (Table 1). In 25.5% an oversizing of the templated size was observed. In 34.5%, the templated stem size was smaller than the implanted stem size.

3.3. Short Stem Total Hip Arthroplasty (STHA)—Conventional Templating in One Plane on the a.p. Pelvic Overview

By using templating based on one radiological plane only, the rate of measurements matching the exact stem size was 36.2% ± 16.9%. By a tolerance of +/−1 stem size, the predictability raised to 86.3% ± 9.5%. A deviation of the implanted and templated stem size of up to +/−2 sizes was observed in 99.7% ± 0.6% of the cases (Table 1)—the remaining 0.3% ± 0.6% of the measurements showed a deviation of ± 3 stem sizes. An oversizing of the templated implant size was found in 31.9%, and an undersizing also in 31.9% of the cases.

3.4. STHA—Templating in Two Planes—a.p. and Lateral View

Adding a second plane (lateral view according to "Lauenstein"), the rate of planning the exact size reached 50.0% ± 27.5%. The predictability was 89.9% ± 12.0% with a tolerance of variation of +/−1 stem size. A variation of the implanted stem size lay within a range of +/−2 sizes in 98.2% ± 3.2% of the cases (Table 1). A deviation of ± 3 stem sizes was observed in the remaining measurement except for one outlier in one patient measured by one rater and showing a deviation of 4 stem sizes. In 31.8%, oversizing and 18.3%, undersizing of the templated size compared to the implanted size was measured.

Overall, the difference between the implanted stem size and the templated size showed a lesser deviation for the STHA planned on two planes compared to one plane, whereas the deviation was rather constant for the CTHA. However, this potential effect did not reach statistical significance. In addition, there was a trend that bigger implant sizes were planned too small, while small stem sizes were planned too big (Figure 4).

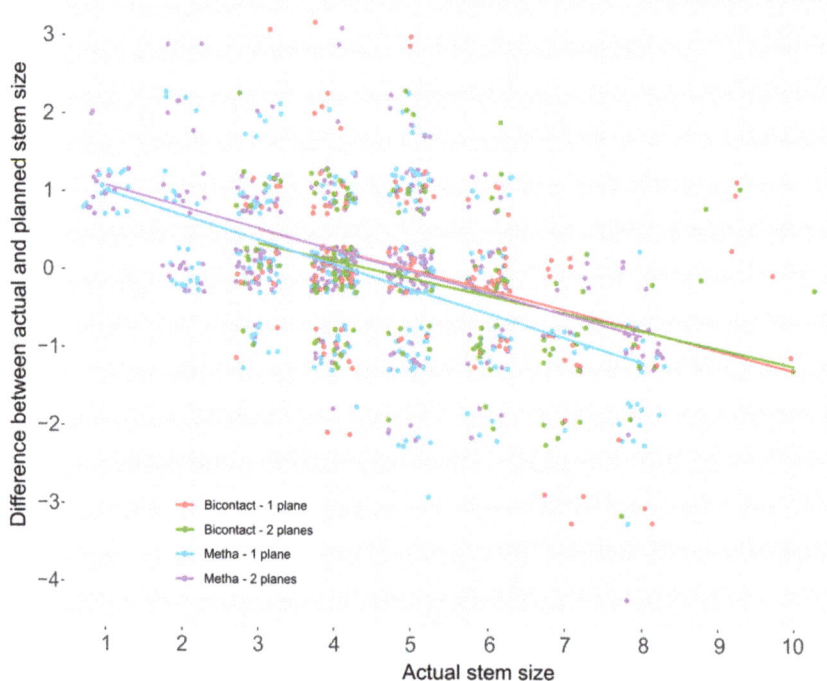

Figure 4. Scatterplots of the difference between actual and planned stem size over the actual stem size. CTHA with one plane planning is displayed in red, two plane planning is displayed in green. STHA with one plane planning is displayed in blue, two plane planning is displayed in purple. Linear regression lines are displayed for all implants and planning methods. For comparability, the implant sizes of the CTHA were substracted by 10.

An additional plane for preoperative stem templating led to an increase in the ICC for the stem size as well as for the difference between the implanted and templated stem size, except for the STHA difference values, where a decrease was observed (Tables 2 and 3).

Table 2. The intra-class correlation ICC (3,1) with a consistency of the values between all three raters.

Stem Size	CTHA	STHA
a.p. planning	0.774	0.736
a.p. + lateral planning	0.838	0.757
Difference to Implanted Size	CTHA	STHA
a.p. planning	0.586	0.483
a.p. + lateral planning	0.623	0.422

Table 3. The ICC (3,k) with conformity of the values between all three raters.

Stem Size	CTHA	STHA
a.p. planning	0.911	0.893
a.p. + lateral planning	0.94	0.903
Difference to Implanted Size	**CTHA**	**STHA**
a.p. planning	0.81	0.737
a.p. + lateral planning	0.832	0.687

The conformity of the three raters was slightly fair according to Landis classification [17] and improved only for the STHA, not for the CTHA (Table 4).

Table 4. Fleiss Kappa as value for the conformity between all the three raters.

Stem Size	CTHA	STHA
a.p. planning	0.411	0.228
a.p. + lateral planning	0.27	0.3
Difference to Implanted Size	**CTHA**	**STHA**
a.p. planning	0.33	0.149
a.p. + lateral planning	0.178	0.16

The consistency of the raters showed a significant correlation for STHA templating in two planes. However, the correlation was for both stem types, and planning conditions were limited (Table 5).

Table 5. Kendall's coefficient of concordance as a value for the consistency between the raters.

	CTHA		STHA	
	r	p	r	p
a.p. planning	0.029	0.266	0.023	0.131
a.p. + lateral planning	0.035	0.196	0.054	0.008

The templated and the implanted stem size showed a significant correlation for both stem types. The addition of an lateral planning plane led to a stronger correlation for CTHA and STHA (Table 6).

Table 6. Spearman's coefficient a value for the correlation between the templated and the implanted stem size.

Stem Size	CTHA		STHA	
	r	p	r	p
a.p. planning	0.74	0.001	0.80	0.001
a.p. + lateral planning	0.79	0.001	0.84	0.001

4. Discussion

Total hip arthroplasty using short stem implants has grown up to a popular technique beside the successful conventional procedure. Short stem devices, such as the METHA stem, show promising short-term results [18,19]. Prior to implantation of the stem, digital preoperative templating is a common and routinely used tool that has not yet been determined with regards to its benefit and exactitude [11,13]. So far, nothing is known about the benefit in terms of the rate of correctly planned sizes when using additional X-rays in a second radiological plane.

This study confirms on the one hand that there is no significant difference between templating STHA in comparison to CTHA, as former studies have shown [11,13,20,21]. On the other hand, the current study indicates that the exactitude can possibly be increased by using a second radiological plane for templating. Although this effect did not reach statistical significance for neither the CTHA nor the STHA group, the tendency of the effect could be observed especially for the short stem implant.

Matching exactly the same stem size as predicted by preoperative templating occurred in 44.4% ± 6.8% with CTHA when using one plane radiographs. Other studies on conventional implants have shown an exact rate of correctly planned sizes between 31% and 58% of cases [6,11,13,22,23]. By tolerating a variation of +/− one size between templating and implantation, the data of this study showed a predictability of 88.4% ± 6.0%, again in good conformity to other studies that have reported a predictability of 71.0%–94.0% under these circumstances.

By the use of a second radiological plane, the lateral view, according to Lauenstein, in addition to the a.p. pelvic overview, a comparable rate of exact matching between templated and implanted size of 40.0% ± 20.8% was determined. With an allowed measuring tolerance of +/− one stem size, a slightly increased accordance of 89.4% ± 9.8% was reached, although the difference was not significant. A variation of more than +/−2 stem sizes between templating and implanted size occurred in 0.7% of the cases when using two radiological planes compared to 6.2% when using only one plane ($p = 0.18$). This reduced range of dispersion indicates a higher accuracy when using two planes, although the difference was not significant.

Results analyzing the rate of correctly planned size of preoperative templating of short stem implants are less documented in the literature. There are only two studies dealing with this question: on the one hand, for the METHA short stem by Schmidutz et al. [11] and on the other hand, for the MAYO short stem (Zimmer, Warsaw, IN, USA) by Wedemeyer et al. [24]. Both of these short stem designs aim at a metaphyseal anchorage. Wedemeyer et al. reported an exact match without size tolerance in 38% of the cases. Schmidutz et al. found for the METHA short stem an exactitude of 49% of preoperative templating. In our study, we found similar results with up to 36.2% ± 16.9%. The MAYO device showed predictability of 95%, Schmidutz et al. reported 89% for the METHA stem, and our study reports a comparable matching rate of 86.3% ± 9.5% when tolerating a difference of one size.

In analogy to the CTHA group, the second plane (lateral view) led to a smaller range of dispersion, matching the exact size in 50% ± 27.5%, and in 89.9% ± 12% with a tolerance of +/−1 stem size.

When comparing the STHA and CTHA groups, adding the second radiological plane increased the probability of matching the exact size in the STHA group (50.0% vs. 36.2%), but not in the CTHA group (40.0% vs. 44.4%). When tolerating a difference of +/− one stem size, templating with two planes revealed comparable results between the groups that were not statistically significant (89.9% for STHA vs. 89.4% for CTHA). Although none of these results reached statistical significance, these data and the graphical illustration (Figure 4) imply that using two planes for preoperative templating is more likely to have a beneficial effect with regard to a short stem than to a conventional stem.

In general, preoperative templating is important with regard to the risk of an intraoperative fracture of the femur that is a common complication in a non-cemented THA [25]. On the other hand, the undersizing of the implant may lead to early implant migration [26] that may, in turn, impair osseointegration and lead to early aseptic loosening [27].

Less experienced surgeons especially benefit from a profound preparation by means of preoperative templating that helps them to improve their orientation and to feel safer during bone preparation. The information derived from this study that the planned size tends to be too big for small implant sizes and too small for big implant sizes might be especially helpful for them.

In this study, all templating was performed by digital techniques, but there are alternative analog techniques using plastic templates. Higher exactitude for digital templating was described in studies of The et al. and Widdon et al. [12,28]. On the other hand, there are also studies that come to the conclusion that analog templating might have a higher rate of correctly planned size [23,29]. All studies showed that templating is a beneficial tool to avoid intraoperative complications.

In particular, templating in two radiological planes may also be very helpful with regard to the preoperative detection of possible contraindications for a certain implant, e.g., a retro torsion or an excessive ante torsion (Figure 5) of the femoral neck when planning the implantation of a short stem device with primary metaphyseal anchorage along the femoral neck.

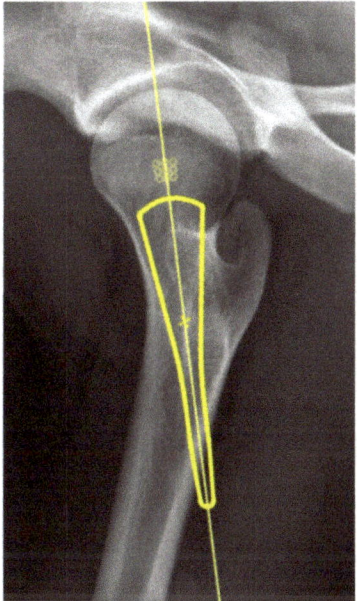

Figure 5. Digital templating of a STHA (lateral view) in a patient with excessive ante torsion of the femoral neck is an obvious contraindication for an implant with orientation parallel to the femoral neck.

This study has some limitations. Although the external calibration marker had been positioned in a standardized way for all patients, an imprecise positioning may influence the correct scaling of the X-rays and the results of THA templating [30]. A high body mass index (BMI) that was not recorded in this study may complicate the exact positioning of the calibration marker. However, the correlation between BMI and magnification has been shown to be weak so that a major bias can be ruled out [31].

Second, due to the retrospective design, the study was not able to analyze whether templating with two radiological planes would have led to a measurable effect on complication rates within this particular study population.

Furthermore, the study had an asymmetrical distribution between the CTHA and STHA groups (50 vs. 100 cases). This rather unconventional study design was chosen due to the fact that the rate of correctly planned size of digital templating of conventional stems has already been well analyzed by other studies, whereas there are very little data about short stems that were put into the focus of this study.

5. Conclusions

In conclusion, the current study indicates that preoperative templating using two radiological planes might at least have a slight, yet not significant, beneficial effect on the accuracy of the preoperative planning of short stem implants. Since contraindications for the use of a short stem can be identified more reliably and since this templating technique is easy to practice without additional expenses, its routine use can be recommended prior to surgery.

Author Contributions: Conceptualization, H.W., T.F., G.v.L.; methodology, H.W., T.F., S.B., G.v.L.; software, J.K.B., M.S., N.W., T.F., S.B.; formal analysis, M.S., N.W.; investigation, J.K.B., T.F., N.W.; data curation, J.K.B., S.B.; writing—original draft preparation, J.K.B., S.B.; writing—review and editing, M.S., N.W., S.B.; visualization, M.S., N.W., S.B.; supervision, H.W., T.F., S.B., G.v.L.; project administration, H.W., S.B.; All authors have read and agreed to the published version of the manuscript.

Funding: This research received no external funding.

Institutional Review Board Statement: Ethical review and approval were waived for this study due to the retrospective design of the study, analyzing X-rays with digital templating and comparing them to data derived from the surgery protocols.

Informed Consent Statement: Patient consent was waived due to the retrospective and anonymized design of the study.

Data Availability Statement: The data presented in this study are available on request from the corresponding author.

Conflicts of Interest: Three authors (G.v.L., H.W., and T.F.) are instructors for minimal-invasive surgery courses using the METHA stem (Aesculap).

References

1. Efe, T.; El Zayat, B.F.; Heyse, T.J.; Timmesfeld, N.; Fuchs-Winkelmann, S.; Schmitt, J. Precision of preoperative digital templating in total hip arthroplasty. *Acta Orthop. Belg.* **2011**, *77*, 616–621. [PubMed]
2. Haddad, F.S.; Masri, B.A.; Garbuz, D.S.; Duncan, C.P. The prevention of periprosthetic fractures in total hip and knee arthroplasty. *Orthop. Clin. N. Am.* **1999**, *30*, 191–207. [CrossRef]
3. Haddad, F.S.; Masri, B.A.; Garbuz, D.S.; Duncan, C.P. Femoral bone loss in total hip arthroplasty: Classification and preoperative planning. *Instr. Course Lect.* **2000**, *49*, 83–96. [PubMed]
4. Muller, M.E. Lessons of 30 years of total hip arthroplasty. *Clin. Orthop. Relat. Res.* **1992**, 12–21.
5. Bono, J.V. Digital templating in total hip arthroplasty. *J. Bone Jt. Surg. Am.* **2004**, *86* (Suppl. 2), 118–122. [CrossRef]
6. Della Valle, A.G.; Padgett, D.E.; Salvati, E.A. Preoperative planning for primary total hip arthroplasty. *J. Am. Acad. Orthop. Surg.* **2005**, *13*, 455–462. [CrossRef]
7. Fottner, A.; Steinbruck, A.; Sadoghi, P.; Mazoochian, F.; Jansson, V. Digital comparison of planned and implanted stem position in total hip replacement using a program form migration analysis. *Arch. Orthop. Trauma Surg.* **2011**, *131*, 1013–1019. [CrossRef]
8. Lecerf, G.; Fessy, M.H.; Philippot, R.; Massin, P.; Giraud, F.; Flecher, X.; Girard, J.; Mertl, P.; Marchetti, E.; Stindel, E. Femoral offset: Anatomical concept, definition, assessment, implications for preoperative templating and hip arthroplasty. *Orthop. Traumatol. Surg. Res.* **2009**, *95*, 210–219. [CrossRef]
9. Kamada, S.; Naito, M.; Nakamura, Y.; Kiyama, T. Hip abductor muscle strength after total hip arthroplasty with short stems. *Arch. Orthop. Trauma Surg.* **2011**, *131*, 1723–1729. [CrossRef]
10. Suh, K.T.; Cheon, S.J.; Kim, D.W. Comparison of preoperative templating with postoperative assessment in cementless total hip arthroplasty. *Acta Orthop. Scand.* **2004**, *75*, 40–44. [CrossRef]
11. Schmidutz, F.; Steinbruck, A.; Wanke-Jellinek, L.; Pietschmann, M.; Jansson, V.; Fottner, A. The accuracy of digital templating: A comparison of short-stem total hip arthroplasty and conventional total hip arthroplasty. *Int. Orthop.* **2012**, *36*, 1767–1772. [CrossRef]
12. The, B.; Verdonschot, N.; van Horn, J.R.; van Ooijen, P.M.; Diercks, R.L. Digital versus analogue preoperative planning of total hip arthroplasties: A randomized clinical trial of 210 total hip arthroplasties. *J. Arthroplast.* **2007**, *22*, 866–870. [CrossRef]
13. Gamble, P.; de Beer, J.; Petruccelli, D.; Winemaker, M. The accuracy of digital templating in uncemented total hip arthroplasty. *J Arthroplast.* **2010**, *25*, 529–532. [CrossRef]
14. Schiffner, E.; Latz, D.; Jungbluth, P.; Grassmann, J.P.; Tanner, S.; Karbowski, A.; Windolf, J.; Schneppendahl, J. Is computerised 3D templating more accurate than 2D templating to predict size of components in primary total hip arthroplasty? *Hip Int.* **2019**, *29*, 270–275. [CrossRef]

15. R Core Team. *R: A Language and Environment for Statistical Computing*; R Foundation for Statistical Computing: Vienna, Austria, 2020; Available online: http://www.R-project.org (accessed on 27 April 2021).
16. Wickham, H. *ggplot2: Elegant Graphics for Data Analysis*; Springer: New York, NY, USA, 2009.
17. Landis, J.R.; Koch, G.G. The measurement of observer agreement for categorical data. *Biometrics* **1977**, *33*, 159–174. [CrossRef]
18. Lerch, M.; von der Haar-Tran, A.; Windhagen, H.; Behrens, B.A.; Wefstaedt, P.; Stukenborg-Colsman, C.M. Bone remodelling around the Metha short stem in total hip arthroplasty: A prospective dual-energy X-ray absorptiometry study. *Int. Orthop.* **2012**, *36*, 533–538. [CrossRef]
19. Thorey, F.; Hoefer, C.; Abdi-Tabari, N.; Lerch, M.; Budde, S.; Windhagen, H. Clinical results of the metha short hip stem: A perspective for younger patients? *Orthop. Rev.* **2013**, *5*, e34. [CrossRef]
20. Iorio, R.; Siegel, J.; Specht, L.M.; Tilzey, J.F.; Hartman, A.; Healy, W.L. A comparison of acetate vs digital templating for preoperative planning of total hip arthroplasty: Is digital templating accurate and safe? *J. Arthroplast.* **2009**, *24*, 175–179. [CrossRef]
21. Morrey, B.F.; Adams, R.A.; Kessler, M. A conservative femoral replacement for total hip arthroplasty. A prospective study. *J. Bone Jt. Surg. Br.* **2000**, *82*, 952–958. [CrossRef]
22. Crooijmans, H.J.; Laumen, A.M.; van Pul, C.; van Mourik, J.B. A new digital preoperative planning method for total hip arthroplasties. *Clin. Orthop. Relat. Res.* **2009**, *467*, 909–916. [CrossRef]
23. Hsu, A.R.; Kim, J.D.; Bhatia, S.; Levine, B.R. Effect of training level on accuracy of digital templating in primary total hip and knee arthroplasty. *Orthopedics* **2012**, *35*, e179–e183. [CrossRef] [PubMed]
24. Wedemeyer, C.; Quitmann, H.; Xu, J.; Heep, H.; von Knoch, M.; Saxler, G. Digital templating in total hip arthroplasty with the Mayo stem. *Arch. Orthop. Trauma Surg.* **2008**, *128*, 1023–1029. [CrossRef] [PubMed]
25. Jakubowitz, E.; Seeger, J.B.; Lee, C.; Heisel, C.; Kretzer, J.P.; Thomsen, M.N. Do short-stemmed-prostheses induce periprosthetic fractures earlier than standard hip stems? A biomechanical ex-vivo study of two different stem designs. *Arch. Orthop. Trauma Surg.* **2009**, *129*, 849–855. [CrossRef] [PubMed]
26. Braun, A.; Sabah, A. Two-year results of a modular short hip stem prosthesis—A prospective study. *Z. Orthop. Unfall* **2009**, *147*, 700–706. [CrossRef]
27. Von Lewinski, G.; Floerkemeier, T. 10-year experience with short stem total hip arthroplasty. *Orthopedics* **2015**, *38*, S51–S56. [CrossRef]
28. Whiddon, D.R.; Bono, J.V.; Lang, J.E.; Smith, E.L.; Salyapongse, A.K. Accuracy of digital templating in total hip arthroplasty. *Am. J. Orthop.* **2011**, *40*, 395–398.
29. Gonzalez Della Valle, A.; Comba, F.; Taveras, N.; Salvati, E.A. The utility and precision of analogue and digital preoperative planning for total hip arthroplasty. *Int. Orthop.* **2008**, *32*, 289–294. [CrossRef]
30. Boese, C.K.; Wilhelm, S.; Haneder, S.; Lechler, P.; Eysel, P.; Bredow, J. Influence of calibration on digital templating of hip arthroplasty. *Int. Orthop.* **2019**, *43*, 1799–1805. [CrossRef]
31. Boese, C.K.; Lechler, P.; Rose, L.; Dargel, J.; Oppermann, J.; Eysel, P.; Geiges, H.; Bredow, J. Calibration Markers for Digital Templating in Total Hip Arthroplasty. *PLoS ONE* **2015**, *10*, e0128529. [CrossRef]

Article

Biomechanical Analysis of Sagittal Plane Pin Placement Configurations for Pediatric Supracondylar Humerus Fractures

Witit Pothong [1], Phichayut Phinyo [2,3], Yuddhasert Sirirungruangsarn [1], Kriengkrai Nabudda [4], Nattamon Wongba [5], Chatchawarl Sarntipiphat [5] and Dumnoensun Pruksakorn [1,6,7,*]

1. Department of Orthopedics, Faculty of Medicine, Chiang Mai University, Chiang Mai 50200, Thailand; wertybooky@gmail.com (W.P.); yuddasert@hotmail.com (Y.S.)
2. Department of Family Medicine, Faculty of Medicine, Chiang Mai University, Chiang Mai 50200, Thailand; phichayutphinyo@gmail.com
3. Center for Clinical Epidemiology and Clinical Statistics, Faculty of Medicine, Chiang Mai University, Chiang Mai 50200, Thailand
4. Research Center for Orthopedics Biomechanics, Khon Kaen University, Khon Kaen 40002, Thailand; kriang_36@hotmail.com
5. Department of Orthopedics, Faculty of Medicine, Khon Kaen University, Khon Kaen 40002, Thailand; mo_nattan@hotmail.com (N.W.); chat-sarn@hotmail.com (C.S.)
6. Musculoskeletal Science and Translational Research Center, Chiang Mai University, Chiang Mai 50200, Thailand
7. Biomedical Engineering Institute, Chiang Mai University, Chiang Mai 50200, Thailand
* Correspondence: dumnoensun.p@cmu.ac.th; Tel.: +66-53-935-540

Abstract: Anterior to posterior (AP) pinning is the recommended sagittal pin configuration in divergent lateral entry coronal pinning of pediatrics supracondylar fractures. However, there was still a lack of evidence regarding alternative sagittal pins configurations. We aimed to compare the construct stiffness of alternative sagittal pin configurations by using synthetic bone models. Sixty synthetic pediatric humeri were osteotomized to create a supracondylar fracture. After the fracture reduction, all specimens were fixed in the coronal plane with divergent lateral entry pin configurations in four different patterns in the sagittal plane: AP, crossed, divergent and parallel sagittal pin configuration. Each configuration was tested with five loading patterns. The AP sagittal pin had significantly lower construct stiffness than the divergent ($p = 0.003$) and the parallel sagittal pin configuration ($p = 0.005$) in external rotation loading tests. The divergent sagittal pin had the highest construct stiffness in extension, valgus, and external rotation loads, but the parallel sagittal pin had lower construct stiffness under extension load than the divergent and crossed sagittal pin configurations. The divergent sagittal pin configuration provides greater construct stiffness than other sagittal pin configurations due to the maximal pin spreading distance at the fracture site and the pin angle lock mechanism.

Keywords: supracondylar humeral fracture; biomechanical study; sagittal pinning; Kirschner wires

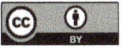

1. Introduction

Supracondylar fractures of the distal humerus are the most common fractures in children, with the peak incidence at age 4–7 years [1]. Many treatment methods have been described, e.g., closed reduction with a long-arm cast, skin traction, axial skeletal traction, and flexible nailing. In the 1940s, publication on closed reduction and percutaneous pinning [2] described the currently preferred surgical treatment for displaced supracondylar fractures [3–6]. The crossed medial-lateral and lateral entry pin configuration in the coronal plane have been favored as an effective pinning technique [7–14]. Biomechanical studies have reported that crossed medial-lateral pins provide greater torsional stiffness than lateral entry pin fixation [15–18] but no clinical difference in treatment outcome [19–22]. We considered two pins with divergent lateral entry to be the most appropriate configuration in the coronal plane because the crossed medial-lateral pin configuration is associated with a higher risk of iatrogenic ulnar nerve injury [6,7,9,21,23].

In contrast to the coronal plane, the construct stiffness of each pin configuration in the sagittal plane has not been extensively evaluated, with few biomechanical or clinical studies on the issue. Anterior to posterior (AP) pinning is currently the most common recommendation for sagittal pin configuration. Ariño suggested using two Kirschner wires (K-wire) with either parallel or crossed pin configuration in both the coronal and sagittal plains [24]. Kallio and Skaggs suggested the appropriate inclination for sagittal pin insertion is from the anterior part of the distal fragment to the posterior part of the diaphyseal cortex [25,26]. Recently, Wallace designed a biomechanical torsion test for sagittal pin configurations [27]. However, no statistically significant difference in torsional stiffness among the three types of sagittal pin configurations was found in the study.

This study aimed to use biomechanical tests to compare the construct stiffness of various types of sagittal pin configurations for pediatrics supracondylar fractures using controlled fixation with two divergent lateral entry pin configurations in the coronal plane under axial torsion and displacement loads.

2. Materials and Methods

2.1. Materials

We conducted a biomechanical analysis of sagittal pin placement configurations for pediatric supracondylar humerus fractures. The research ethics committee of the Faculty of Medicine, Chiang Mai University, approved the study protocol (ORT 2562 06622). Sixty Sawbones pediatric synthetic humeri (Sawbones model #1052, Pacific Research Laboratories, Vashon Island, WA, USA) were obtained using the same model in previous pediatrics supracondylar humerus fracture biomechanics studies [27,28]. These synthetic humeri are made of a rigid foam shell with inner cancellous material and are anatomically correct pediatric bone dimensions.

2.2. Methods

We controlled coronal plane pinning with two divergent lateral entry pin configurations following the technique of Hamdi [29]. Different pin placement configurations in the sagittal plane were evaluated for feasibility, given the limited area/size of pediatric bones. All configurations were bicortical medial and lateral cortex fixation. We established zones of pin entry and exit using the transverse diaphyseal diameter of the humeral shaft in the sagittal plane as reference. We first divided the anterior and posterior with an anatomical axis line, after which we drew a vertical line separating the cortical bone and the intramedullary canal. Then we designated four zones where pins would penetrate the bone cortex: zone 1 = the anterior diaphyseal cortex, zone 2 = the anterior diaphyseal medullary canal, zone 3 = the posterior diaphyseal medullary canal, and zone 4 = the posterior diaphyseal cortex (Figure 1). In each case, both pins were started from the lateral part of the distal fragment to the medial diaphyseal cortex. Pin trajectories were labeled numerically by entry and exit zone, e.g., 2–3 represents pin entry at the lateral part of the distal fragment (zone 2) and exit at the medial diaphyseal cortex (zone 3). In the coronal plane: the first pin was proximal and was parallel to the lateral metaphyseal flare of the humeral cortex; the second pin was distal and crossed the fracture site at the medial edge of the coronoid fossa. In the sagittal plane: the combined pin configuration designation listed the proximal pin trajectory first and distal pin trajectory second. For example, if the first proximal pin trajectory was 2-2 and the second distal pin trajectory was 1-1, the pin configuration was represented as [2-2,1-1]. Finally, four different pin configurations were chosen for study: the AP sagittal pin configuration [2-3,1-3] (currently the standard recommendation), the crossed sagittal pin configuration [2-4,4-2], the divergent sagittal pin configuration [3-3,3-1], and parallel sagittal pin configuration [3-3,2-2].

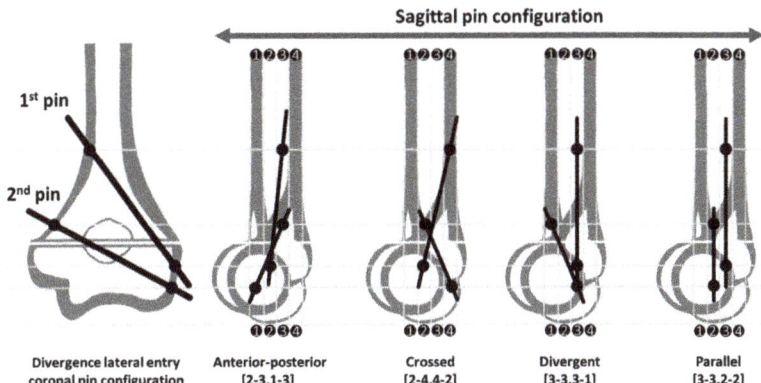

Figure 1. Schematic showing the orientation of the four sagittal pin configurations in the controlled divergence lateral entry coronal pin configurations. The black dots represent the location of pin penetration through the bone cortex.

Four pin targeting guides were created from an epoxy resin casting to provide pin placement consistency and reproducibility. The specimens were securely encased in the epoxy mold and 1.5 mm holes were predrilled using the pin targeting guide. Transverse osteotomies were made at the level of the epicondyle (mid olecranon fossa) perpendicular to the anatomic axis of the humerus (28 mm from the distal end of the trochlea humerus) with a 0.5-mm cutting blade and the custom-built guide cutting. After fracture reduction, two pieces of 1.6 mm diameter Kirchner wire were inserted through the predrilled in the center of each of the four zones. After pinning, a fluoroscopic evaluation was accomplished to confirm the placement of all wires. Bone specimens underwent axial torsion and displacement load tests using an Instron ElectroPuls™ E10000 (Instron, Norwood, MA, USA).

In external and internal torsion tests, we created an epoxy resin mold jig system consisting of outer and inner parts (Figure 2). The outer mold jig was attached permanently to the testing machine at the center of rotation of the long anatomical axis of the humerus to ensure that the position did not vary between specimens. The inner part could be moved into and out of the outer mold jig. After the bone specimen was inserted into the proximal and distal parts of the inner mold jig, it was mounted vertically on an outer jig and secured tightly with multiple bolts and nuts. Loads were applied to the proximal part of the bone by an actuator. The actuator allowed 0–25° of internal and external rotation, and samples were tested at a rate of 0.5 degrees/second. Torque (Nm/degrees) and degrees of rotation were recorded. Based on previous studies, rotational testing beyond 25–30° resulted in a plastic deformation or failure of the construct [16,18]. Thus, in this study, we limited the degree for rotational testing at 25 degrees.

For extension, varus, and valgus displacement tests, the proximal part of the specimen was secured in a horizontal cylindrical metal tube (Figure 3). The anatomical axis of the humerus was set at the center of the cylindrical tube for all specimens. Load displacement was applied by the actuator of the machine via the 8 mm diameter cylindrical rod at a level 1 cm distal to the fracture site. The load was applied at the distal part, increasing displacement from 0 to 7 mm at a rate of 0.5 mm/second. Displacement (mm) and force (N/mm) were recorded. We used a maximal translational displacement of 7 mm as this point was the maximal point for all previous biomechanical analyses for the construct stiffness of supracondylar fracture.

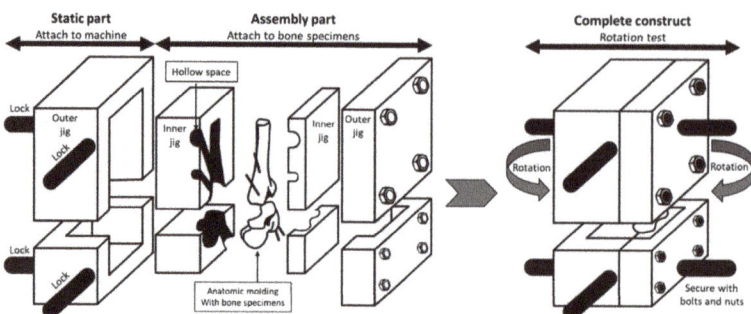

Figure 2. Schematic presentation of the two layers of the axial torsional mold jig. The outer layer was statically attached to the testing machine. The inner layer containing the bone specimen could be moved into and out of the assembly. The portion of the pins extending beyond the bone was accommodated in hollow spaces of the mold jig without impingement. All constructs were secured tightly with multiple bolts and nuts.

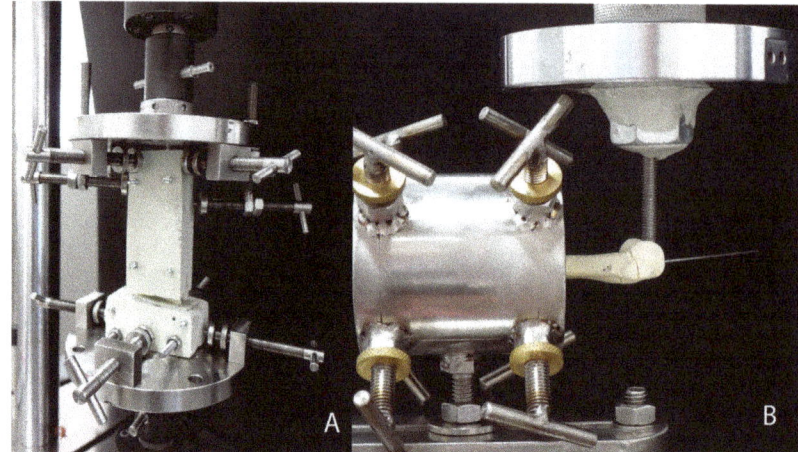

Figure 3. A specimen mounted in the testing machine: (**A**) axial torsion test (internal and external rotation) using the custom epoxy resin fixation jig and (**B**) load displacement test (extension, valgus and varus) using the fixed metal tube.

A total of 60 humeri were prepared in four different pin configurations (15 specimens per configuration). Three specimens of each configuration were used in each loading test. Specimens were tested only once to avoid potential measurement errors due to bone destruction during the previous experiment.

2.3. Statistical Analysis

One-way analysis of variance with repeated measures was used to compare the construct stiffness of the four different pin configurations for each of the five modes of applied force. Statistical significance was set at $p < 0.05$. Post hoc Bonferroni comparison was conducted to determine the specific difference between the pin configurations in cases where one-way analysis of variance detected differences. Data analysis was conducted using STATA version 16 (StataCorp, College Station, TX, USA).

3. Results

There were no permanent construct failures due to bone specimen fracture, pin deformation, or loss of fixation in any loading conditions.

Construct stiffness (Figure 4) was calculated from the slope of the load–displacement curve that best fit the data with the linear portion between 2 and 7 mm of the load–displacement curve and torsional stiffness was measured between 5 and 25 degrees of the load–displacement curve.

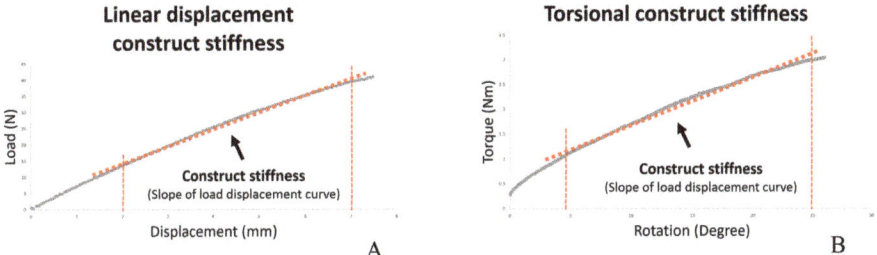

Figure 4. Load–displacement curve generated during sagittal pin configurations stiffness assessment. The construct stiffness was calculated from the slope of the load–displacement curve best fitting the data between 2 and 7 mm of displacement (**A**). Torsional stiffness was measured between 5 and 25 degrees of rotation (**B**).

Figures 5 and 6 show a torsional and linear load–displacement curve and slope load–displacement curve (construct stiffness) of all 4 pins configurations under external rotation, internal rotation, extension, valgus, and varus load.

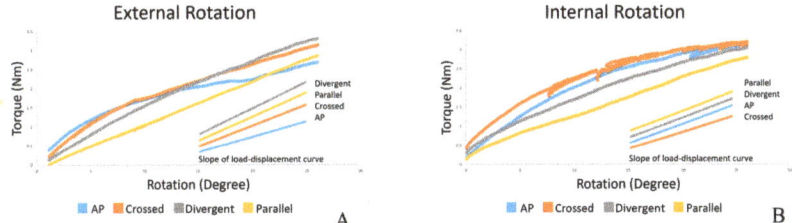

Figure 5. Comparison between the torsional load–displacement curve and slope of the load–displacement curve between different sagittal pin configuration in external rotation load (**A**) and internal rotation load (**B**).

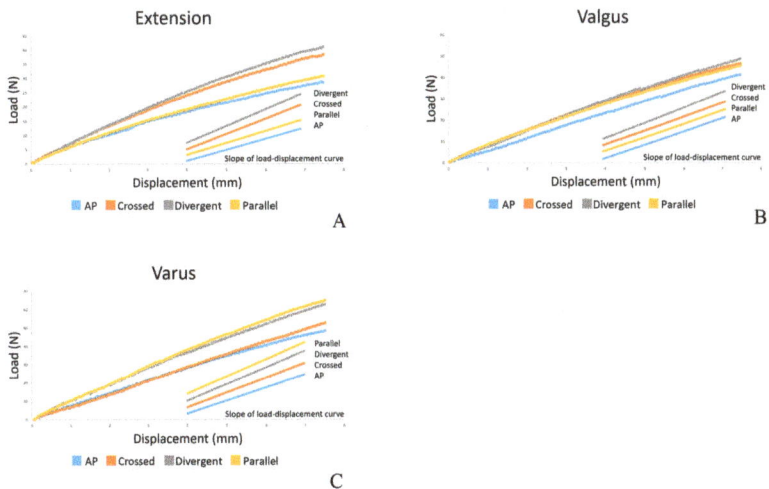

Figure 6. Comparison between linear load–displacement curve and slope of the straight line of different sagittal pin configuration in extension load (**A**) and valgus load (**B**) and varus load (**C**).

There was no statistically significant difference among the four-pin configurations in extension, valgus, varus, and internal rotation loading (Table 1).

Table 1. Comparison of construct stiffness of different pin configurations in the sagittal plane.

Loading Condition	AP	Crossed	Divergent	Parallel	ANOVA p-Values
	Mean ± SD	Mean ± SD	Mean ± SD	Mean ± SD	
Extension (N/mm)	3.38 ± 1.25	4.73 ± 0.79	5.20 ± 0.45	3.68 ± 0.21	0.066
Valgus (N/mm)	5.54 ± 0.72	5.79 ± 0.75	6.21 ± 0.78	5.63 ± 0.77	0.726
Varus (N/mm)	6.36 ± 1.64	7.13 ± 0.97	8.01 ± 0.57	8.46 ± 0.40	0.132
Internal rotation (Nm/deg)	0.085 ± 0.006	0.073 ± 0.006	0.093 ± 0.020	0.098 ± 0.010	0.134
External rotation (Nm/deg)	0.063 ± 0.008	0.093 ± 0.017	0.120 ± 0.012	0.115 ± 0.010	0.002

Abbreviations: AP, anterior to posterior pinning; ANOVA, analysis of variance.

For external rotation loading, anterior to posterior pinning gave the lowest construct stiffness (0.063 ± 0.008 Nm/deg). This was significantly lower than for both divergent pinning (0.120 ± 0.012 Nm/deg) and parallel pinning (0.115 ± 0.010 Nm/deg) ($p = 0.003$ and $p = 0.005$, respectively) (Table 2).

Table 2. Post hoc comparison of external rotation loading of different pin configurations.

External Rotation (Nm/deg)	AP	Crossed	Divergent
Crossed	$p = 0.096$		
Divergence	$p = 0.003$	$p = 0.165$	
Parallel	$p = 0.005$	$p = 0.359$	$p = 1.000$

Abbreviations: AP, anterior to posterior pinning; ANOVA, analysis of variance. Statistically significant figures are shown in bold figures.

4. Discussion

Adequate fixation stability is the key measure of success in the treatment of displaced pediatric supracondylar fractures. Closed reduction and percutaneous pinning is a standard technique for fixation, especially for Gartland type 2 and type 3 fractures [6,30]. Low construct stiffness is an important factor in the loss of fracture reduction. Many previous studies have discussed construct stiffness in the coronal pin configuration. The divergent lateral entry pin technique has been recommended in many institutes because of the lower risk of iatrogenic ulnar nerve injury than the medial-lateral crossed pin technique [7,31]. In contrast, there have been few studies in biomechanical and clinical evidence about the sagittal pin configuration. Our study aimed to biomechanically evaluate which of the sagittal pin configuration has the strongest construct stiffness in two controlled divergence lateral entry coronal pin configurations.

The sagittal pin configuration in this study was based on two considerations: first, limitations on the use of K-wire in small pediatric bones, and second, the K-wire must penetrate only the lateral and medial cortex of the bones. K-wire inserted into the medullary canal must travel without cutting through the bone cortex. For each test, a newly synthetic specimen was used instead of reused specimen because the initial procedure could potentially have damaged the outer cortical and inner cancellous structure of the synthetic bone after previous testing and thus destroyed or changed its material construction.

This study investigated three interesting areas. The first area is the weakness of the AP sagittal pin configuration. Although AP is the standard recommendation for sagittal pin configuration, there are many alternative pin configurations for fixation, which have not yet been thoroughly evaluated. The present study found that the AP sagittal pin configuration had the lowest construct stiffness under many load types. We used previous studies associated with coronal pin configuration to explain the lack of this construct stiffness.

Kallio suggested that the pins cross each other in the lateral entry pin configuration at the fracture site level [25], resulting in horizontal malrotation and the development of cubitus varus. Ziont showed that the two coronal lateral entry pinning, which crosses at the fracture site, has very low construct stiffness [18]. Sankar et al. suggested that loss of reduction occurs when the pins are too close to each other at the fracture site level [20]. We assumed that the construct weakness in the coronal plane is the result of two pins starting from the same side and crossing near the fracture site level. We applied this assumption to the AP sagittal pin configuration, where two pins also start from the same anterior side and cross near the fracture site, which might explain why the AP sagittal pin configuration has lower construct stiffness than the other sagittal pin configurations.

The second area is the divergent sagittal pin had the maximum pin spread at the fracture site, which the highest construct stiffness in extension, valgus, and external rotation loads. Skaggs recommended that both divergent and parallel coronal pins should be maximally separated at the fracture site for maximal stability [26]. Sankar suggested that loss of reduction occurs when the pin spread is less than 2 mm at the fracture site level [20]. Kocher divided the distal humerus into medial, central, and lateral columns. Then, it suggested that the divergent configuration should provide adequate spread between pins and engage both the lateral and central columns of the distal humerus [21]. Pennock conducted a retrospective review and suggested the pins should be spread at least 13 mm or more than one-third of humeral width at the fracture site to minimize the loss of reduction [32].

The third area is the weakness of the parallel sagittal pin configuration under extension loads despite the fact that it carried significantly high construct stiffness in external rotation loading as divergent sagittal pin configuration. Lee studied the biomechanics of construct stiffness between divergent and parallel pin configurations in the coronal plane [17]. His results showed significantly lower construct stiffness with the parallel compared to divergent pinning. That explains the "lock" and "unlock" effect of the angle between the two pins, which concurs with our finding that with the divergent sagittal pin configuration, the two pins act together to create a "lock" effect, while parallel pins create an "unlock" effect under extension load.

There were some limitations to our study. The first and most important limitation was the limited number of specimens ($n = 3$) used for each loading test. According to the power analysis, our study would require at least eight specimens in each loading test to achieve 80% power to detect a significantly large effect size (Cohen's d 2.0) accounting for multiplicity. Thus, our results might be considered only for hypothesis-generating. Further research with an adequate study size is still needed to confirm our findings. Second, the material used was not an authentic human bone. Thus, it lacks natural pediatric bone properties such as soft tissue tensioning, periosteal effect, and cartilaginous physis. Pediatrics cadavers are very rare and are more expensive than artificial bone. However, a synthetic model does have advantages, e.g., the realistic anatomy truly represents the limitations of pin placement in pediatric bone, the specimens are homogeneous, and the results are reproducible. Real pediatric human bone varies in bone quality, bone density, and periosteal thickening, confounding factors avoided by using the pediatric synthetic bone.

5. Conclusions

For the fixation of pediatrics supracondylar fractures with controlled divergent lateral entry coronal pin configuration, the divergent sagittal pin configuration is recommended as it provides the highest construct stiffness under various loads compared to other sagittal pin configurations. The superiority of the divergent sagittal pin configuration could be explained by the maximal pin spreading distance at the fracture site and the pin angle lock mechanism.

Author Contributions: Conceptualization, W.P., Y.S., and D.P.; methodology, W.P., K.N., and D.P.; software, W.P., P.P., and K.N.; validation P.P. and D.P.; formal analysis, W.P. and P.P.; investigation, W.P., K.N., N.W., and C.S.; resources, D.P.; data curation, W.P.; writing—original draft preparation, W.P. and Y.S.; writing—review and editing, P.P. and D.P.; visualization, W.P.; supervision, D.P.; project administration, D.P.; funding acquisition, D.P. All authors have read and agreed to the published version of the manuscript.

Funding: This research received no external funding.

Institutional Review Board Statement: The research ethics committee of the Faculty of Medicine, Chiang Mai University, approved the study protocol (ORT 2562 06622).

Informed Consent Statement: Not Applicable.

Data Availability Statement: The datasets used and/or analyzed during the current study are available from the corresponding author on reasonable request.

Acknowledgments: We would like to express our sincere thanks to G Lamar Robert and Chongchit Sripun Robert for English editing the manuscript, and Areerak Phanphaisarn for her useful and encouraging supports during the research and publication process. This work was partially supported by the Faculty of Medicine, Chiang Mai University.

Conflicts of Interest: The authors declare no conflict of interest.

References

1. Farnsworth, C.L.; Silva, P.D.; Mubarak, S.J. Etiology of Supracondylar Humerus Fractures. *J. Pediatr. Orthop.* **1998**, *18*, 38–42. [CrossRef] [PubMed]
2. Swenson, A.L. The Treatment of Supracondylar Fractures of the Humerus by Kirschner-Wire Transfixion. *J. Bone Jt. Surg. Am.* **1948**, *30A*, 993–997. [CrossRef]
3. Omid, R.; Choi, P.D.; Skaggs, D.L. Supracondylar Humeral Fractures in Children. *J. Bone Jt. Surg. Am.* **2008**, *90*, 1121–1132. [CrossRef]
4. Ym, Y.; Ms, K. Lateral Entry Compared with Medial and Lateral Entry Pin Fixation for Completely Displaced Supracondylar Humeral Fractures in Children. Surgical Technique. *J. Bone Jt. Surg. Am.* **2008**, *90 Pt 1* (Suppl. 2), 20–30. [CrossRef]
5. Leitch, K.K.; Kay, R.M.; Femino, J.D.; Tolo, V.T.; Storer, S.K.; Skaggs, D.L. Treatment of Multidirectionally Unstable Supracondylar Humeral Fractures in Children. A Modified Gartland Type-IV Fracture. *J. Bone Jt. Surg. Am.* **2006**, *88*, 980–985. [CrossRef]
6. Skaggs, D.L. Elbow Fractures in Children: Diagnosis and Management. *J. Am. Acad. Orthop. Surg.* **1997**, *5*, 303–312. [CrossRef]
7. Topping, R.E.; Blanco, J.S.; Davis, T.J. Clinical Evaluation of Crossed-Pin versus Lateral-Pin Fixation in Displaced Supracondylar Humerus Fractures. *J. Pediatr. Orthop.* **1995**, *15*, 435–439. [CrossRef]
8. Nacht, J.L.; Ecker, M.L.; Chung, S.M.; Lotke, P.A.; Das, M. Supracondylar Fractures of the Humerus in Children Treated by Closed Reduction and Percutaneous Pinning. *Clin. Orthop.* **1983**, 203–209. [CrossRef]
9. Flynn, J.C.; Matthews, J.G.; Benoit, R.L. Blind Pinning of Displaced Supracondylar Fractures of the Humerus in Children. Sixteen Years' Experience with Long-Term Follow-Up. *J. Bone Jt. Surg. Am.* **1974**, *56*, 263–272. [CrossRef]
10. Mehserle, W.L.; Meehan, P.L. Treatment of the Displaced Supracondylar Fracture of the Humerus (Type III) with Closed Reduction and Percutaneous Cross-Pin Fixation. *J. Pediatr. Orthop.* **1991**, *11*, 705–711. [CrossRef] [PubMed]
11. Mehlman, C.T.; Crawford, A.H.; McMillion, T.L.; Roy, D.R. Operative Treatment of Supracondylar Fractures of the Humerus in Children: The Cincinnati Experience. *Acta Orthop. Belg.* **1996**, *62* (Suppl. 1), 41–50.
12. Cheng, J.C.; Lam, T.P.; Shen, W.Y. Closed Reduction and Percutaneous Pinning for Type III Displaced Supracondylar Fractures of the Humerus in Children. *J. Orthop. Trauma* **1995**, *9*, 511–515. [CrossRef]
13. Foead, A.; Penafort, R.; Saw, A.; Sengupta, S. Comparison of Two Methods of Percutaneous Pin Fixation in Displaced Supracondylar Fractures of the Humerus in Children. *J. Orthop. Surg. Hong Kong* **2004**, *12*, 76–82. [CrossRef]
14. Mazda, K.; Boggione, C.; Fitoussi, F.; Pennecot, G.F. Systematic Pinning of Displaced Extension-Type Supracondylar Fractures of the Humerus in Children. A Prospective Study of 116 Consecutive Patients. *J. Bone Jt. Surg. Br.* **2001**, *83*, 888–893. [CrossRef]
15. Herzenberg, J.E.; Koreska, J.; Carroll, N.C.; Rang, M. Biomechanical Testing of Pin Fixation Techniques for Pediatric Supracondylar Elbow Fractures. *Orthop. Trans.* **1988**, *12*, 678–679.
16. Larson, L.; Firoozbakhsh, K.; Passarelli, R.; Bosch, P. Biomechanical Analysis of Pinning Techniques for Pediatric Supracondylar Humerus Fractures. *J. Pediatr. Orthop.* **2006**, *26*, 573–578. [CrossRef] [PubMed]
17. Lee, S.S.; Mahar, A.T.; Miesen, D.; Newton, P.O. Displaced Pediatric Supracondylar Humerus Fractures: Biomechanical Analysis of Percutaneous Pinning Techniques. *J. Pediatr. Orthop.* **2002**, *22*, 440–443. [CrossRef] [PubMed]
18. Zionts, L.E.; McKellop, H.A.; Hathaway, R. Torsional Strength of Pin Configurations Used to Fix Supracondylar Fractures of the Humerus in Children. *J. Bone Jt. Surg. Am.* **1994**, *76*, 253–256. [CrossRef]

19. Gaston, R.G.; Cates, T.B.; Devito, D.; Schmitz, M.; Schrader, T.; Busch, M.; Fabregas, J.; Rosenberg, E.; Blanco, J. Medial and Lateral Pin versus Lateral-Entry Pin Fixation for Type 3 Supracondylar Fractures in Children: A Prospective, Surgeon-Randomized Study. *J. Pediatr. Orthop.* **2010**, *30*, 799–806. [CrossRef]
20. Sankar, W.N.; Hebela, N.M.; Skaggs, D.L.; Flynn, J.M. Loss of Pin Fixation in Displaced Supracondylar Humeral Fractures in Children: Causes and Prevention. *J. Bone Jt. Surg. Am.* **2007**, *89*, 713–717. [CrossRef]
21. Kocher, M.S.; Kasser, J.R.; Waters, P.M.; Bae, D.; Snyder, B.D.; Hresko, M.T.; Hedequist, D.; Karlin, L.; Kim, Y.-J.; Murray, M.M.; et al. Lateral Entry Compared with Medial and Lateral Entry Pin Fixation for Completely Displaced Supracondylar Humeral Fractures in Children. A Randomized Clinical Trial. *J. Bone Jt. Surg. Am.* **2007**, *89*, 706–712. [CrossRef]
22. Woratanarat, P.; Angsanuntsukh, C.; Rattanasiri, S.; Attia, J.; Woratanarat, T.; Thakkinstian, A. Meta-Analysis of Pinning in Supracondylar Fracture of the Humerus in Children. *J. Orthop. Trauma* **2012**, *26*, 48–53. [CrossRef] [PubMed]
23. Lyons, J.P.; Ashley, E.; Hoffer, M.M. Ulnar Nerve Palsies after Percutaneous Cross-Pinning of Supracondylar Fractures in Children's Elbows. *J. Pediatr. Orthop.* **1998**, *18*, 43–45. [CrossRef]
24. Ariño, V.L.; Lluch, E.E.; Ramirez, A.M.; Ferrer, J.; Rodriguez, L.; Baixauli, F. Percutaneous Fixation of Supracondylar Fractures of the Humerus in Children. *J. Bone Jt. Surg. Am.* **1977**, *59*, 914–916. [CrossRef]
25. Kallio, P.E.; Foster, B.K.; Paterson, D.C. Difficult Supracondylar Elbow Fractures in Children: Analysis of Percutaneous Pinning Technique. *J. Pediatr. Orthop.* **1992**, *12*, 11–15. [CrossRef]
26. Skaggs, D.L.; Cluck, M.W.; Mostofi, A.; Flynn, J.M.; Kay, R.M. Lateral-Entry Pin Fixation in the Management of Supracondylar Fractures in Children. *J. Bone Jt. Surg. Am.* **2004**, *86*, 702–707. [CrossRef] [PubMed]
27. Wallace, M.; Johnson, D.B.; Pierce, W.; Iobst, C.; Riccio, A.; Wimberly, R.L. Biomechanical Assessment of Torsional Stiffness in a Supracondylar Humerus Fracture Model. *J. Pediatr. Orthop.* **2019**, *39*, e210–e215. [CrossRef]
28. Jaeblon, T.; Anthony, S.; Ogden, A.; Andary, J.J. Pediatric Supracondylar Fractures: Variation in Fracture Patterns and the Biomechanical Effects of Pin Configuration. *J. Pediatr. Orthop.* **2016**, *36*, 787–792. [CrossRef]
29. Hamdi, A.; Poitras, P.; Louati, H.; Dagenais, S.; Masquijo, J.J.; Kontio, K. Biomechanical Analysis of Lateral Pin Placements for Pediatric Supracondylar Humerus Fractures. *J. Pediatr. Orthop.* **2010**, *30*, 135–139. [CrossRef]
30. Otsuka, N.Y.; Kasser, J.R. Supracondylar Fractures of the Humerus in Children. *J. Am. Acad. Orthop. Surg.* **1997**, *5*, 19–26. [CrossRef]
31. Skaggs, D.L.; Hale, J.M.; Bassett, J.; Kaminsky, C.; Kay, R.M.; Tolo, V.T. Operative Treatment of Supracondylar Fractures of the Humerus in Children. The Consequences of Pin Placement. *J. Bone Jt. Surg. Am.* **2001**, *83*, 735–740. [CrossRef]
32. Pennock, A.T.; Charles, M.; Moor, M.; Bastrom, T.P.; Newton, P.O. Potential Causes of Loss of Reduction in Supracondylar Humerus Fractures. *J. Pediatr. Orthop.* **2014**, *34*, 691–697. [CrossRef] [PubMed]

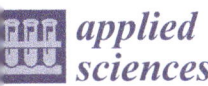

Article

Different ISO Standards' Wear Kinematic Profiles Change the TKA Inlay Load

Leandra Bauer, Manuel Kistler, Arnd Steinbrück, Katrin Ingr, Peter E. Müller, Volkmar Jansson, Christian Schröder and Matthias Woiczinski *

Department of Orthopedic Surgery, Physical Medicine and Rehabilitation, Campus Grosshadern, University Hospital of Munich (LMU), Marchioninistr. 15, 81377 Munich, Germany; Leandra.bauer@med.uni-muenchen.de (L.B.); manuel.kistler@med.uni-muenchen.de (M.K.); arnd.steinbrueck@med.uni-muenchen.de (A.S.); katrin.ingr@med.uni-muenchen.de (K.I.); peter.mueller@med.uni-muenchen.de (P.E.M.); volkmar.jansson@med.uni-muenchen.de (V.J.); christian.schroeder@med.uni-muenchen.de (C.S.)
* Correspondence: matthias.woiczinski@med.uni-muenchen.de; Tel.: +49-89-4400-74859

Abstract: Wear is an important factor in the long-term success of total knee arthroplasty (TKA). Therefore, wear testing methods have become standard in implant research and development. In the EU, these are based on two simulation concepts, which are defined in standards ISO 14243-1 and 14243-3, differentiated by the control mode—force-controlled or displacement-controlled. The aim of this study was to compare the mechanical stresses within the different ISO concepts using a finite element model (the newest displacement-controlled norm from 2014 compared with force-controlled). The in silico model showed strong correlation with the experimental data (r > 0.8). The adapted force-controlled ISO showed higher mechanical stress during the gait cycle, which also might lead to higher wear rates (14243-1 (2009): 11.15 MPa, 10.15 MPa and 9.16 MPa). The displacement-controlled ISO led to higher mechanical stress because of the constraint at the end of the stance phase (14243-3: 20.59 MPa and 17.19 MPa). Future studies should analyse different inlay designs within the same ISO standards to guarantee comparability.

Keywords: TKA; wear simulator; ISO standard; FEM; finite element

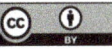

1. Introduction

Total knee arthroplasty (TKA) has been established as an operative procedure for osteoarthrosis with good to very good clinical outcomes and long-term success for patients [1,2]. Nevertheless, in some cases revision surgery is necessary, and in some patients the main reason for implant loosening is osteolysis possibly caused by wear particles [3,4]. Therefore, experimental wear testing in a laboratory environment has become an important tool for evaluating new TKA designs and new materials. Furthermore, these tests are also necessary for the approval of newly developed knee implant designs through the notified body. To generate experiments that are comparable across several research groups and companies, standards have been developed.

The International Organization for Standardization (ISO) has two main concepts established: the force-controlled (FC, 14243-1) and displacement-controlled (DC, 14243-3) standards. These standards are reviewed and renewed at regular intervals. The 2002 version was renewed in 2009; the DC norm in 2014. Both standards are used for the wear testing of different TKA designs, with one exception. The displacement-controlled norm states that completely congruent TKA designs *may not be tested* with this standard. When comparing these two different control modes, they share the same force profile for the axial (femorotibial) compression force and the same flexion/extension profile of the femoral component. The differences are in the control mode of the anterior/posterior translation and internal/external rotation of the tibia component relative to its counterpart, the femoral component. The force-controlled norm induces this movement with a load profile on the components, and the displacement-controlled standard therefore uses fixed translational and rotational values. Interestingly, for the displacement standard, the anterior/posterior movement of the tibia and the rotational profile were changed in 2014 to the opposite way around because Sutton et al. showed that the load-controlled standard was not consistent with the displacement-controlled standard in human specimens [5].

Various working groups have been working on similar issues. Mell et al. compared the DC norm of 2004 with the changed one of 2014 [6]. By means of computer simulation, the kinematic inputs, contact condition, and wear of both standards were investigated. They showed a lower wear rate for the newer version, but at the same time a higher wear area. Overall, they were able to show a difference between the two standards and advised that historical wear results be compared with newer results only with caution [6]. In another study, the ISO standard 14342-1 was compared with American Society for Testing and Materials (ASTM) F3141. They found a very similar overall wear rate (13.64–54.9 mm^3/million vs. 13.48–55.26 mm^3/million) but different wear contours and wear depth [7].

These differences in wear may result in problems for medical companies. For example, for the approval of a new medical device, the new European Medical Device Regulation (MDR) or American Food and Drug Administration (FDA) provides the possibility of using clinical data related to an equivalent device, sometimes called a "predicate device", in the clinical evaluation process. For the MDR, this is only possible if the technical, biological, and clinical characteristics are equivalent; therefore, full access to the technical documentation of the medical device is needed, which will lead in many cases to a situation where results may only be compared within inhouse products. However, if the differences in the load and motion profiles across different ISO standard versions are too great, and knowing that these kinematic profiles and loads strongly influence the generation of wear, comparisons will be difficult [8]. This leads to problems in the certification process of new implants, because if experimental wear tests are no longer comparable due to major changes over the years, companies lose the possibility of comparing results to their old result database.

The aim of this study was therefore to compare the different ISO standards across different publication years and loading concepts and to gain a deeper insight into the resulting kinematics and differences in stress in the polyethylene insert. To discover whether low congruence inlay designs are more affected by different loading conditions, the differences in inlay design across the standards should be analysed.

We hypothesise that (1) each norm will result in different inlay stresses (three norms tested: ISO 14243-1:2002, ISO 14243-1:2009, and ISO 14243-3:2014) within the same inlay design, and (2) the force-controlled norm will differ in stress and kinematics between 2002 and 2009. The comparison of the kinematics and the stress behaviour is investigated using finite element methods.

2. Materials and Methods
2.1. General

Nine different finite element models were constructed for the different inlay designs of one prosthesis (Aesculap, Tuttlingen, Germany) and the different ISO standards tested in this study (Table 1). A validation between the experimental wear tests and the in silico model was established. Therefore, the boundary conditions of ISO 14243-1:2002 (force-controlled) and the deep dish inlay design were used. Based on this validated computer model, different modifications corresponding to the different ISO standards or inlay designs were established. In this study, three different inlay designs were used: cruciate-retaining (CR), deep dish (DD), and ultra-congruent (UC). All inlays were compatible with the Columbus® knee system (Aesculap, Tuttlingen, Germany).

Table 1. Overview of the different model conditions for ISO norms 14243-1:2002 force-controlled (FC), 14243-1:2009 FC (without posterior cruciate ligament (PCL) and with PCL), and 14243-3:2014 displacement-controlled (DC).

Inlay Design	ISO Norm 14243-1:2002 (FC)	ISO Norm 14243-1:2009 (FC)		ISO Norm 14243-3:2014 (DC)
		Without PCL	With PCL	
Cruciate-Retaining (CR)	anterior/posterior spring: 30 N/mm torsional spring: 600 Nmm/°	-	anterior spring: 44 N/mm posterior spring: 9.3 N/mm torsional spring: 360 Nmm/° Note: First ±2.5 mm (a/p spring) and ±6° (torsional spring) without constraint	No spring—defined via displacement control
Deep Dish (DD)	anterior/posterior spring: 30 N/mm torsional spring: 600 Nmm/°	-	anterior spring: 44 N/mm posterior spring: 9.3 N/mm torsional spring: 360 Nmm/° Note: First ±2.5 mm (a/p spring) and ±6° (torsional spring) without constraint	No spring—defined via displacement control
Ultra-Congruent (UC)	anterior/posterior spring: 30 N/mm torsional spring: 600 Nmm/°	anterior spring: 9.3 N/mm posterior spring: 9.3 N/mm torsional spring: 360 Nmm/° Note: First ±2.5 mm (a/p spring) and ±6° (torsional spring) without constraint	-	No spring—defined via displacement control

2.2. Experimental Setup of the Wear Simulator for Validation of the Finite Element Model

An experimental wear simulator test to validate the in silico model was performed on a servo-hydraulic knee wear simulator (EndoLab GmbH, Rohrdorf, Germany). The kinematic and force patterns for the mechanical simulator were based on level walking according to ISO standard 14243-1:2002 (force-controlled standard) [9]. Internal/external rotational torque, anterior/posterior force, and axial force were generated by hydraulic cylinders accordingly. The axial force was applied in a medio-lateral compartment ratio of 60% to 40%; therefore, a lateral implantation offset of 5.6 mm (0.07 times the width of the tibial component) was implemented. To simulate the knee ligaments, the wear simulator included spring restraints of 30 N/mm in anterior/posterior translation and 600 Nmm/° in internal/external rotation, also defined in the ISO standard.

The movement constraints of the various components of the knee system in the wear simulator were as follows: The femoral component was restricted to move in anterior/posterior, medial/lateral, axial translation, internal/external rotation, and varus/valgus rotation. Flexion/extension was free, and the axis of the J-curved femoral component was developed according to the ISO standard. In two positions, 30° of flexion and 60° of flexion viewed on the sagittal plane, a line was drawn perpendicular to the ground and through the contact point of the femoral condyles. The crossover point of these two lines was defined as the flexion/extension axis. The tibial component was only restricted in flexional rotation. Anterior/posterior, medial/lateral, and axial movement were free, while varus/valgus and internal/external rotation were possible. For comparison with the in silico model, the kinematic data of the experimental setup were processed after 5000 cycles to ensure that the same surface geometry was maintained between the in silico model (no wear simulated) and the experiment due to the changing surface during the experimental wear test.

2.3. Computational Model

Kinematic Validation and Basic Model for ISO 14243-1:2002 (Force-Controlled)

The validation computer model was based on the ISO standard 14243-1:2002 (force-controlled standard), and for the equal inlay design which was used in the experimental setup, a deep dish (DD) design was used. The CAD file was imported into Ansys Workbench software (V16; Ansys, Inc., Canonsburg, PA, USA). The femoral component, inlay, and tibial baseplate were positioned in a neutral starting position to conform with the ISO standard [9]. The tibial base plate was embedded in a round rigid body according to the ISO standard with a lateralisation of 7% of the width, equivalent to that in the experimental tests. Flexion/extension was free, and the axis of the J-curved femoral component was developed according to the experimental setup.

The boundary conditions of the tibial baseplate were established on the bottom of the rigid body representing the embedded tibial component in resin (Figure 1). For translational movement, it was free to move in the medial/lateral, anterior/posterior, and proximal/distal (axial) directions. For rotational movement, it was free to rotate internally/externally and was free in varus/valgus rotation. Rotation around the *x*-axis, which represented the slope axis, was restricted during the whole simulation according to the ISO standard and the experimental setup.

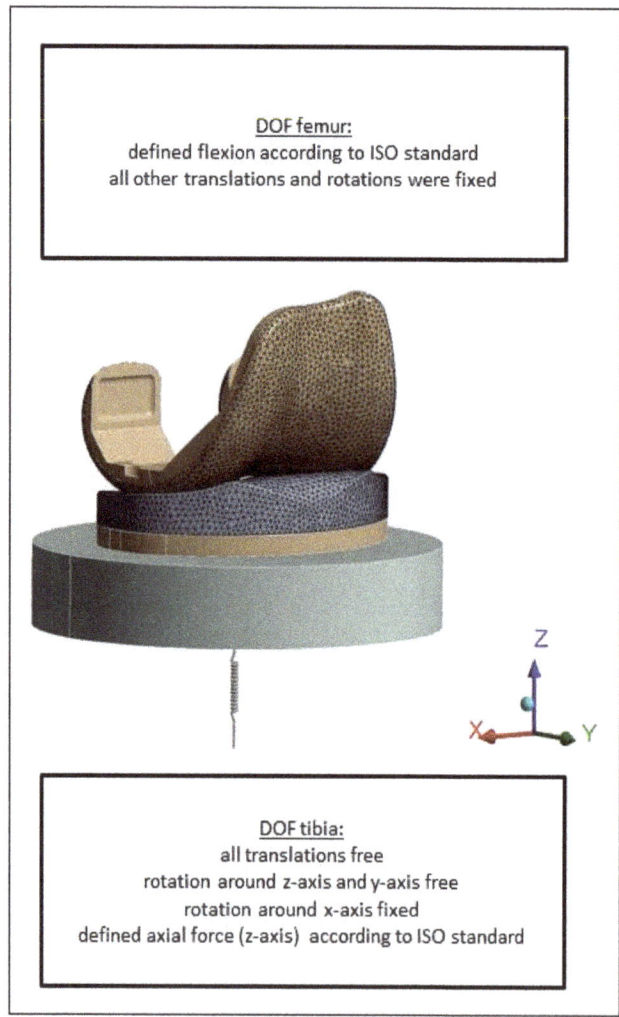

Figure 1. Structure of the finite element (FE) model with the degrees of freedom (DOF) for femur and tibia according to the International Organization for Standardization (ISO).

Forces for anterior/posterior translation, internal/external rotation (torque), and axial force were also established on the resin body. The anterior/posterior force was applied to the posterior part, while the axial force and the rotational torque were applied to the bottom part of the resin body. Due to the 7% lateral translation of the tibia and inlay component during implantation, the line of action of the forces was secured according to the ISO standard.

Restraint system-simulating ligaments and a capsule environment were added to the simulation with a linear spring according to the ISO standard with 30 N/mm in the anterior/posterior direction with a linear spring element. A restraint system for internal/external rotation of the tibia was also implemented via a linear spring element, i.e., a torsional spring element with 600 Nmm/°.

Femorotibial contact was established in the finite element model using an augmented Lagrange algorithm and a basic frictional coefficient of 0.05 [10,11]. To confirm the frictional coefficient, variations of 0.01, 0.03, and 0.08 were calculated and compared with the experimental kinematic data. The contacts between the inlay, tibial base plate, and the rigid body representing the embedded resin were defined as fixed joints in the simulation, which means no separation was possible, and all bodies except the inlay were not deformable. One hundred and four load steps were implemented in the in silico model to simulate the gait cycle. The first four loading steps were used to establish the initial contact between the femoral component and the inlay of the prosthesis, which is necessary in a computer model. The remaining 100 loading steps were the gait cycle steps, which are specified by the ISO standard.

2.4. Numerical Model Validation

The model validation was performed with the DD inlay using the described experimental wear simulator. For kinematic comparison, the Pearson correlation coefficient (r) was used and secured with different frictional coefficients within the simulation. For finite element models, it is necessary to conduct a mesh validation, which is known as a convergence study. Since the TKA design was also used in an earlier validated study, the mesh size was identical to that used in a validation study by Woiczinski et al. [12]. The correlation for the kinematic comparision was calculated by using the following formula (1):

$$r = \frac{\sum_{i=1}^{n}(x_i - \bar{x}) * (y_i - \bar{y})}{\sqrt{\sum_{i=1}^{n}(x_i - \bar{x})^2 * \sum_{i=1}^{n}(y_i - \bar{y})^2}} \quad (1)$$

2.5. Model Variation 1: New ISO 14243-1:2009 (Force-Controlled)

The newer ISO standard was adapted and compared to the version from the year 2002. In the new standard, some boundary conditions differ between the different inlay designs. For example, there is a difference in the restraint system for cruciate-retaining inlays compared to that for ultra-high-congruence inlays. To represent these changing boundary conditions, the initial numerical model (ISO 14243:2002) was adapted accordingly to meet the newer standard [13]. For the CR computer model, the spring elements were changed to tension-only elements. In the resin body, an anterior-positioned spring, which restrains posterior movement of the tibia, was added with a spring rate of 44 N/mm, simulating a posterior cruciate ligament according to the ISO standard. In contrast, in the resin body, a posterior-positioned spring with a rate of 9.3 N/mm was added to restrain anterior movement of the tibia, simulating only the capsule of the knee, because no anterior cruciate ligament is currently present in this type of prosthesis design. Furthermore, both spring elements had no restraint in ±2.5 mm anterior/posterior movement from a neutral position, also according to the ISO standard. The torsional spring was adapted to the new standard with a restraint force of 360 Nmm/° and no restraint up to ±6° starting at a neutral position. The boundary conditions and forces within the norm were equal to those in the old ISO standard and therefore were not changed in this in silico model.

2.6. ISO 14243-3:2014 Model (Displacement-Controlled)

In contrast to the force-controlled standard, there is no anterior/posterior force or internal/external torque defined in ISO 14243-3:2014. The movements in these directions are displacement-controlled. These boundary conditions were changed in the computer model according to the ISO standard [14]. Furthermore, no restraint system is required due to the displacement-controlled movement, which is why the spring elements were removed in the in silico model. The axial force and flexion profile were not changed in the model because they are equal to those in the force-constrained ISO standard.

3. Results

3.1. Validation

All different friction models showed a good comparison with the experimental movement tests (Figure 2). The correlation coefficients for the anterior/posterior movement ranged from r = 0.91 for the model with a frictional coefficient of 0.01 and r = 0.87 for a frictional coefficient of 0.08. For the rotational data, also, all in silico models presented a good trend compared to the experimental data. The correlation coefficients ranged from r = 0.80 for a 0.01 friction coefficient and r = 0.81 for a 0.08 friction coefficient.

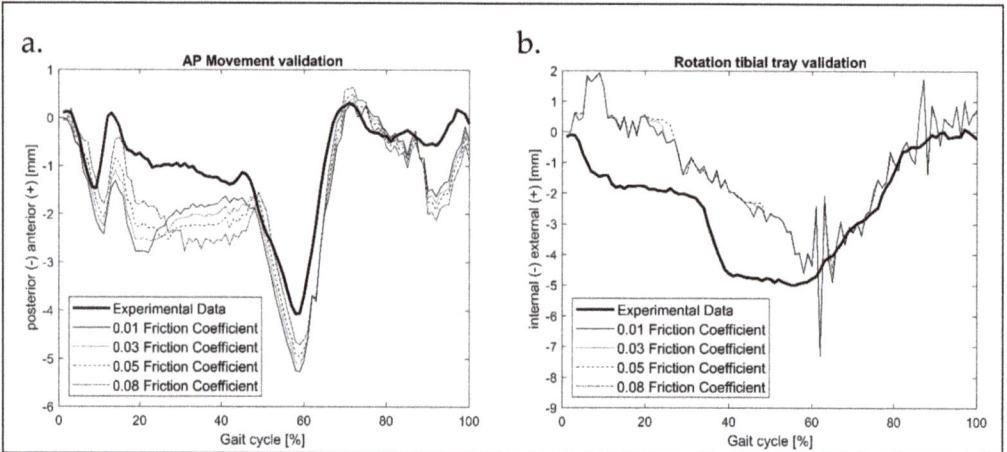

Figure 2. Validation with the deep dish (DD) inlay with different friction coefficients; (**a**) anterior/posterior (AP) movement, (**b**) tibia rotation.

3.2. Comparison of FC-2002, FC-2009, and DC-2014 with the CR Inlay

The results of this comparison are presented in Figure 3. Stress in the CR inlay during the gait cycle showed two peaks of 12.38 MPa and 9.27 MPa for FC-2002 and another two of 20.59 MPa and 17.19 MPa for the DC-2014 standard. FC-2009 generated three maxima of 11.15 MPa, 10.15 MPa, and 9.16 MPa. These results are also shown in Figure 4. For the anterior/posterior translation of the tibia, one maximum was seen at 57% of the gait cycle in the posterior direction (4.74 mm) for FC-2002, and a second maximum was observed at 71% of the gait cycle for FC-2009 in the anterior direction (7.51 mm). DC-2014 generated an anterior/posterior movement profile of two maxima in the anterior direction, as predefined at 18% and 57% of the gait cycle, with values of 4.47 mm and 5.13 mm, respectively. Rotational data showed an internally rotating tibia for FC-2002, with a maximum of 6.18° at 54% of the gait cycle, and for FC-2009, with a maximum of 9.00° at 56% of the gait cycle. DC-2014 generated, as predefined, one maximum at the end of the gait cycle of 90% in the 5.72° external direction.

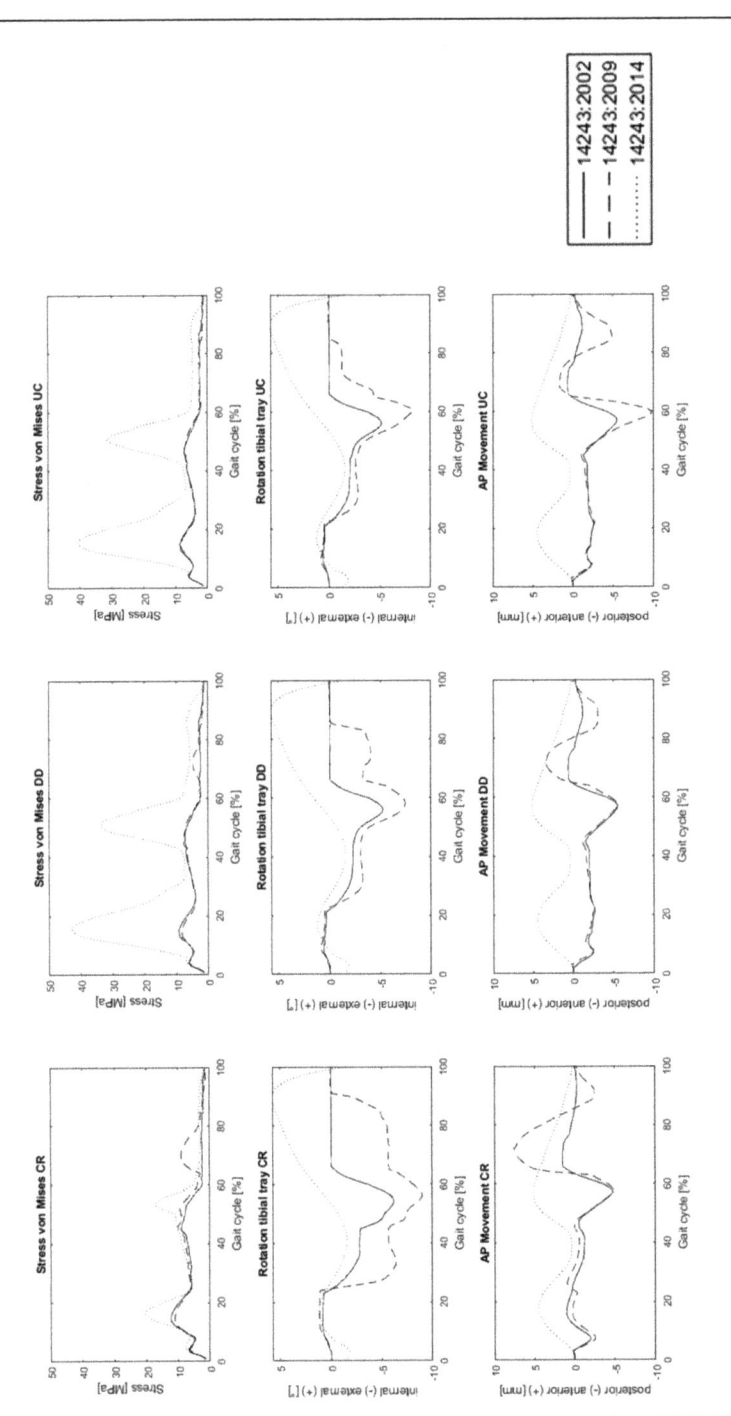

Figure 3. Results of stress and kinematic analysis for different ISO norms (14243-1:2002, 14243-1:2009, 14243-3:2014) and inlays (cruciate-retaining—CR, deep dish—DD, ultra-congruent—UC).

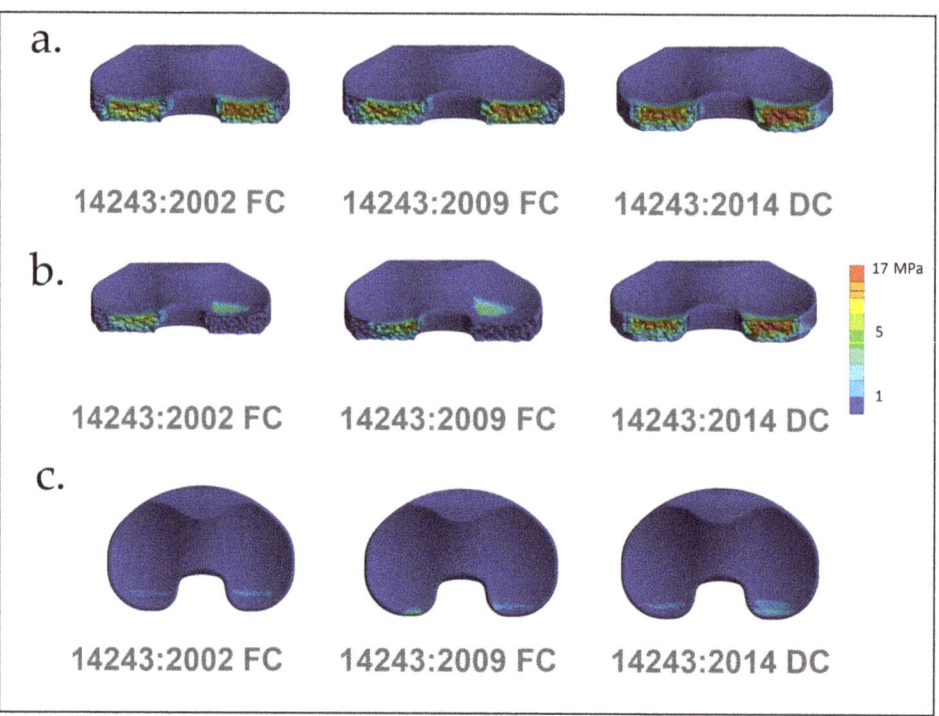

Figure 4. Stress in the cruciate-retaining (CR) inlay for different ISO norms: (**a**) first peak, (**b**) second peak, (**c**) third peak.

3.3. Comparison of Different Inlay Designs

In addition to the main questions, a comparison of different inlays within one standard was carried out. Within FC-2002, the different design variants generated different stresses and different anterior/posterior and rotational movement. The maximum stresses in the CR, DD, and UC inlays were lower in FC-2002 and FC-2009 and higher in DC-2014. Furthermore, FC-2009 generated no third peak value within the UC inlay in the swing phase, unlike the other designs (CR and DD). Kinematic data showed different values for FC-2002 and the CR inlay variant compared to the DD and UC designs. To be more precise, between 20% and 50% of the gait cycle, the CR inlay moved less in the posterior direction in FC-2002 than did the other designs. Anterior/posterior movement was similar in FC-2002 for the DD and UC inlays. In FC-2009, more anterior movement was observed with a maximum of 7.51 mm at 72% of the gait cycle with the CR inlay. The DD and UC inlays showed less anterior movement at the same percentage of the gait cycle. The UC inlay showed greater posterior movement of 9.69 mm at 60% of the gait cycle in FC-2009. Rotational data showed no difference between the inlay designs for FC-2002 and DC-2014. More internal rotation was seen for the CR inlay in FC-2009 compared to the DD and UC inlays.

4. Discussion

The main important finding of this study is that the force-controlled norms of 2002 and 2009 are different in the resulting femorotibial kinematics and von Mises stress behaviour within the inlay over the gait cycle. Moreover, the displacement-controlled standard from 2014 generated up to four times more von Mises stress in all three tested inlay designs.

There were differences between FC-2002 and FC-2009 regarding the kinematic results within the CR inlay. FC-2009 led to more internal rotation in all inlays than FC-2002. Furthermore, at about 75% of the gait cycle, increased anterior movement was observed with the FC-2009 norm compared to FC-2002. The ISO standard changed from 2002 to 2009 by modifying the anterior/posterior and torsional springs (30 to 44 N/mm and 600 to 360 Nmm/°) and adding a slack condition for ±2.5 mm (a/p spring) and ±6° (torsional spring). As a result, the movement experiences less resistance. This might explain the increased anterior movement and internal rotation of the tibia in the model with the ISO 2009 standard for all inlays. The adapted force-controlled ISO from 2009 showed higher mechanical stress during the gait cycle in the CR and DD designs, which might also lead to higher wear rates. In general, the changes in the standard from 2002 to 2009 show an increase in the range of motion. This can have a negative effect on the wear contact area of both components in the form of increased wear. Studies by Grupp et al. and Kretzer et al. were also able to confirm this observation with an increased amount of abrasion particles found across different ISO norms [8,15,16]. Grupp et al. compared the kinematics of posterior-stabilised inlays produced according to the standard protocol ISO 14243-1 versions from 2002 and 2009. In agreement with our results, they found a change in anterior/posterior (AP) translation and internal/external rotation, which resulted in a 3.2 times higher wear rate. They came to the conclusion that a change in the kinematics has a strong influence on the wear behaviour in TKA [16].

Compared to FC-2009, the displacement-controlled ISO standard (2014) can lead to a higher mechanical load due to displacement-controlled movement. In the FC-2009 norm, an additional peak at about 70% of the gait cycle occurred for CR and DD designs compared to the older version. The maximum contact pressure occurred as expected with each inlay on the medial side. However, DC-2014 showed a more dorsal distribution of the pressure, resulting in a smaller surface. This can be explained by the fact that displacement control dictates anterior movement of the inlay, whereas force control is directed both anteriorly and posteriorly. The DC-2014 standard is controlled by a defined path. This control mechanism does not account for possible resistance in the joint. Therefore, the standard automatically leads to more movement in the prosthetic joint and creates more von Mises stress. Increased stress in the inlay can also lead to increased wear of the prosthesis. This fact leads to the problem that if the prostheses are tested with different standards, higher wear cannot automatically be attributed to the type of prosthesis. The different results of the tested standards are extremely limited in terms of comparability.

In a comparison of different inlay designs, increased movement in the posterior direction with a maximum at the beginning of the swing phase was only seen in the UC inlay for FC-2009. The more paradoxical posterior displacement of the UC inlay can be explained by the different definition of the restraint spring system (9.3 N/mm vs. 44 N/mm). The maximum total rotation increased from 7.0° to 10.1° for the UC inlay. A similar increase from 5.2° to 12.0° was also determined by Grupp et al., who investigated the renewal of the norm using a posterior stabilised inlay [16]. Kretzer et al. found an increase from 4.1° to 7.7°, where only the change in the nonlinear spring constraint was congruent with this experiment, since the level of resistance of the springs remained the same [8]. Regarding the stress in the DC norm, the DD and UC inlays for the displacement-controlled standard had the highest values. The DC norm forces the inlay to a specified position, so that the strong curvature of the inlay acts as a resistance to the femur and thus leads to an increased pressure load on the inlay surface. Barnett et al., Knight et al., and McEwen et al. also came to the conclusion in previous work that different kinematic conditions specified by different ISO standards lead to changes in wear [17–19]. Wear was demonstrably decreased when AP movements and internal/external rotation were reduced. Zietz et al. confirmed as much [20]. Even the definition of the ISO standard states that "(..) this part of ISO 14243 may not be applicable to knee designs with a high degree of constraints (..)" [14]. This statement can be interpreted as a warning that inlays like UC and possibly DD should not be tested with this standard; however, it does not prohibit it.

This explains the extremely high values and deviations in standards for the UC and DD inlays compared to the CR inlay.

The created finite element model (FEM) was first validated using existing experimental data for the DD inlay. A mean value of 0.05 for the coefficient of friction seemed appropriate for further calculations. Godest et al. used a similar approach in their work and achieved comparable results [21].

Of course, our study has some limitations. One is that the calculations are based on a computer model. A model can only ever give an approximation of the actual results in humans. Furthermore, it must be noted that this is not an in vivo study. Moreover, a computer model always brings a certain amount of error into the calculations. Components that are not represented within the simulation compared to the experiment may influence results. Therefore, a validation process is mandatory for each in silico computer model to ensure slight and unrecognised different loadings. Another limitation is that our computer model did not measure the wear, so due to the changed kinematics and contact stress only a tendency can be expressed.

5. Conclusions

In conclusion, it can be stated that all ISO standards induced different stresses, AP movement, and tibia rotation in all inlay designs. The adapted force-controlled ISO from the year 2009 showed higher mechanical stress and AP motion during the gait cycle because of the different spring system. The displacement-controlled ISO led to higher mechanical stress. If the results of the present study are considered in light of the new MDR, it becomes clear that not only must the same standard (force-controlled vs. displacement-controlled) basis be used for testing new products, but the same version must also be used (2002 vs. 2009 vs. 2014). If older, already-approved medical devices are tested using an older ISO standard version, the results of kinematics and pressure behaviour are not comparable. Thus, approval of a medical product by the MDR should only be given if the test requirements are the same. Future studies should analyse different inlay designs within the same ISO standards to guarantee comparability.

Author Contributions: Conceptualisation, C.S., M.W., and L.B.; methodology, M.K., K.I.; data citation, L.B.; validation, K.I., C.S. and M.W.; formal analysis, L.B.; writing—original draft preparation, L.B., A.S. and M.W.; writing—review and editing, P.E.M., V.J.; visualisation, L.B., M.W.; supervision, M.W.; project administration, M.W., P.E.M. and V.J. All authors have read and agreed to the published version of the manuscript.

Funding: This research received no external funding.

Institutional Review Board Statement: Not applicable.

Informed Consent Statement: Not applicable.

Data Availability Statement: The data cannot be made available for company law reasons.

Acknowledgments: The authors wish to thank Aesculap for providing the prosthesis system.

Conflicts of Interest: The authors declare no conflict of interest.

References

1. Grimberg, A.; Volkmar, J.; Melsheimer, O. *Jahresbericht 2019*; EPRD Deutsche Endoprothesenregister: Berlin, Germany, 2019.
2. Kurtz, S.; Ong, K.; Lau, E.; Mowat, F.; Halpern, M. Projections of primary and revision hip and knee arthroplasty in the United States from 2005 to 2030. *J. Bone Jt. Surg. Am.* **2007**, *89*, 780–785. [CrossRef]
3. Schwenke, T.; Orozco, D.; Schneider, E.; Wimmer, M. Differences in wear between load and displacement control tested total knee replacements. *Wear* **2009**, *267*, 757–762. [CrossRef]
4. Brockett, C.L.; Abdelgaied, A.; Haythornthwaite, T.; Hardaker, C.; Fisher, J.; Jennings, L.M. The influence of simulator input conditions on the wear of total knee replacements: An experimental and computational study. *Proc. Inst. Mech. Eng. Part H J. Eng. Med.* **2016**, *230*, 429–439. [CrossRef] [PubMed]
5. Sutton, L.G.; Werner, F.W.; Haider, H.; Hamblin, T.; Clabeaux, J.J. In vitro response of the natural cadaver knee to the loading profiles specified in a standard for knee implant wear testing. *J. Biomech.* **2010**, *43*, 2203–2207. [CrossRef] [PubMed]

6. Mell, S.P.; Fullam, S.; Wimmer, M.A.; Lundberg, H.J. Finite element evaluation of the newest ISO testing standard for polyethylene total knee replacement liners. *Proc. Inst. Mech. Eng. Part H J. Eng. Med.* **2018**, *23*, 545–552. [CrossRef] [PubMed]
7. Wang, X.-H.; Li, H.; Dong, X.; Zhao, F.; Cheng, C.-K. Comparison of ISO 14243-1 to ASTM F3141 in terms of wearing of knee prostheses. *Clin. Biomech.* **2019**, *63*, 34–40. [CrossRef] [PubMed]
8. Kretzer, J.P.; Jakubowitz, E.; Sonntag, R.; Hofmann, K.; Heisel, C.; Thomsen, M. Effect of joint laxity on polyethylene wear in total knee replacement. *J. Biomech.* **2010**, *43*, 1092–1096. [CrossRef] [PubMed]
9. International Organization for Standardization. *International Standard, Implants for Surgery—Wear of Total Knee-Joint Prostheses—Part 1: Loading and Displacement Parameters for Wear-Testing Machines with Load Control and Corresponding Environmental Conditions for Test*; ISO: Geneva, Switzerland, 2002.
10. Gispert, M.; Serro, A.; Colaco, R.; Saramago, B. Friction and wear mechanisms in hip prosthesis: Comparison of joint materials behaviour in several lubricants. *Wear* **2006**, *260*, 149–158. [CrossRef]
11. Kyomoto, M.; Iwasaki, Y.; Moro, T.; Konno, T.; Miyaji, F.; Kawaguchi, H.; Takatori, Y.; Nakamura, K.; Ishihara, K. High lubricious surface of cobalt–chromium–molybdenum alloy prepared by grafting poly (2-methacryloyloxyethyl phosphorylcholine). *Biomaterials* **2007**, *28*, 3121–3130. [CrossRef] [PubMed]
12. Woiczinski, M.; Steinbrück, A.; Weber, P.; Müller, P.E.; Jansson, V.; Schröder, C. Development and validation of a weight-bearing finite element model for total knee replacement. *Comput. Methods Biomech. Biomed. Engin.* **2016**, *19*, 1033–1045. [CrossRef] [PubMed]
13. International Organization for Standardization. *International Standard, Implants for Surgery—Wear of Total Knee-Joint Prostheses—Part 1: Loading and Displacement Parameters for Wear-Testing Machines with Displacement Control and Corresponding Environmental Conditions for Test*; ISO: Geneva, Switzerland, 2009.
14. International Organization for Standardization. *International Standard, Implants for Surgery—Wear of Total Knee-Joint Prostheses—Part 3: Loading and Displacement Parameters for Wear-Testing Machines with Displacement Control and Corresponding Environmental Conditions for Test*; ISO: Geneva, Switzerland, 2014.
15. Grupp, T.M.; Saleh, K.J.; Mihalko, W.M.; Hintner, M.; Fritz, B.; Schilling, C.; Schwiesau, J.; Kaddick, C. Effect of anterior–posterior and internal–external motion restraint during knee wear simulation on a posterior stabilised knee design. *J. Biomech.* **2013**, *46*, 491–497. [CrossRef] [PubMed]
16. Grupp, T.M.; Schroeder, C.; Kim, T.K.; Miehlke, R.K.; Fritz, B.; Jansson, V.; Utzschneider, S. Biotribology of a mobile bearing posterior stabilised knee design-effect of motion restraint on wear, tibio-femoral kinematics and particles. *J. Biomech.* **2014**, *47*, 2415–2423. [CrossRef] [PubMed]
17. Barnett, P.I.; Fisher, J.; Auger, D.D.; Stone, M.H.; Ingham, E. Comparison of wear in a total knee replacement under different kinematic conditions. *J. Mater. Sci. Mater. Med.* **2001**, *12*, 1039–1042. [CrossRef] [PubMed]
18. Knight, L.A.; McEwen, H.M.; Farrar, R.; Stone, M.H.; Fisher, J.; Taylor, M. The Influence of the Wear Path on the Wear Rates in Total Knee Replacement. In Proceedings of the 2003 Summer Bioengineering Conference, Key Biscayne, FL, USA, 25–29 June 2003.
19. McEwen, H.M.; Barnett, P.I.; Bell, C.J.; Farrar, R.; Auger, D.D.; Stone, M.H.; Fisher, J. The influence of design, materials and kinematics on the in vitro wear of total knee replacements. *J. Biomech.* **2005**, *38*, 357–365. [CrossRef]
20. Zietz, C.; Reinders, J.; Schwiesau, J.; Paulus, A.; Kretzer, J.; Grupp, T.; Utzschneider, S.; Bader, R. Experimental testing of total knee replacements with UHMW-PE inserts: Impact of severe wear test conditions. *J. Mater. Sci. Mater. Med.* **2015**, *26*, 1–13. [CrossRef] [PubMed]
21. Godest, A.C.; Beaugonin, M.; Haug, E.; Taylor, M.; Gregson, P.J. Simulation of a knee joint replacement during a gait cycle using explicit finite element analysis. *J. Biomech.* **2002**, *35*, 267–275. [CrossRef]

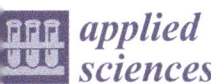

Article

An MRI-Based Patient-Specific Computational Framework for the Calculation of Range of Motion of Total Hip Replacements

Maeruan Kebbach [1,*], Christian Schulze [1], Christian Meyenburg [1], Daniel Kluess [1], Mevluet Sungu [2], Albrecht Hartmann [3], Klaus-Peter Günther [3] and Rainer Bader [1]

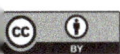

1 Biomechanics and Implant Technology Research Laboratory, Department of Orthopaedics, University Medicine Rostock, Doberaner Str. 142, 18057 Rostock, Germany; Christian.Schulze2@med.uni-rostock.de (C.S.); christian.meyenburg@gmail.com (C.M.); daniel.kluess@med.uni-rostock.de (D.K.); rainer.bader@med.uni-rostock.de (R.B.)
2 Aesculap AG Research and Development, 78532 Tuttlingen, Germany; mevluet.sungu@aesculap.de
3 Department of Orthopedic Surgery, University Hospital Carl Gustav Carus, Technische Universität Dresden, 01307 Dresden, Germany; Albrecht.Hartmann@uniklinikum-dresden.de (A.H.); Klaus-Peter.Guenther@uniklinikum-dresden.de (K.-P.G.)
* Correspondence: maeruan.kebbach@med.uni-rostock.de; Tel.: +49-381-498-8985

Abstract: The calculation of range of motion (ROM) is a key factor during preoperative planning of total hip replacements (THR), to reduce the risk of impingement and dislocation of the artificial hip joint. To support the preoperative assessment of THR, a magnetic resonance imaging (MRI)-based computational framework was generated; this enabled the estimation of patient-specific ROM and type of impingement (bone-to-bone, implant-to-bone, and implant-to-implant) postoperatively, using a three-dimensional computer-aided design (CAD) to visualize typical clinical joint movements. Hence, patient-specific CAD models from 19 patients were generated from MRI scans and a conventional total hip system (Bicontact® hip stem and Plasmacup® SC acetabular cup with a ceramic-on-ceramic bearing) was implanted virtually. As a verification of the framework, the ROM was compared between preoperatively planned and the postoperatively reconstructed situations; this was derived based on postoperative radiographs (n = 6 patients) during different clinically relevant movements. The data analysis revealed there was no significant difference between preoperatively planned and postoperatively reconstructed ROM (Δ_{ROM}) of maximum flexion ($\Delta_{ROM} = 0°$, $p = 0.854$) and internal rotation ($\Delta_{ROM} = 1.8°$, $p = 0.917$). Contrarily, minor differences were observed for the ROM during maximum external rotation ($\Delta_{ROM} = 9°$, $p = 0.046$). Impingement, of all three types, was in good agreement with the preoperatively planned and postoperatively reconstructed scenarios during all movements. The calculated ROM reached physiological levels during flexion and internal rotation movement; however, it exceeded physiological levels during external rotation. Patients, where implant-to-implant impingement was detected, reached higher ROMs than patients with bone-to-bone impingement. The proposed framework provides the capability to predict postoperative ROM of THRs.

Keywords: joint replacement; hip joint; range of motion; impingement

1. Introduction

Total hip replacement (THR) constitutes the gold standard for the treatment of end-stage hip osteoarthritis and is currently performed more than 230,000 times per year in Germany [1,2]. In 2015, the incidence of THR surgery was 166 per 100,000 cases in the OECD34 region [3]. This number is expected to rise [4–6] due to an increase in life expectancy of a globally aging population [5,7]. In this context, complications after THR represent an economic burden for the world healthcare system, which is primarily owing to an increasing number of primary and revision operations [5].

Despite improvements in surgical techniques and implant designs, impingement and dislocation constitute a crucial cause of failure of THR; this is due to a limited postoperative range of motion (ROM) during activities of daily living [7,8]. Besides aseptic loosening, dislocation is one of the major complications of hip replacement [1,9–11]. In the USA, dislocation is considered as the most common indication for revision surgery [8]. A high ROM is essential, especially for patients with extreme movements in different populations worldwide as well as for young and more active patients [9,10]. Besides bone and prosthetic impingement, the ROM of THRs may also be limited due to the surrounding soft-tissue structures [11]. The impingement process and, thus, the resulting ROM are dependent on patient-specific anatomy, the implant design, and intraoperative implant position, as well as the condition of the surrounding patient-specific soft-tissue structures [12–20]. Additionally, impingement can cause hip joint instability, induce wear or damage to the articulating implant surfaces, reduce the implant fixation, and cause total hip dislocation [16,21,22]. Moreover, impingement of the femoral neck on the acetabular cup can result in increased wear and liner damage due to higher contact pressure at the contact point, presenting a higher risk for subluxation or dislocation [21]. Hereby, impingement is responsible for the lever arm to lever out the prosthetic head from the acetabular cup.

Currently, the occurrence of impingement is manually assessed by an orthopedic surgeon, by intraoperatively imposing specific motion patterns while the impingement is detected [23]. To analyze the maximum ROM of different implant designs, several experimental [24–29] and computational studies [13,18,20,21,23,30–38], using computer-aided design (CAD), finite element analyses, or multibody simulations, have been conducted. Previous studies described the effect of the orientation of the acetabular cup, prosthetic head size on the impingement, and risk of dislocation [21,39,40]. A recent computational study conducted by Widmer et al. [41] optimized the recommendations to reach the largest impingement-free ROM, by finding optimal target zones for implant positioning; this was achieved by using 3D kinematic hip motion analyses with respect to the contribution of various intraoperative positioning and implant design parameters. In a retrospective study, the sagittal orientation of the pelvis after THR was investigated, which is an important factor for functional cup orientation [42]. However, most of the studies did not consider real patient-specific data or were mostly based on computed tomography (CT) scans, which were hazardous for the patient, and, therefore, not the first choice in a preoperative planning scenario. The ROM is linked to the postoperative outcome and has attracted attention from the research community by using experimental and numerical methods [21,30,38,41,43–52]. Despite these studies, there is, to our knowledge, no approach that can be used to assess ROM in preoperative planning without subjecting the patient to additional radiation by CT scanning. In this regard, due to the high anatomical variability of hip joint geometry, patient-specific geometries are needed to perform more realistic computational preoperative analysis [23,32].

We aimed to prove the feasibility of investigating ROM, based on patient data, using the proposed methodology which enables the computational prediction of postoperative ROM, depending on the component selection and alignment. Therefore, we introduce a magnetic resonance imaging (MRI)–based computational framework to support the preoperative assessment of THRs. In this context, MRI allows computational reconstruction of the bone structures, enabling the virtual implantation of different endoprosthetic designs and various implant positioning. Moreover, this ensures that patients undergoing a computational assessment of ROM using the proposed methodology are not exposed to additional amounts of radiation. The framework will be subjected to verification steps, to enable the estimation of the patient-specific ROM and type of impingement (bone-to-bone, implant-to-bone, and implant-to-implant) postoperatively by using three-dimensional CAD, which will visualize typical clinical movement maneuvers. Hence, we generated patient-specific CAD models from THR patients from MRI scans (n = 19) and calculated the ROM of a virtually implanted and commercially available THR system for this patient cohort. Additionally, the ROM was compared between the preoperatively planned and the postoperatively reconstructed situation; the latter was derived from postoperative radiographs. Finally, we used the proposed framework to evaluate the effect of different implant-specific parameters (size of the prosthetic head and acetabular cup) on the estimated postoperative ROM of the patients.

2. Materials and Methods

2.1. Overview of the Deployed Framework

In this study, we introduce a new computational framework (Figure 1), which is based on non-invasive MRI data of patients, and a previously described method of CAD modeling [18,24,30,53]; this enables the estimation of the patient-specific ROM for THRs during the movements similar to ISO-21535 and clinical joint movements [54–57].

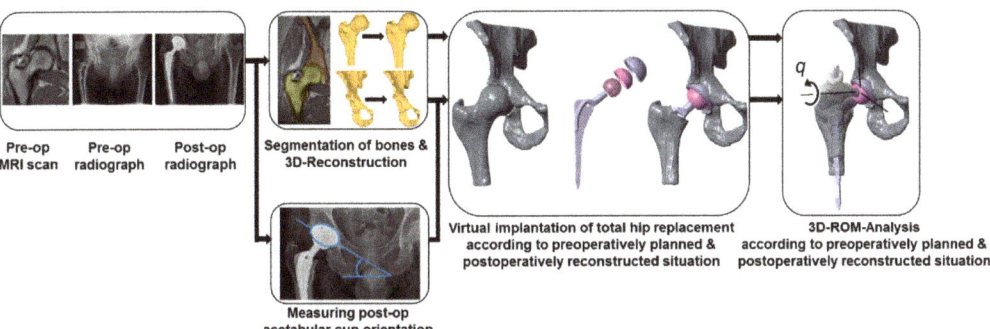

Figure 1. The computational framework for the preoperative calculation of the patient-specific range of motion (ROM) after subjection to virtually performed total hip arthroplasty. Note that the postoperative radiograph is solely used to generate the postoperatively reconstructed situation, which is intended to be used to compare the ROM with the preoperatively planned situation. Therefore, this is not necessary for the intended framework, i.e., the estimation of the postoperative ROM during preoperative planning based on MRI data.

On the one hand, the implant component alignment was derived from the preoperatively planned situation. On the other hand, the alignment was derived from the postoperatively reconstructed situation, enabling comparison between both situations. In this context, 19 patients (8 females and 11 males) suffering from hip osteoarthritis and scheduled for THR (Universitätsklinikum, Dresden, Germany) were selected to investigate the ROM of the artificial joint after virtual implantation of a THR (Figure 1). The mean age of the 19 patients was 52.1 ± 7.2 years. More precisely, six of these patients received surgical treatment with a Bicontact hip stem system (Aesculap AG, Tuttlingen, Germany), where the implant component alignment was virtually reconstructed using postoperative radiographs by the method of Liaw et al. [58]. The Bicontact hip stem (size from 10 to 16), with different centrum–collum–diaphyseal (CCD) angles (128° and 135°), was combined with a ceramic ball head (diameter 28 to 36 mm, cone 12/14 mm) consisting of BIOLOX®delta (CeramTec, Plochingen, Germany). Furthermore, the acetabular cup (outer diameter 46 to 60 mm, Plasmacup® SC) (Aesculap AG, Tuttlingen, Germany) was equipped with the Plasmacup® delta ceramic liner (BIOLOX®delta, inner diameter 28 to 36 mm). All the patient cases with the implant-specific parameters are presented in Table 1. Note that intraoperative deviations from preoperative planning have occurred and, therefore, some patients have been treated with different implant component sizes. Regarding the THR design, different implant-specific design parameters for the examined THR are depicted in Figure 2.

Table 1. Implant-specific parameters (cup size, head size, centrum–collum–diaphyseal (CCD) angles) virtually implanted for each patient case for the preoperatively planned situation and postoperatively reconstructed situation.

Patient No.	Preoperatively Planned Situation					Postoperatively Reconstructed Situation				
	Liner (Inner-Ø in mm)	Cup (Outer-Ø in mm)	Stem (CCD in °)	Head (Ø in mm; Head Offset Type)	Head-to-Neck Ratio	Liner (Inner-Ø in mm)	Cup (Outer-Ø in mm)	Stem (CCD in °)	Head (Ø in mm; Head Offset Type)	Head-to-Neck Ratio
210	36	52	NK113T (128)	36S	2.67	–	–	–	–	–
212	32	50	NK510T (135)	32S	2.37	–	–	–	–	–
216	32	48	NK110T (128)	32S	2.37	–	–	–	–	–
219	28	46	NK111T (128)	28M	2.07	–	–	–	–	–
253	36	52	NK112T (128)	36L	2.67	–	–	–	–	–
256	36	52	NK512T (135)	36M	2.67	–	–	–	–	–
259	36	52	NK112T (128)	36XL	2.67	–	–	–	–	–
260	28	46	NK110T (128)	28S	2.07	–	–	–	–	–
208	36	52	NK112T (128)	36L	2.67	52	NK112T (128)	36XL	2.67
213	32	48	NK110T (128)	32L	2.37	48	NK112T (128)	32L	2.37
214	36	52	NK113T (128)	36M	2.67	52	NK112T (128)	36M	2.67
217	36	60	NK114T (128)	36M	2.67	56	NK114T (128)	36S	2.67
252	36	58	NK516T (135)	36S	2.67	56	NK516T (135)	36M	2.67
254	32	48	NK113T (128)	32L	2.37	50	NK112T (128)	32L	2.37
106	32	50	NK511T (135)	32S	2.37	–	–	–	–	–
107	36	52	NK512T (135)	36M	2.67	–	–	–	–	–
108	36	56	NK114T (128)	36L	2.67	–	–	–	–	–
109	36	58	NK114T (128)	36XL	2.67	–	–	–	–	–
110	36	54	NK112T (128)	36XL	2.67	–	–	–	–	–

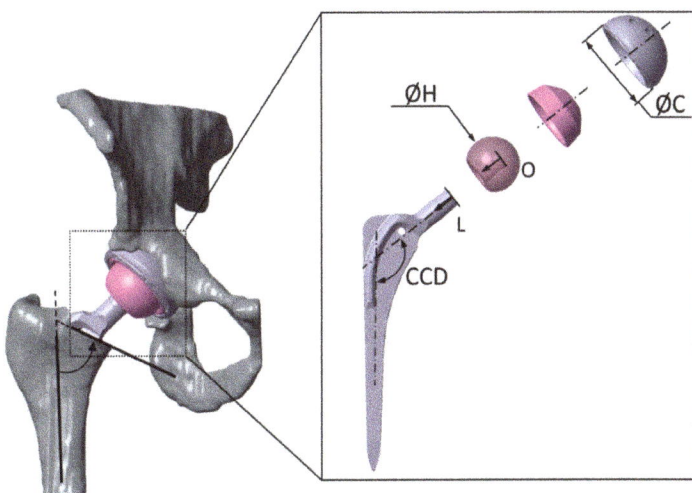

Figure 2. Virtually implanted total hip replacement (Bicontact® hip stem and Plasmacup® SC acetabular cup with a ceramic-on-ceramic bearing). The virtual implantation was carried out by an experienced orthopedic surgeon. Implant design parameters are subject to variation for the implant shaft (neck-to-shaft angle CCD, neck length L, head offset O, neck length L, and head diameter H) as well as for the acetabular cup (diameter C) of the analyzed total hip replacement.

2.2. Geometry Data Acquisition

For each patient, preoperative MRI scans of the native hip joint (hi-res, voxel-size 1.8 mm) and an overview MRI of the distal femur and the pelvis were conducted. Additionally, standard pre- and postoperative radiographs (anterior–posterior projection) of the hip joint treated with THR were acquired. The study was approved by the local ethics committee (EK 175052011). Written informed consent was obtained from all patients before participation.

The MRI files of the patients were imported in the software package Amira (v.5.4.1, Zuse Institute Berlin, Berlin, Germany; Thermo Fisher Scientific, Waltham, MA, USA), to reconstruct the 3D bone surface models using triangulated surfaces. The 3D surface models of the bony structure of the femur and acetabulum were obtained (Figure 1) by manually segmenting the bony structures slice per slice. Subsequently, the resulting 3D surface models were smoothed and converted into surfaces of mathematically defined non-uniform rational B-splines (NURBS) using Geomagic Studio (v.2013, 3D Systems, Rock Hill, SC, USA) [59]. In this manner, we enabled the subsequent virtual implantation of THR implants.

Accordingly, an established joint coordinate system of the pelvis was generated according to Kluess et al. [18]. The pelvic coordinate system was created, originating out of the center of rotation of the hip joint, by fitting a sphere into the articulating joint surface of the acetabulum and defining its orientation using anatomical landmarks. The x-axis connected the right and left spinae iliacae anterior superior; the z-axis touched the pubic symphysis and was directed cranially. Consequently, the y-axis was defined perpendicular to the x- and z-axis. The axes were translated into the center of rotation, and the Cartesian coordinate system, which refers to the anterior pelvic plane, was set up. In anatomical terms, this means that the x-axis represents the medio-lateral direction; the y-axis, the anterior–posterior direction; and the z-axis, the inferior–superior direction.

The femoral coordinate system was generated using the anatomical frontal, sagittal, and transversal planes, which were defined by anatomical landmarks [18]. The frontal plane was defined as being tangential to three points: the most posterior points of the medial and lateral femoral condyles, and the most posterior point of the trochanter minor. The sagittal plane was perpendicular to the frontal plane and contained the most lateral points of the condylus lateralis and trochanter major. Additionally, the transversal plane was perpendicular to the frontal and sagittal plane and contained the most distal point of the femoral condyles. Additionally, the condylar notch was marked to allow reconstruction of the mechanical axis after virtual implantation. The defined planes were transformed into the center of rotation of the hip joint, which was defined using a spherical best-fit algorithm at the femoral head and acetabulum.

The virtual implantation of the THR and the ROM analyses were conducted with the CAD software Creo Parametric (v.2.0, Parametric Technology Corporation, Boston, MA, USA) according to the preoperatively planned and postoperatively reconstructed situation, where the components were aligned under the supervision of one experienced orthopedic surgeon using clinical imaging data.

2.3. Preoperatively Planned Situation

To represent the ideal configuration of the THR, implants were positioned according to the surgical technique of the manufacturer and preoperative planning. Prior to the placement of the femoral hip stem, virtual resection of the femoral head was performed using Boolean operations, resembling the principle of step osteotomy and an osteotomy plane angle of 55° relative to the femoral shaft axis (Figure 2). After virtual osteotomy, the hip stem equipped with the prosthetic head was aligned parallel to the shaft axis of the proximal femoral bone. The placement of both the THR components aimed for the best possible restoration of the preoperative center of rotation of the hip joint. Furthermore, the prosthetic shaft was well centered in the medullary femoral canal. Finally, the acetabular cup was aligned with 45° of inclination and 15° anteversion referenced to the anterior pelvic plane.

2.4. Postoperatively Reconstructed Situation

The postoperative situation of the THR was reconstructed by virtual implantation based on postoperative radiographs of the hip joint. Due to metallic artifacts in the postoperative MRI data, the preoperative MRI scans were also used for virtual implantation. In particular, the postoperative acetabular cup position was derived from two-dimensional anterior–posterior radiographs of six patients who received the Bicontact hip system (Table 1). The definitions for radiological inclination and anteversion were adopted from Murray et al. [60]. Therefore, radiologic inclination angle α was derived from the postoperative radiograph, measuring the angle between a line defined by the lowest points of both ischiadic bones and a line defined by the two edges of the acetabular cup. The anteversion angle β was determined according to Liaw et al. [58], where α is the inclination angle, μ is the correction angle, S is the short axis of the ellipse, and L is the long axis of the ellipse, which is derived from the projection circular opening of the acetabular cup in the two-dimensional radiograph.

$$\beta = \tan^{-1}\left(\tan\left(\tan^{-1}\left(\tan\left(\sin^{-1}\left(\frac{S}{L}\right)\right) * \left(\frac{1}{\sin(\alpha)}\right)\right) + \mu\right) * \sin(\alpha)\right) \quad (1)$$

The correction angle μ reduces the error due to the perspective projection. It was determined with the following equations using anatomical landmarks [61]:

$$u = \tan^{-1}\left(\left(\frac{x}{2} + \Delta x\right)/z\right) \quad (2)$$

$$z = \frac{x}{2} / \tan 5.46° \quad (3)$$

where Δx represents the distance between the symphysis pubis and a perpendicular line in the middle of the radiograph, x is the distance between the left and right acetabular center of rotation, and z is the distance of the radiation source from the image plane [61].

Similarly, the virtual implantation of the THR was conducted analogously to the procedure during the configuration, according to the preoperatively planned situation. The acetabular cup was aligned using the inclination and anteversion angles derived previously from the anterior–posterior radiographs, and the femoral stem was implanted using postoperative radiographs for deriving the alignment. The antetorsion of the native femur and the virtually implanted femoral hip stem was determined according to the method of Dunlap et al. [62]. First, the transepicondylar axis on the distal femur of each case was determined using the Amira software (v.5.4.1, Zuse Institute Berlin, Berlin, Germany; Thermo Fisher Scientific, Waltham, MA, USA). The transepicondylar axis, femoral neck axis, and implant neck axis were projected to the horizontal plane perpendicular to the femoral shaft axis for each case. Based on the horizontal plane, the anteversion of the virtually implanted hip stems was determined. The final positions of the implant components after virtual implantation, according to the data described above, were verified for each case by an experienced orthopedic surgeon.

2.5. Analysis of Range of Motion

The ROM analysis was conducted with Creo Parametric (v.2.0, Parametric Technology Corporation, Boston, MA, USA) by deploying a kinematic motion analysis, using a kinematic chain. In this manner, a predefined motion until impingement was applied to the hip joint. The coordinate systems of the femur and acetabulum, respectively, were translated to the center of rotation of the virtually implanted acetabular cup and into the center of rotation of the virtually implanted femoral head. Subsequently, the initial positioning of the pelvic bone and the femur to each other was performed according to the anatomical positional relationships. The collision detection routine of Creo Parametric was considered to detect the occurrence of impingement situations [18]. For this, the contact was defined between the external surfaces of the femur and the pelvis, between the femoral hip stem and the acetabular cup, and between the femoral hip stem and the liner. The motion was stopped when a collision between bone and bone, implant and bone, or implant and implant was detected.

The rigid bodies of bones and implant components were connected by ideal joints to set up a kinematic chain. The acetabulum was assumed to be ground fixed, followed by the acetabular cup and liner, which were also fixed to the pelvic bone. The prosthetic head, together with the hip stem, was fixed to the femoral bone and these were connected to the acetabular cup and liner fixed to the pelvic bone by a spherical joint, with a fixed center of rotation. The kinematic chain represents an open-loop mechanism. A virtual servomotor with a constant angular velocity was used to impose a specific motion in one degree of freedom between the two bodies along a predefined fixed rotational axis of the joint.

Generally, the motion was started at the initial configuration for each load case and continued until impingement [23,63] was detected. In our approach, impingement between femoral configuration—consisting of the femoral bone, stem, and prosthetic head—and pelvic configuration—consisting of the pelvic bone, acetabular cup, and liner—was recognized. The definition of contact in this algorithm is the occurrence of the intersection between pelvic and femoral configuration. The hip joint angle at this specific position was then recorded as the functional ROM of the THR. Within the ROM analysis, three different movements similar to ISO-21535 and typical clinical joint movements [54–57] were considered (Figure 3): maximum flexion from neutral (maxFlex), combined internal rotation at 90° flexion (IR@90Flex), and combined external rotation at 90° flexion (ER@90Flex).

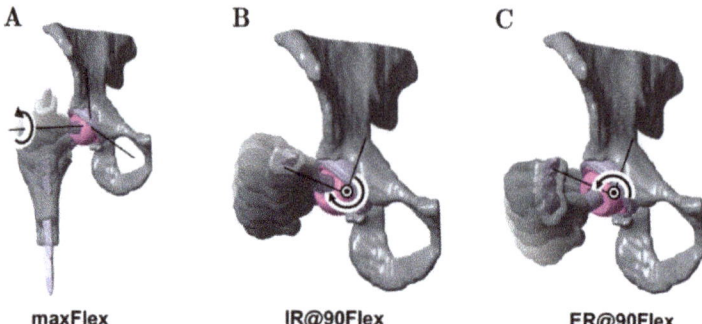

Figure 3. Depiction of the analyzed movements considered in the ROM analyses: maximum flexion starting from neutral (maxFlex) (**A**), internal rotation at 90° flexion (IR@90Flex) (**B**), and external rotation at 90° flexion (ER@90Flex) (**C**).

The neutral position of the hip joint for the maxFlex movement is defined by bringing the sagittal plane and transversal plane of the pelvis into coincidence with the sagittal plane and transversal plane of the femur. The flexion axis is defined by the intersection of the transversal and frontal plane. A flexion rotation was applied until impingement was detected.

For IR@90Flex and ER@90Flex, the mechanical axis of the femur, which is defined by the condylar notch and the center of rotation of the femoral head, was used as a femoral rotational axis. The initial configurations of these motions were generated by applying 90° of flexion, using the neutral position of the maxFlex motion. Subsequently, internal rotation or external rotation started and was performed until impingement was detected.

Finally, the resulting ROM and type of impingement (bone-to-bone, implant-to-implant, and implant-to-bone) were analyzed during the three movements.

2.6. Analyzed Parameters

Within the framework of the study, the results for the preoperatively planned situation were compared with the postoperatively reconstructed situation for the n = 6 patients (13 patients had to be excluded due to different treatment options with other THR designs), who received the Bicontact total hip replacement system as planned. The mean ROM and the achieved ROM, depending on the type of impingement, were evaluated during flexion, internal rotation, and external rotation. Moreover, the quantity for each of the three impingement types was also evaluated.

The influence of the design-specific parameters of the Bicontact implant system for n = 9 patients on the resulting ROM was investigated in terms of the CCD angle, acetabular cup size, prosthetic head size, and head offset. These implant configurations were derived from a preoperative surgery planning tool by an orthopedic surgeon.

2.7. Statistical Metrics

All data given in the diagrams are expressed as mean values ± standard deviation (SD). The deviation in ROM (Δ_{ROM}) between the postoperatively reconstructed and preoperatively planned situation was calculated using the median of differences. Statistical analyses were performed using SPSS V27.0 (SPSS® Inc., Chicago, IL, USA), to determine statistically significant differences in the ROM of the preoperatively planned situation and postoperatively reconstructed situation for each of the three movements. Both situation groups within the movements, maxFlex, IR@90Flex, and ER@90Flex, were examined for statistically significant differences with the Wilcoxon test. The preoperatively planned situation and postoperatively reconstructed situation of the same patient were assumed to be combined samples. A level of $p \leq 0.05$ was considered statistically significant.

3. Results

3.1. Comparison of ROM and Predominant Impingement Type between the Preoperatively Planned and Postoperatively Reconstructed Situation

The maximum ROM until impingement was evaluated for all patients according to the preoperatively planned and postoperatively reconstructed situation. Concerning the postoperatively reconstructed situation, n = 6 patients were compared with the respective preoperatively planned situation (Figure 4).

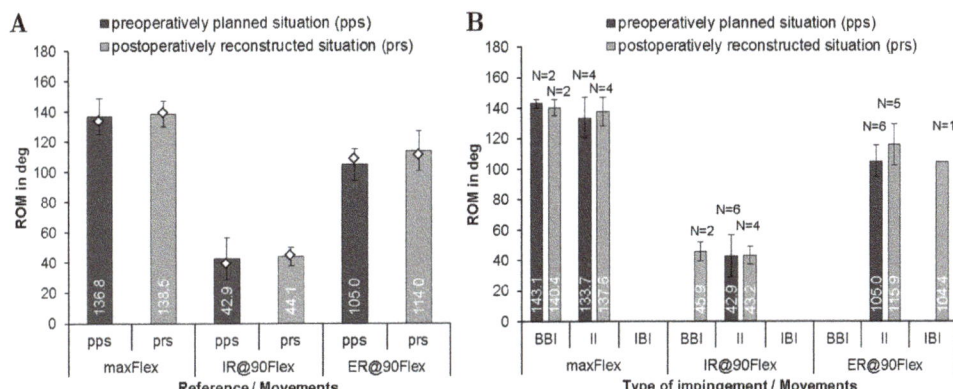

Figure 4. Comparison of the range of motion using implantation according to preoperatively planned situation (pps) and postoperatively reconstructed situation (prs) for each patient during maximum flexion (maxFlex), internal rotation at 90° of flexion (IR@90Flex), and external rotation at 90° flexion (ER@90Flex) for n = 6 patients. (**A**) Mean range of motion with standard deviations until impingement during the three movements for n = 6 patients. Note that the median of range of motion values are depicted as diamonds. (**B**) Quantity N of the impingement type (BBI, bone-to-bone impingement; II, implant-to-implant impingement; IBI, implant-to-bone impingement).

The mean femoral stem antetorsion was 6.9° ± 9.1° for preoperatively planned situation and 4.5° ± 4.6° for the postoperatively reconstructed situation. Regarding the acetabular component, the cup was implanted with 45° inclination and 15° anteversion for the preoperatively planned situation and 39.7° ± 4.7° inclination and 22.9° ± 6.6° anteversion for the postoperatively reconstructed situation. The ROM analysis (Figure 4A) showed no significant difference between both groups for flexion (Δ_{ROM} = 0°, p = 0.854) and internal rotation movement (Δ_{ROM} = 1.8°, p = 0.917). Contrarily, a significant difference was detected during external rotation (Δ_{ROM} = 9°, p = 0.046). Regarding the impingement, the postoperatively reconstructed situation showed a shift to more implant-to-implant impingement for internal rotation. During flexion and external rotation, larger angles up to the implant-to-implant impingement were determined in the analysis of the postoperatively reconstructed situation (Figure 4B). In the case of bone-to-bone impingement, the flexion angles of 143.1 ± 2.7° and 140.4 ± 5.4° were determined in the preoperatively planned and postoperatively reconstructed situation, respectively.

3.2. Investigation of ROM and Predominant Impingement Type for the Preoperatively Planned Situation

The femoral stem antetorsion, which included n = 19 patients, preoperatively ranged from 0.4° to 40°. The comparison of the ROM for the three motions is depicted in Figure 5A. After virtual implantation, 124.3° ± 14.5° of mean flexion was reached. Internal rotation averaged at 37.5° ± 12.9° and external rotation at 102.6° ± 13.6°. Compared to physiological ROMs [18,64], similar values were observed for flexion and internal rotation. Contrarily, the ROM for external rotation of the patients treated with THR exceeded the physiological ROM [54]. Within the ROM analysis, the different types of impingement at maximum ROM was detected depending on the movement (Figure 5B). Regarding the type of impingement, a maximum flexion of 128.7 ± 13.0° up to the implant impingement was detected. In the case of bone-to-bone impingement, the ROM slightly decreased to 122.3° ± 14.7°. The predominant type of impingement at the flexion movement (Figure 5B) was bone-to-bone impingement with N = 13, followed by implant-to-implant impingement with N = 6, while for internal rotation, implant-to-implant impingement with N = 10 was followed by bone-to-bone impingement with N = 8. Implant-to-implant impingement was the most dominant type of impingement during external rotation, which occurred in 17 out of 19 patients. It is apparent (Figure 5B) that bone impingement restricted the ROM more than implant impingement during all movements. It is also noteworthy that implant-to-bone impingement occurred only once in all 19 patients.

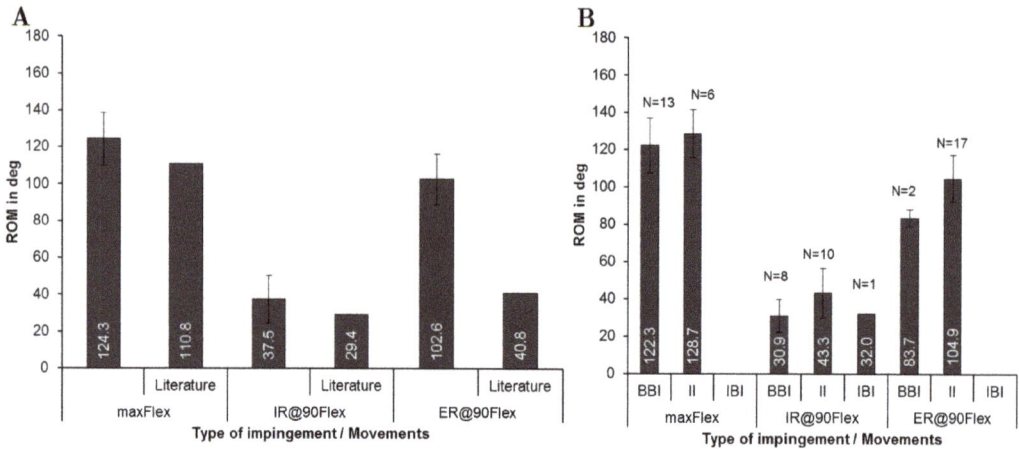

Figure 5. Comparison of the range of motion using implantation according to preoperatively planned situation for each patient (n = 19) during maximum flexion (maxFlex), internal rotation at 90° of flexion (IR@90Flex), and external rotation at 90° flexion (ER@90Flex). (**A**) Mean range of motion with standard deviations until impingement during the three movements. Physiological ROM are represented from literature studies for maxFlex and IR@90Flex [18,64], and ER@90Flex [54]. (**B**) Quantity N of impingement type (BBI, bone-to-bone-impingement; II, implant-to-implant-impingement; IBI, implant-to-bone-impingement).

3.3. Influence of Implant Related Factors on ROM for the Preoperatively Planned Situation

Figure 6 gives an overview of the ROM concerning the implant-specific design parameters–stem size, CCD-angle, acetabular cup size, prosthetic head size, and femoral neck length for the preoperatively planned situation (n = 19 patients). The results in relation to CCD-angle (Figure 6A) showed that there was a minor decrease in ROM using a higher CCD-angle during flexion (125.3 ± 16.1° for 128° CCD-angle and 120.6 ± 2.5° for 135° CCD-angle). Contrarily, the ROM was slightly higher when CCD-angle was increased (101.3° ± 14.7° for 128° CCD-angle and 107.6 ± 6.0° for 135° CCD-angle) during external rotation.

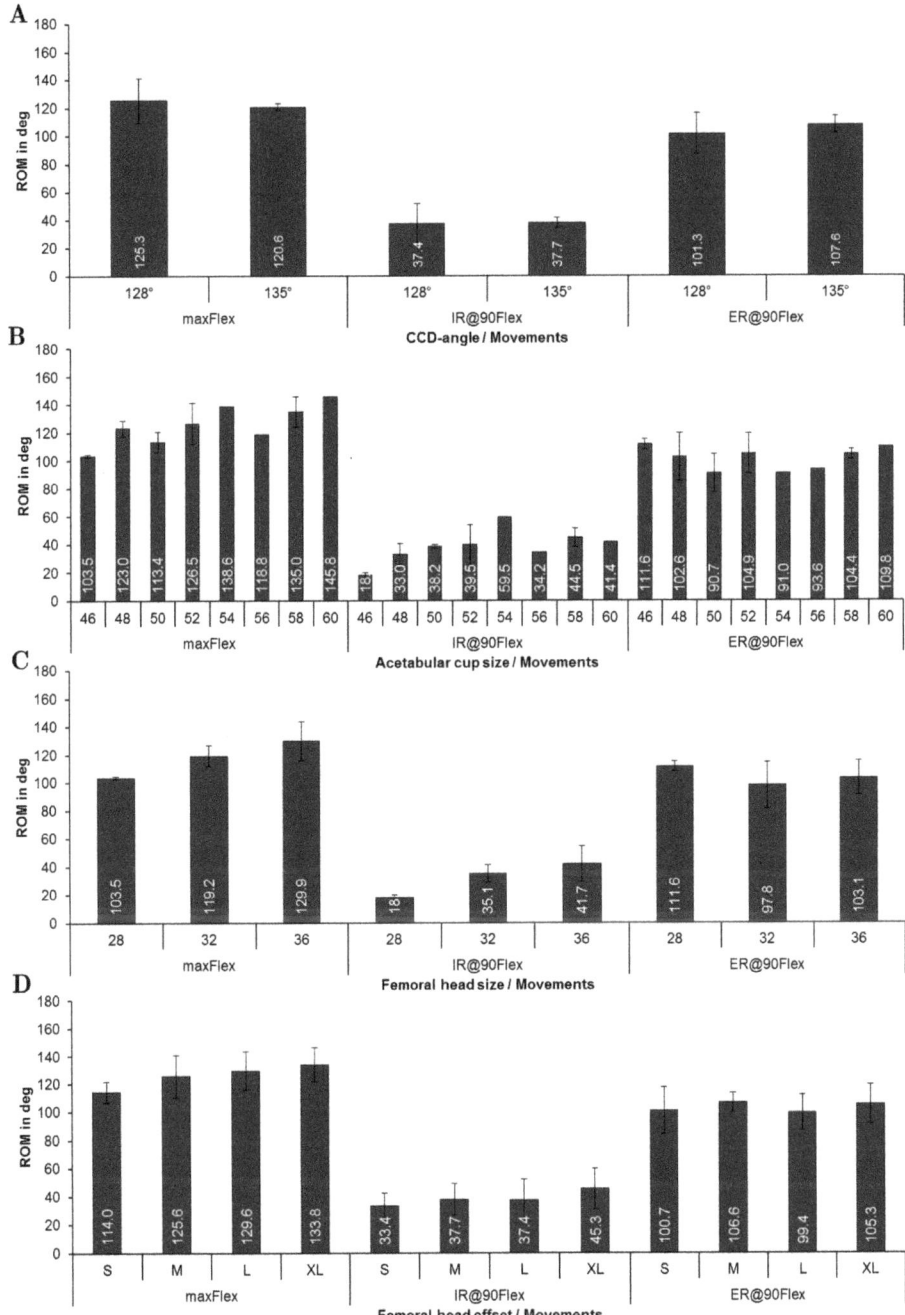

Figure 6. Results of the ROM analysis depending on implant-specific design parameters during maximum flexion (maxFlex), internal rotation at 90° flexion (IR@90Flex), and external rotation at 90° flexion (ER@90Flex): (**A**) CCD-angle; (**B**) acetabular cup size; (**C**) prosthetic head size; (**D**) prosthetic head offset.

It was observed that as the acetabular cup size was increased, progressively more ROM during flexion was achieved (Figure 6B). For instance, impingement occurred at 103.5° ± 0.9° during flexion in case of a 46 mm cup, while impingement occurred at 145.8° of flexion in case of a 60 mm cup. A larger cup was also related to a higher maximum internal rotation at 90° of flexion (increased by up to 130%), whereas no clear trend was observed during external rotation. Figure 6C depicts the ROM depending on the head size, where each patient received a femoral stem equipped with a taper 12/14, which establishes the connection between stem and head. Every stem had, therefore, the same neck diameter, which links the prosthetic head size directly to the head-to-neck ratio. For this patient group, the head-to-neck ratio ranged from 2.07 for a 28 mm head to 2.67 for a 36 mm head (reported in Table 1 for all patients). The ROM until impingement increased with increasing head size. Accordingly, the head size of 28 mm resulted in 103.5° ± 0.9° and a head size of 36 mm resulted in 129.9° ± 13.9° during flexion. During internal rotation, the ROM rose from 18° ± 1.8° (28 mm head size) to 41.7° ± 12.7° (36 mm head size). A higher head offset (Figure 6D), which was defined by the design of the prosthetic head, was paired with a higher ROM during flexion (114° ± 7.5° on average for type S vs. 133.8° ± 12.2° for type XL) with a mean improvement of 19.8°. Likewise, this finding could be observed during internal rotation (33.4° ± 8.7° on an average for type S and 45.3° ± 14.6° on an average for type XL) with a mean improvement of 11.9°. Similar to the behavior observed for the prosthetic head size, no influence of the femoral neck length was detected during external rotation.

4. Discussion

After THR, the ROM is an important factor for patient satisfaction, as it is a major parameter that can restrict activities of daily living, especially in cultures where a higher ROM is demanded [9,10]. Additionally, impingement limits the ROM and is a common cause of postoperative instability [47,65]. ROM analyses have raised much attention from the research community using experimental [24–29] and numerical methods [21,30,43,44,46–50]. However, to the best of our knowledge, there is no approach published to assess ROM after THR in surgery planning without applying additional radiation to the patient; for example, by CT scanning. To fill this gap and to provide a tool for computational assessment of ROM, we developed a framework for ROM analysis, based on preoperative MRI data and anterior–posterior radiographs, the latter being usually performed before THR for preoperative planning. Similar to the approach of Gilles et al. [66], we used preoperative MRI data to derive the CAD model of the bony structures. In contrast to their study, we manually segmented the MRI data to get our patient-specific volume models. This time-consuming approach needs to be replaced by more efficient and automatic methods like statistical shape modeling [67,68]. The main advantage of our method is that bone geometries from real patients scheduled for THR and the real implant geometry were used for the analyses.

Another advantage is that no patient undergoing computational assessment of ROM with the proposed methodology will be subjected to additional radiation. Hence, our MRI-based framework is capable of estimating postoperative ROM in a realistic manner and, thus, may support clinical decision-making in the future.

The positioning of the implant components between the preoperatively planned and postoperatively reconstructed situation showed an acceptable agreement in terms of the acetabular cup inclination and anteversion. However, it should be noted that the MRI scans and radiographs were acquired in the supine position of the patient. In this context, it is important to emphasize that there is a change in pelvic tilt between the supine and standing positions [69]. Further, in the literature, average changes of the pelvic tilt from preoperative supine to the standing position between 2° and 7° in posterior direction were reported [70], while with each degree of pelvic tilt, the radiographic cup anteversion changes nearly by 0.7° [69]. However, neither the pelvic tilt during MRI nor the supine position on the operating table accurately reflects the functional pelvic tilt for all patients, resulting in a difference in functional cup orientation between the supine and standing positions. Comparing the preoperatively planned ROM with the postoperatively reconstructed one, no significant differences were observed for flexion and internal rotation, while a significant difference was detected for external rotation. The detection of the type of impingement agreed well between preoperatively planned and postoperatively reconstructed situations, except in one case for external rotation and two cases for internal rotation. The ROM reached physiological levels during flexion and internal rotation, which is in agreement with previous studies [18,44,46,47,54]. This supports the reliability of our results, which are based on the previously described CAD methods [18,30,38,53]. Regarding the observed impingement type, our results showed that the ROM in flexion was more likely restricted by bone-to-bone impingement, whereas internal and external rotations were more likely restricted by implant-to-implant impingement. Therefore, restriction of flexion is not only caused by implant-to-implant geometry but mostly by the alignment of the implant components in femoral and pelvic bone [33]. The ROM for bone-to-bone impingement, which is known as a major cause of limited ROM of the hip joint, was lower compared to implant-to-implant impingement, which is in line with the literature [23,32,71]. However, it should be carefully noted that the virtual ROMs during external rotation exceeded the clinical expectations [35,55,57], most likely due to the neglected active and passive parts of the soft-tissue structures, which are known to limit the ROM. This is also supported by the study of Tannast et al. [64], where they have investigated the impingement on cadaver specimens and reported that computational assessment of ROM tended to overestimate the values due to the absence of soft-tissue structures. Moreover, our results are in excellent agreement with a recent study conducted by Han et al. [54], where they reported that neglecting soft-tissue structures in computer simulations led to significant overestimation of hip ROM up to 68.1° for external rotation at 90° flexion (more than 60° in our results). Therefore, the ROM for such movement is not only controlled by bone-to-bone or implant-to-implant impingement but also limited by the surrounding soft-tissue structures of the hip joint, i.e., muscles, capsule, labrum, and ligaments [54,64]. Hence, the results for external rotation at 90° flexion should not be taken for direct comparison with data from clinical examinations of patients.

Regarding the influence of THR design parameters, we observed a minor influence of the CCD angle on ROM for all movements, which is in accordance to the study by Widmer et al. [51]. It is also known that a change in CCD angles requires adaption of cup anteversion, to overcome the reduction of ROM caused by increased CCD angle [41], which we also observed during flexion movement. However, inaccuracy of the manually performed alignment of the femoral hip stem is a factor that influences the ROM as a function of the CCD angle. Considering the acetabular cup, increasing the cup size led to higher ROM in the flexion and internal rotation movements. Since prosthetic impingement was mostly between the neck and the liner, the cross-interference of other parameters can influence the ROM. The underlying factor in the increased ROM may be the prosthetic head diameter because the patients with a larger cup also received a larger head (Table 1). Therefore, the increase of ROM is most likely caused by the resulting higher head-to-neck ratio. Additionally, there is no systematic methodology available to assess stem antetorsion from radiographs, which also complicates the efforts to reconstruct postoperative alignment. A second limitation is the fact that the bone geometries of 19 patients were used for this investigation, which leads to the additional cross-interference of varying bone geometry. With respect to parameter studies, our MRI-based framework could be used for analyzing the interplay between implant positioning and design parameters, such as head-to-neck ratio, CCD angle, head size, and stem antetorsion as well as cup anteversion and inclination as previously shown in the comprehensive computational study conducted by Widmer et al. [41]. Moreover, our framework may contribute to an improved preoperative planning in the future by virtually testing off-the-shelf endoprosthetic designs, thus assisting an orthopedic surgeon to select a proper implant design in terms of personalized component positioning based on the patient's requirements, i.e., to maximize the impingement-free

ROM. Another limitation was that the hip joint was assumed to have a fixed center of rotation during motion. In fact, the prosthetic head and liner are not perfectly congruent due to the clearance between head and acetabular cup, allowing translational degrees of freedom [27]. Additionally, we observed that an increased head size allowed more ROM during flexion and internal rotation, which was shown to extend the range for orienting the acetabular cup [41]; this is in agreement with previous studies [21,25,30,41,43]. The increase in ROM owing to the higher head size can be explained with the higher head-to-neck ratio, which causes delayed contact between the femoral neck and the acetabular cup [72]. We observed a similar tendency for internal rotation as Kluess et al. [21], where increasing head diameter led to more ROM. It is also noteworthy that increasing the head size would decrease the contact stresses at the liner during subluxation as well as lower component damage and the risk of dislocation [21,25,41], which is supported by clinical experience [73,74]. It has to be taken into account that increasing the head size not always increased ROM. The reached ROM is also dependent on the femoral neck configuration, which can lead to the unexpected event of reduced ROM despite larger head sizes for very short neck length, caused by loss of femoral offset [49]. On the other hand, we observed higher ROM for an increased head offset, which was also observed by other research groups [25,41,49]. Our findings confirm this well-known correlation as well as the clinical experience that increasing the offset reduces the risk for dislocation in THR [18,41,52,53,75]. Furthermore, this is also in good agreement with the study by Matsushita et al. [52], who reported an improved flexion of more than 20° and an improved internal rotation of more than 13°, which corresponds well with our data (19.8° for flexion and 11.9° for internal rotation). A shorter neck, caused by a reduced head offset, is known to result in earlier contact between the proximal stem built-up and the liner component. Therefore, increasing the head offset is an option for the surgeon to mitigate issues with insufficient ROM intraoperatively, but this also causes an increased leg length and change in soft-tissue condition [25,49]. Additionally, the femoral offset can also change the strain/stress pattern in the surrounding bone.

Despite the progress in methodology for computational ROM analysis, our approach has some limitations. Firstly, the geometry generation is time-consuming and unacceptable in the clinical setting in its current state; however, this can be mitigated by using more advanced techniques in medical imaging data or with statistical shape models, which turned out as feasible for femoral and acetabular bones [67,68,76,77]. Additionally, due to the rather limited resolution of MRI, segmentation, and deviations because of surface triangulation, a difference between the bony geometry and the derived model is unavoidable, which can influence the ROM, especially when bone-to-bone impingement or implant-to-bone impingement occurs. However, current methods for shape modeling [67,68,76] can be used in future studies to also mitigate discretization, but this may be associated with a less accurate representation of the patient's bone geometry, leading to less reliable results in terms of bone-to-bone or bone-to-implant impingement. This and the more favorable time effectivity gained by more sophisticated approaches in obtaining patient individual bone geometry will make the proposed framework more attractive as a preoperative analysis tool. Secondly, due to the lack of soft-tissue structures in the presented numerical model, the real ROM is likely to be smaller [11,36,47]. However, this is a typical assumption for studies investigating the ROM [18,21,32,33,64,78]. Due to the fact that physiological ROM was achieved during flexion and internal rotation movements, we can assume that this limitation only affects the results for external rotation, where the detected ROM exceeded the physiological ROM. For the reconstruction of the postoperative cases, the postoperative anterior–posterior radiograph was used to derive the alignment of the femoral stem and the acetabular cup, which is less accurate than a 3D assessment of the postoperative alignment using x-ray stereophotogrammetric analysis or postoperative CT imaging [61]. However, this would expose patients to additional radiation. Regarding the measurement error of our method, there is a difference between the radiologic and anatomic inclination and anteversion of the acetabular cup. The difference between anatomic and radiologic anteversion can be neglected in our study because the measured radiologic anteversion was lower than 25° for most of the patients, which would lead to a deviation between anatomic and radiologic anteversion of less than 10% [58,79,80]. A further limitation is that due to the necessities of the treatment of real patients, no real parameter study was conducted, where systematically only one parameter was changed at one time. In our study, more than one design parameter was changed for each patient, committing the limitation of cross-interference between distinct parameters. To overcome these limitations, further studies where only one parameter will be changed need to be conducted.

Due to the fact that the analyses were only conducted for one distinct implant design, our results may not be fully applicable for other implant designs developed by other manufacturers. Further studies, therefore, investigating other implant designs should follow. Furthermore, total hip impingement represents a multifactorial process within the musculoskeletal system. Our new framework provides a convenient alternative to estimate the patient-specific ROM in a preoperative manner, where neither forces and torques nor complex constraints are of interest and the result is the geometric interference [33,38]. Therefore, it may be beneficial to consider the active muscle forces and real contact behavior of the implant components, which was previously performed on the example of the hip and knee joint, using a robot-assisted test method based on a musculoskeletal multibody model that can also provide data with respect to resulting joint forces [27,81].

5. Conclusions

Our present study aimed to propose and introduce a computational framework for preoperative and postoperative assessment of ROM, without subjecting patients to additional doses of radiation for acquisition of bony geometry. To fulfill this goal, we used an approach starting with the preoperative acquisition of MRI data in addition to pre- and postoperative radiographs performed as a standard measure in THR. We used the MRI data to derive a CAD model of the bone structure and the anatomical landmarks necessary for virtual implantation of the implant system, which is aligned resembling the preoperatively planned and the postoperatively reconstructed situation. We used the CAD modeling method, with the virtually implanted model, to conduct ROM analyses of three movements, whose results were in line with the literature. Major patterns when changing design features of THR reported by the literature were also observed in the current study using our proposed methodology. Therefore, the proof of principle was achieved, showing the feasibility of the proposed framework for future studies relying on patients' individual morphology and implantation technique of different THR designs.

Author Contributions: Conceptualization, D.K., M.S., A.H., K.-P.G. and R.B.; methodology, M.K., C.S., C.M.; software, M.K., C.S., C.M.; validation, M.K., C.S. and C.M.; formal analysis, C.S. and C.M.; investigation, M.K., C.S. and C.M.; resources, A.H., K.-P.G. and R.B.; data curation, M.K., C.S. and C.M.; writing—original draft preparation, M.K. and C.S.; writing—review and editing, M.K., C.S., C.M., D.K., M.S., A.H., K.-P.G. and R.B.; visualization, M.K., C.S. and C.M.; supervision, D.K., M.S., A.H., K.-P.G. and R.B.; project administration, D.K., M.S., A.H., K.-P.G. and R.B.; funding acquisition, D.K., A.H., K.-P.G. and R.B. All authors have read and agreed to the published version of the manuscript.

Funding: This research project was funded by Aesculap AG Research and Development, Tuttlingen, Germany.

Institutional Review Board Statement: The study was conducted according to the guidelines of the Declaration of Helsinki, and approved by the Institutional Ethics Committee of Technische Universität Dresden, Germany (EK 175052011).

Informed Consent Statement: An informed consent was obtained from all subjects involved in the study. A written informed consent has been obtained from the patient(s) to publish this paper.

Data Availability Statement: Data are contained within the article.

Acknowledgments: We would like to thank Enrico Mick and Andreas Wolf for preparing the raw data. We thank Martin Weser for segmenting the image data and deriving the surface models. We also would like to thank the Department of Radiology, Universitätsklinikum Dresden, Germany for providing the medical image data.

Conflicts of Interest: Mevluet Sungu is an employee of Aesculap AG Tuttlingen, a manufacturer of orthopedic implants. All other authors have no competing interests to disclose.

References

1. Brown, T.D.; Elkins, J.M.; Pedersen, D.R.; Callaghan, J.J. Impingement and Dislocation in Total HIP Arthroplasty: Mechanisms and Consequences. *Iowa Orthop. J.* **2014**, *34*, 1–15.
2. Klauber, J.; Geraedts, M.; Friedrich, J.; Wasem, J. *Krankenhaus-Report 2019*; Springer: Berlin/Heidelberg, Germany, 2019; ISBN 978-3-662-58224-4.
3. Organisation for Economic Co-operation and Development. *Health at a Glance 2017: OECD Indicators*; OECD Publishing: Paris, France, 2017; ISBN 9264280405.
4. Maradit Kremers, H.; Larson, D.R.; Crowson, C.S.; Kremers, W.K.; Washington, R.E.; Steiner, C.A.; Jiranek, W.A.; Berry, D.J. Prevalence of Total Hip and Knee Replacement in the United States. *J. Bone Jt. Surg. Am.* **2015**, *97*, 1386–1397. [CrossRef]
5. Kurtz, S.M.; Ong, K.L.; Lau, E.; Bozic, K.J. Impact of the economic downturn on total joint replacement demand in the United States: Updated projections to 2021. *J. Bone Jt. Surg. Am.* **2014**, *96*, 624–630. [CrossRef] [PubMed]
6. Wolford, M.L.; Palso, K.; Bercovitz, A. *Hospitalization for Total Hip Replacement Among Inpatients Aged 45 and Over: United States, 2000–2010*; Data Brief; Centers for Disease Control & Prevention: Atlanta, GA, USA, 2015; pp. 1–8.
7. Pilz, V.; Hanstein, T.; Skripitz, R. Projections of primary hip arthroplasty in Germany until 2040. *Acta Orthop.* **2018**, *89*, 308–313. [CrossRef]
8. Gwam, C.U.; Mistry, J.B.; Mohamed, N.S.; Thomas, M.; Bigart, K.C.; Mont, M.A.; Delanois, R.E. Current Epidemiology of Revision Total Hip Arthroplasty in the United States: National Inpatient Sample 2009 to 2013. *J. Arthroplast.* **2017**, *32*, 2088–2092. [CrossRef] [PubMed]
9. Jamari, J.; Anwar, I.B.; Saputra, E.; van der Heide, E. Range of Motion Simulation of Hip Joint Movement during Salat Activity. *J. Arthroplast.* **2017**, *32*, 2898–2904. [CrossRef]
10. Sugano, N.; Tsuda, K.; Miki, H.; Takao, M.; Suzuki, N.; Nakamura, N. Dynamic measurements of hip movement in deep bending activities after total hip arthroplasty using a 4-dimensional motion analysis system. *J. Arthroplast.* **2012**, *27*, 1562–1568. [CrossRef]
11. Nakamura, N.; Maeda, Y.; Hamawaki, M.; Sakai, T.; Sugano, N. Effect of soft-tissue impingement on range of motion during posterior approach Total Hip Arthroplasty: An in vivo measurement study. *Comput. Assist. Surg.* **2016**, *21*, 132–136. [CrossRef]
12. Amstutz, H.C.; Lodwig, R.M.; Schurman, D.J.; Hodgson, A.G. Range of motion studies for total hip replacements. A comparative study with a new experimental apparatus. *Clin. Orthop. Relat. Res.* **1975**, 124–130. [CrossRef] [PubMed]
13. Scifert, C.F.; Brown, T.D.; Pedersen, D.R.; Callaghan, J.J. A finite element analysis of factors influencing total hip dislocation. *Clin. Orthop. Relat. Res.* **1998**, 152–162. [CrossRef] [PubMed]
14. Miki, H.; Kyo, T.; Kuroda, Y.; Nakahara, I.; Sugano, N. Risk of edge-loading and prosthesis impingement due to posterior pelvic tilting after total hip arthroplasty. *Clin. Biomech.* **2014**, *29*, 607–613. [CrossRef]
15. Zhang, J.; Wei, J.; Mao, Y.; Li, H.; Xie, Y.; Zhu, Z. Range of Hip Joint Motion in Developmental Dysplasia of the Hip Patients Following Total Hip Arthroplasty With the Surgical Technique Using the Concept of Combined Anteversion: A Study of Crowe I and II Patients. *J. Arthroplast.* **2015**, *30*, 2248–2255. [CrossRef]
16. Malik, A.; Maheshwari, A.; Dorr, L.D. Impingement with total hip replacement. *J. Bone Jt. Surg. Am.* **2007**, *89*, 1832–1842. [CrossRef] [PubMed]
17. Karachalios, T.; Komnos, G.; Koutalos, A. Total hip arthroplasty: Survival and modes of failure. *EFORT Open Rev.* **2018**, *3*, 232–239. [CrossRef]
18. Kluess, D.; Zietz, C.; Lindner, T.; Mittelmeier, W.; Schmitz, K.-P.; Bader, R. Limited range of motion of hip resurfacing arthroplasty due to unfavorable ratio of prosthetic head size and femoral neck diameter. *Acta Orthop.* **2008**, *79*, 748–754. [CrossRef] [PubMed]
19. Scheerlinck, T. Cup positioning in total hip arthroplasty. *Acta Orthop. Belg.* **2014**, *80*, 336–347. [PubMed]
20. Nadzadi, M.E.; Pedersen, D.R.; Yack, H.J.; Callaghan, J.J.; Brown, T.D. Kinematics, kinetics, and finite element analysis of commonplace maneuvers at risk for total hip dislocation. *J. Biomech.* **2003**, *36*, 577–591. [CrossRef]
21. Kluess, D.; Martin, H.; Mittelmeier, W.; Schmitz, K.-P.; Bader, R. Influence of femoral head size on impingement, dislocation and stress distribution in total hip replacement. *Med. Eng. Phys.* **2007**, *29*, 465–471. [CrossRef]
22. Shon, W.Y.; Baldini, T.; Peterson, M.G.; Wright, T.M.; Salvati, E.A. Impingement in total hip arthroplasty a study of retrieved acetabular components. *J. Arthroplast.* **2005**, *20*, 427–435. [CrossRef]
23. Palit, A.; King, R.; Hart, Z.; Gu, Y.; Pierrepont, J.; Elliott, M.T.; Williams, M.A. Bone-to-Bone and Implant-to-Bone Impingement: A Novel Graphical Representation for Hip Replacement Planning. *Ann. Biomed. Eng.* **2020**. [CrossRef] [PubMed]
24. Bader, R.; Scholz, R.; Steinhauser, E.; Busch, R.; Mittelmeier, W. Methode zur Evaluierung von Einflussfaktoren auf die Luxationsstabilität von künstlichen Hüftgelenken. *Biomed. Tech.* **2004**, *49*, 137–144. [CrossRef]
25. Burroughs, B.R.; Hallstrom, B.; Golladay, G.J.; Hoeffel, D.; Harris, W.H. Range of motion and stability in total hip arthroplasty with 28-, 32-, 38-, and 44-mm femoral head sizes. *J. Arthroplast.* **2005**, *20*, 11–19. [CrossRef]

26. Qurashi, S.; Parr, W.; Jang, B.; Walsh, W.R. Elevated lip liner positions improving stability in total hip arthroplasty. An experimental study. *JISRF* **2017**, *7*. [CrossRef]
27. Geier, A.; Kluess, D.; Grawe, R.; Herrmann, S.; D'Lima, D.; Woernle, C.; Bader, R. Dynamical analysis of dislocation-associated factors in total hip replacements by hardware-in-the-loop simulation. *J. Orthop. Res.* **2017**, *35*, 2557–2566. [CrossRef] [PubMed]
28. Herrmann, S.; Kluess, D.; Kaehler, M.; Grawe, R.; Rachholz, R.; Souffrant, R.; Zierath, J.; Bader, R.; Woernle, C. A Novel Approach for Dynamic Testing of Total Hip Dislocation under Physiological Conditions. *PLoS ONE* **2015**, *10*, e0145798. [CrossRef] [PubMed]
29. Bader, R.; Scholz, R.; Steinhauser, E.; Zimmermann, S.; Busch, R.; Mittelmeier, W. The influence of head and neck geometry on stability of total hip replacement: A mechanical test study. *Acta Orthop. Scand.* **2004**, *75*, 415–421. [CrossRef]
30. Bader, R.; Steinhauser, E.; Gradinger, R.; Willmann, G.; Mittelmeier, W. Computergestützte Bewegungssimulation an Hüftendoprothesen mit Keramik-Keramik-Gleitpaarung. Analyse der Einflussparameter Implantat-Design und Position. *Z. Orthop. Grenzgeb.* **2002**, *140*, 310–316. [CrossRef]
31. Pedersen, D.R.; Callaghan, J.J.; Brown, T.D. Activity-dependence of the "safe zone" for impingement versus dislocation avoidance. *Med. Eng. Phys.* **2005**, *27*, 323–328. [CrossRef]
32. Putame, G.; Pascoletti, G.; Franceschini, G.; Dichio, G.; Terzini, M. Prosthetic Hip ROM from Multibody Software Simulation. In Proceedings of the 2019 41st Annual International Conference of the IEEE Engineering in Medicine and Biology Society (EMBC), Berlin, Germany, 23–27 July 2019; pp. 5386–5389. [CrossRef]
33. Zanetti, E.M.; Bignardi, C.; Terzini, M.; Putame, G.; Audenino, A.L. A multibody model for the optimization of hip arthroplasty in relation to range of movement. *AMJ* **2018**, *11*. [CrossRef]
34. Chang, T.-C.; Kang, H.; Arata, L.; Zhao, W. A pre-operative approach of range of motion simulation and verification for femoroacetabular impingement. *Int. J. Med. Robot.* **2011**, *7*, 318–326. [CrossRef] [PubMed]
35. Miki, H.; Kyo, T.; Sugano, N. Anatomical hip range of motion after implantation during total hip arthroplasty with a large change in pelvic inclination. *J. Arthroplast.* **2012**, *27*, 1641–1650.e1. [CrossRef]
36. Klingenstein, G.G.; Yeager, A.M.; Lipman, J.D.; Westrich, G.H. Computerized range of motion analysis following dual mobility total hip arthroplasty, traditional total hip arthroplasty, and hip resurfacing. *J. Arthroplast.* **2013**, *28*, 1173–1176. [CrossRef]
37. Weber, M.; Woerner, M.; Craiovan, B.; Voellner, F.; Worlicek, M.; Springorum, H.-R.; Grifka, J.; Renkawitz, T. Current standard rules of combined anteversion prevent prosthetic impingement but ignore osseous contact in total hip arthroplasty. *Int. Orthop.* **2016**, *40*, 2495–2504. [CrossRef]
38. Widmer, K.-H. Impingementfreie Bewegung nach Hüft-TEP—Wie realisieren? *Z. Orthop. Unfallchir.* **2016**, *154*, 392–397. [CrossRef] [PubMed]
39. Kummer, F.J.; Shah, S.; Iyer, S.; DiCesare, P.E. The effect of acetabular cup orientations on limiting hip rotation. *J. Arthroplast.* **1999**, *14*, 509–513. [CrossRef]
40. Bader, R.; Willmann, G. Keramische Pfannen für Hüftendoprothesen. Teil 6: Pfannendesign, Inklinations- und Antetorsionswinkel beeinflussen Bewegungsumfang und Impingement. *Biomed. Tech.* **1999**, *44*, 212–219. [CrossRef]
41. Widmer, K.-H. The Impingement-free, Prosthesis-specific, and Anatomy-adjusted Combined Target Zone for Component Positioning in THA Depends on Design and Implantation Parameters of both Components. *Clin. Orthop. Relat. Res.* **2020**, *478*, 1904–1918. [CrossRef]
42. Fischer, M.C.M.; Tokunaga, K.; Okamoto, M.; Habor, J.; Radermacher, K. Preoperative factors improving the prediction of the postoperative sagittal orientation of the pelvis in standing position after total hip arthroplasty. *Sci. Rep.* **2020**, *10*, 15944. [CrossRef] [PubMed]
43. Ezquerra, L.; Quilez, M.P.; Pérez, M.Á.; Albareda, J.; Seral, B. Range of Movement for Impingement and Dislocation Avoidance in Total Hip Replacement Predicted by Finite Element Model. *J. Med. Biol. Eng.* **2017**, *37*, 26–34. [CrossRef] [PubMed]
44. Kliewe, C.; Souffrant, R.; Kluess, D.; Woernle, C.; Brökel, K.; Bader, R. Analytisches Berechnungsmodell zur Bestimmung des Einflusses konstruktiver und operativer Faktoren auf den Bewegungsumfang von Hüftendoprothesen. *Biomed. Tech.* **2010**, *55*, 47–55. [CrossRef] [PubMed]
45. Yoshimine, F. The safe-zones for combined cup and neck anteversions that fulfill the essential range of motion and their optimum combination in total hip replacements. *J. Biomech.* **2006**, *39*, 1315–1323. [CrossRef]
46. Rodriguez-Elizalde, S.; Yeager, A.M.; Ravi, B.; Lipman, J.D.; Salvati, E.A.; Westrich, G.H. Computerized virtual surgery demonstrates where acetabular rim osteophytes most reduce range of motion following total hip arthroplasty. *HSS J.* **2013**, *9*, 223–228. [CrossRef]
47. Shoji, T.; Yasunaga, Y.; Yamasaki, T.; Izumi, S.; Hachisuka, S.; Ochi, M. Low femoral antetorsion as a risk factor for bony impingement after bipolar hemiarthroplasty. *J. Orthop. Surg. Res.* **2015**, *10*, 105. [CrossRef]
48. Brown, T.D.; Callaghan, J.J. Impingement in Total Hip Replacement: Mechanisms and Consequences. *Curr. Orthop.* **2008**, *22*, 376–391. [CrossRef] [PubMed]
49. Hariri, S.; Chun, S.; Cowan, J.B.; Bragdon, C.; Malchau, H.; Rubash, H.E. Range of motion in a modular femoral stem system with a variety of neck options. *J. Arthroplast.* **2013**, *28*, 1625–1633. [CrossRef]
50. Herrlin, K.; Selvik, G.; Pettersson, H.; Lidgren, L. Range of motion caused by design of the total hip prosthesis. *Acta Radiologica* **1988**, *29*, 701–704. [CrossRef] [PubMed]
51. Widmer, K.-H.; Majewski, M. The impact of the CCD-angle on range of motion and cup positioning in total hip arthroplasty. *Clin. Biomech.* **2005**, *20*, 723–728. [CrossRef]

52. Matsushita, A.; Nakashima, Y.; Jingushi, S.; Yamamoto, T.; Kuraoka, A.; Iwamoto, Y. Effects of the femoral offset and the head size on the safe range of motion in total hip arthroplasty. *J. Arthroplast.* **2009**, *24*, 646–651. [CrossRef] [PubMed]
53. Bader, R.; Klüss, D.; Gerdesmeyer, L.; Steinhauser, E. Biomechanische Aspekte zur Implantatverankerung und Kinematik von Oberflächenersatzhüftendoprothesen. *Der Orthopäde* **2008**, *37*, 634–643. [CrossRef]
54. Han, S.; Owens, V.L.; Patel, R.V.; Ismaily, S.K.; Harrington, M.A.; Incavo, S.J.; Noble, P.C. The continuum of hip range of motion: From soft-tissue restriction to bony impingement. *J. Orthop. Res.* **2020**, *38*, 1779–1786. [CrossRef]
55. Kouyoumdjian, P.; Coulomb, R.; Sanchez, T.; Asencio, G. Clinical evaluation of hip joint rotation range of motion in adults. *Orthop. Traumatol. Surg. Res.* **2012**, *98*, 17–23. [CrossRef]
56. Wilson, J.J.; Furukawa, M. Evaluation of the patient with hip pain. *Am. Fam. Physician* **2014**, *89*, 27–34.
57. Kataoka, T.; Oshima, Y.; Iizawa, N.; Majima, T.; Takai, S. Influence of Total Knee Arthroplasty on Hip Rotational Range of Motion. *J. Nippon Med. Sch.* **2020**, *87*, 191–196. [CrossRef] [PubMed]
58. Liaw, C.-K.; Yang, R.-S.; Hou, S.-M.; Wu, T.-Y.; Fuh, C.-S. Measurement of the acetabular cup anteversion on simulated radiographs. *J. Arthroplast.* **2009**, *24*, 468–474. [CrossRef] [PubMed]
59. Kluess, D.; Souffrant, R.; Mittelmeier, W.; Wree, A.; Schmitz, K.-P.; Bader, R. A convenient approach for finite-element-analyses of orthopaedic implants in bone contact: Modeling and experimental validation. *Comput. Methods Programs Biomed.* **2009**, *95*, 23–30. [CrossRef] [PubMed]
60. Murray, D.W. The definition and measurement of acetabular orientation. *J. Bone Jt. Surg. Br. Vol.* **1993**, *75*, 228–232. [CrossRef] [PubMed]
61. Widmer, K.-H. A simplified method to determine acetabular cup anteversion from plain radiographs. *J. Arthroplast.* **2004**, *19*, 387–390. [CrossRef] [PubMed]
62. Dunlap, K.; Shands, A.R.; Hollister, L.C.; Gaul, J.S.; Streit, H.A. A new method for determination of torsion of the femur. *J. Bone Jt. Surg. Am.* **1953**, *35*, 289–311. [CrossRef]
63. Bartz, R.L.; Nobel, P.C.; Kadakia, N.R.; Tullos, H.S. The effect of femoral component head size on posterior dislocation of the artificial hip joint. *J. Bone Jt. Surg. Am.* **2000**, *82*, 1300–1307. [CrossRef]
64. Tannast, M.; Kubiak-Langer, M.; Langlotz, F.; Puls, M.; Murphy, S.B.; Siebenrock, K.A. Noninvasive three-dimensional assessment of femoroacetabular impingement. *J. Orthop. Res.* **2007**, *25*, 122–131. [CrossRef]
65. Mulholland, S.J.; Wyss, U.P. Activities of daily living in non-Western cultures: Range of motion requirements for hip and knee joint implants. *Int. J. Rehabil. Res.* **2001**, *24*, 191–198. [CrossRef]
66. Gilles, B.; Christophe, F.K.; Magnenat-Thalmann, N.; Becker, C.D.; Duc, S.R.; Menetrey, J.; Hoffmeyer, P. MRI-based assessment of hip joint translations. *J. Biomech.* **2009**, *42*, 1201–1205. [CrossRef]
67. Zheng, G.; von Recum, J.; Nolte, L.-P.; Grützner, P.A.; Steppacher, S.D.; Franke, J. Validation of a statistical shape model-based 2D/3D reconstruction method for determination of cup orientation after THA. *Int. J. Comput. Assist. Radiol. Surg.* **2012**, *7*, 225–231. [CrossRef]
68. Zheng, G. Statistical shape model-based reconstruction of a scaled, patient-specific surface model of the pelvis from a single standard AP x-ray radiograph. *Med. Phys.* **2010**, *37*, 1424–1439. [CrossRef] [PubMed]
69. Shon, W.Y.; Gupta, S.; Biswal, S.; Hur, C.Y.; Jajodia, N.; Hong, S.J.; Myung, J.S. Validation of a simple radiographic method to determine variations in pelvic and acetabular cup sagittal plane alignment after total hip arthroplasty. *Skelet. Radiol.* **2008**, *37*, 1119–1127. [CrossRef] [PubMed]
70. Yun, H.; Murphy, W.S.; Ward, D.M.; Zheng, G.; Hayden, B.L.; Murphy, S.B. Effect of Pelvic Tilt and Rotation on Cup Orientation in Both Supine and Standing Positions. *J. Arthroplast.* **2018**, *33*, 1442–1448. [CrossRef] [PubMed]
71. Wu, C.-H.; Lin, C.-C.; Lu, T.-W.; Hou, S.-M.; Hu, C.-C.; Yeh, L.-S. Evaluation of ranges of motion of a new constrained acetabular prosthesis for canine total hip replacement. *Biomed. Eng. Online* **2013**, *12*, 116. [CrossRef] [PubMed]
72. Cross, M.B.; Nam, D.; Mayman, D.J. Ideal femoral head size in total hip arthroplasty balances stability and volumetric wear. *HSS J.* **2012**, *8*, 270–274. [CrossRef]
73. Howie, D.W.; Holubowycz, O.T.; Middleton, R. Large femoral heads decrease the incidence of dislocation after total hip arthroplasty: A randomized controlled trial. *J. Bone Jt. Surg. Am.* **2012**, *94*, 1095–1102. [CrossRef]
74. Hummel, M.T.; Malkani, A.L.; Yakkanti, M.R.; Baker, D.L. Decreased dislocation after revision total hip arthroplasty using larger femoral head size and posterior capsular repair. *J. Arthroplast.* **2009**, *24*, 73–76. [CrossRef]
75. Scifert, C.F.; Noble, P.C.; Brown, T.D.; Bartz, R.L.; Kadakia, N.; Sugano, N.; Johnston, R.C.; Pedersen, D.R.; Callaghan, J.J. Experimental and computational simulation of total hip arthroplasty dislocation. *Orthop. Clin. N. Am.* **2001**, *32*, 553–567. [CrossRef]
76. Hettich, G.; Schierjott, R.A.; Ramm, H.; Graichen, H.; Jansson, V.; Rudert, M.; Traina, F.; Grupp, T.M. Method for quantitative assessment of acetabular bone defects. *J. Orthop. Res.* **2019**, *37*, 181–189. [CrossRef] [PubMed]
77. Schierjott, R.A.; Hettich, G.; Ringkamp, A.; Baxmann, M.; Morosato, F.; Damm, P.; Grupp, T.M. A method to assess primary stability of acetabular components in association with bone defects. *J. Orthop. Res.* **2020**. [CrossRef] [PubMed]
78. Gu, Y.; Pierrepont, J.; Stambouzou, C.; Li, Q.; Baré, J. A Preoperative Analytical Model for Patient-Specific Impingement Analysis in Total Hip Arthroplasty. *Adv. Orthop.* **2019**, *2019*, 6293916. [CrossRef] [PubMed]

79. Schwarz, T.J.; Weber, M.; Renkawitz, T.; Greimel, F.; Leiss, F.; Grifka, J.; Schaumburger, J. Diskrepanz zwischen radiographischer und tatsächlicher Pfannenstellung bei der Hüft-TEP-Versorgung: Interpretieren wir unsere radiologischen Qualitätsindikatoren richtig? Videobeitrag. *Der Orthopäde* **2020**, *49*, 226–229. [CrossRef]
80. Visser, J.D.; Konings, J.G. A new method for measuring angles after total hip arthroplasty. A study of the acetabular cup and femoral component. *J. Bone Jt. Surg. Br. Vol.* **1981**, *63B*, 556–559. [CrossRef]
81. Kebbach, M.; Grawe, R.; Geier, A.; Winter, E.; Bergschmidt, P.; Kluess, D.; D'Lima, D.; Woernle, C.; Bader, R. Effect of surgical parameters on the biomechanical behaviour of bicondylar total knee endoprostheses—A robot-assisted test method based on a musculoskeletal model. *Sci. Rep.* **2019**, *9*, 14504. [CrossRef]

Article

The Effect of Cement Aging on the Stability of a Cement-in-Cement Revision Construct

Mareike Schonhoff [1,*], Therese Bormann [1], Kevin Knappe [2], Tobias Reiner [2], Linda Stange [1] and Sebastian Jaeger [1,*]

1. Laboratory of Biomechanics and Implant Research, Clinic for Orthopedics and Trauma Surgery, Heidelberg University Hospital, 69118 Heidelberg, Germany; therese.bormann@med.uni-heidelberg.de (T.B.); linda.stange@med.uni-heidelberg.de (L.S.)
2. Clinic for Orthopedics and Trauma Surgery, Heidelberg University Hospital, 69118 Heidelberg, Germany; kevin.knappe@med.uni-heidelberg.de (K.K.); tobias.reiner@med.uni-heidelberg.de (T.R.)
* Correspondence: mareike.schonhoff@med.uni-heidelberg.de (M.S.); sebastian.jaeger@med.uni-heidelberg.de (S.J.)

Abstract: A revision surgery can be a complicated procedure. The prevention of the removal of a well-integrated cement mantle can minimize intraoperative complications. With the cement-in-cement technique, the implant will be fixated with a layer of bone cement onto the remaining cement mantle. In our experimental in vitro study, we investigated the effect of cement aging of a cement-in-cement revision construct and regular cement mantle on the bending strength. Two different types of bone cement were tested at four different stages of aging. The Palacos cement showed no significant difference in bending strength at any aging point, regardless of whether it was used primarily or as a cement-in-cement revision. In contrast, the SmartSet MV cement showed a significant difference between the primary and cement-in-cement applications depending on cement aging time. The comparison of the two cement-in-cement structures investigated showed significant differences between the manufacturers depending on the cement aging.

Keywords: cement-in-cement; revision; aging cement; joint arthroplasty; cement; bending strength

1. Introduction

The number of total joint replacements has increased over the last years, and the number of associated revision surgeries will also increase [1]. Based on register data, aseptic loosening is one of the most common causes for revision surgery [1,2]. In the case of total knee arthroplasty, more than 83% of all implantations performed are cemented [2]. For total hip arthroplasty, there is regional prevalence in relation to implant fixation technique. Thus, according to the Swedish register, 57.5% of primary total hip arthroplasties are cemented [3]. Specifically, the registers for hip arthroplasty vary in percentages between the different fixation techniques [1,2]. In both hip arthroplasty and knee arthroplasty, the hybrid fixation, i.e., the combination of cemented prosthesis parts with uncemented parts, is also a frequently used technique [2]. Especially in elderly people, cement is commonly used.

Revision surgery is a challenging procedure for both the surgeon and the patient. For example, when revising a cemented hip stem, it is common to remove the complete cement mantle from the femur. Different methods can be used to remove the cement, for example, with ultrasonic waves. However, the gold standard is still the mechanical removal of the cement. This, however, can be challenging and can entail some complications in cement removal [4].

Among other things, the risk of blood loss and the risk of bone perforation or even fracture is high [5–7]. Removing the remaining bone cement often is time-consuming, which can lead to intraoperative complications [8]. To improve this, Greenwald et al.

considered a different approach than removing all the existing cement [9]. They suggested to remain the cement and implant the new stem with a thin layer of bone cement on the old cement mantle if the original bone cement mantle is well-fixed and integrated into the femur. This approach is known as the cement-in-cement technique (also known as in-cement or cement-within-cement). After removing the femoral stem, the existing cement mantle is checked for possible damage. If damage is found, a conventional method has to be used. If a fully intact cement mantle is present, the surface is prepared by a burr then cleaned and dried so that the new bone cement has no contamination and a stable connection can be formed. After all these preparations, the new stem can be cemented into the femur. The use of the cement-in-cement technique has increased over the years [10–12]. The advantages of this technique are less host bone stock loss, less blood loss and a lower risk of femoral perforation or even fracture [5–7]. In addition, a cement-in-cement revision needs less time because cement removal is time-consuming [5,13,14]. This is a medical as well as a financial advantage due to a shorter time under narcotics and also the personal and room resources are used less [8]. However, only a few biomechanical studies on the strength between two cement layers exist. Testing the bending strength of different cement combinations was done, concentrated on the shear strength between the two layers [15]. However, the influence of different aging points was not considered. Liddle et al. investigated the shear strength while using different techniques to prepare the cement-in-cement interface [16]. A preparation with an ultrasonic device showed lower shear bond strength. In an experimental in vitro study, we investigated the effect of cement aging on a cement-in-cement revision construct. For this purpose, we used a four-point bending test to compare the bending strength of different cement-in-cement constructs over different times of bone cement aging.

2. Materials and Methods

We analyzed the influence of cement aging on a cement-in-cement revision construct using the bending strength as the evaluation criterion. For the study, we used Palacos R+G (Heraeus, Hanau, Germany) and SmartSet MV (DePuy Synthes, Warsaw, IN, USA) bone cement. The monomer of both cement types contains 98% of methy methacrylate and 2% N,N-dimethyl-p-toluidine. The cement powder of the Palacos R+G bone cement contains 81.9% of poly (methylacrylate, methyl methacrylate), 15% zirconium dioxide, 1% hydrous benzoyl peroxide, and 2.1% gentamicin sulphate. The compositions of the SmartSet MV powder contain 67% Polymetyl Methacrylate, 21.1% Methyl Methaacrylate/Styrene Copolymer, 1.9% Benzoyl Peroxide, and 10% Barium Sulfate. A total amount of 112 samples were prepared and tested from both types of cement. The samples were divided into four groups, and each group was differed into four examination times. In two of the four groups, cement-in-cement revision constructs were applied. This resulted in the groups Palacos–Revision and Smartset–Revision. The groups, Palacos–Reference and SmartSet–Reference, served as aged-only reference groups. The time of examination results from four different aging states. According to ISO 5833:2002-05, the first point in time was 24 ± 2 h after sample preparation [17]. The further examinations were 4 weeks plus 1 day, 4 weeks plus 3 days, and 4 weeks plus 10 days. A set of 7 specimens was tested at each investigation time point for each group.

2.1. Cement Aging

According to ISO 5833:2002-05, the first point in time for testing the bending strength of the samples was 24 ± 2 h (24 h) at room conditions of $23 \pm 1\ °C$ [17]. The specimens were stored under dry conditions also at a room temperature of $23 \pm 1\ °C$. A baseline aging of 4 weeks was performed for all other examination time points. For the baseline aging, the cement samples were stored in an incubator for 4 weeks in a saline solution (0.9% NaCl) at $37 \pm 1\ °C$ [18]. The groups, Palacos–Revision and Smartset–Revision, were removed from the incubator after 4 weeks of base aging, and the cement-in-cement revision construct was applied. Subsequently, the samples were returned to the aging process. The second test time was after 4 weeks base aging plus adding 1 day of aging (4W + 1d), also at 37 ± 1 °C in the saline solution (0.9% NaCl). The third test was after 4 weeks base aging plus 3 days (4W + 3d) of additional aging, and the fourth examination time was after 4 weeks of base aging plus 10 days (4W + 10d). All the groups of revisions and references had an identical aging process (Table 1).

Table 1. Aging times; (+) testing times; (-) no adding/modifications.

	24 h	4 Weeks Base Aging	4W + 1d	4W + 3d	4W + 10d
Palacos–Reference	+	-	+	+	+
Palacos–Revision	+	Adding new layer as revision construct	+	+	+
SmartSet–Reference	+	-	+	+	+
SmartSet–Revision	+	Adding new layer as revision construct	+	+	+

2.2. Cementing Procedure

According to the ISO 5833:2002-05, the specimen size is defined as a rectangular bar with a length of 75 ± 0.2 mm, a width of 10 ± 0.2 mm, and a total thickness of 3.3 ± 0.2 mm [17]. To form the cement specimens, the bone cement was filled into a mold. To smooth the surfaces, the bottom and the top plate of the mold were covered with a heat-stable polyester film (Tartan transparency film 901, 3M, Saint Paul, MN, USA) in combination with a PTFE (polytetrafluoroethylene) plate (Figure 1).

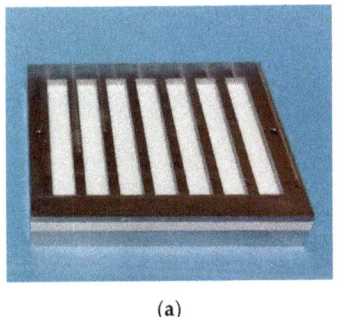
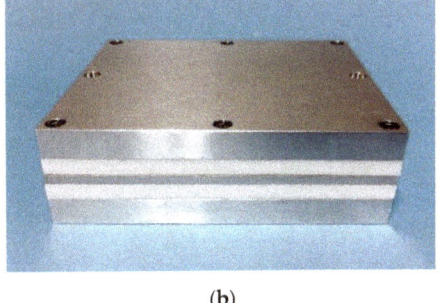

(a)   (b)

Figure 1. The molds to form the specimens, (**a**) Bottom plate, PTFE (polytetrafluoroethylene) plate, polyester film, and molds plate, (**b**) closed form adding another PTFE plate and the top plate.

For the cement-in-cement revision construct, a mold with half-thickness (1.65 mm) was used. For cementing the revision group, after cement base aging, the cement specimens were placed in the full-thickness mold and cemented to their full thickness of 3.3 mm. A single cement unit was used for each group and each aging time. Each cementing procedure strictly followed the manufacturer's instructions. All cement-mixing procedures were performed under vacuum (Vacuum mixing system, Optivac, Biomet, Warsaw, IN, USA) at a room temperature of 23 ± 1 °C and humidity of at least 40%. At the beginning of the application phase, the bone cement was applied into the molds. The time for application varied between the two kinds of cement (Palacos R+G 00:50 min; SmartSet MV 03:40 min). A cement gun was used to dispense the cement into the mold. A polyester film and the top plate with a PTFE plate were added, and then the molds were clamped for over an hour for fully curing the bone cement. After one hour in the clamping system, the top and bottom plates of the molds, including the polyester film, were removed, and the specimens were taken out of the molds. In the case of the revision groups, before adding the new layer of cement, the samples were dried with a compress. After the curing, all cement specimens were wet ground at the edges and top faces using 400-grade emery paper (Hermes, Hamburg, Germany). All cement samples were examined radiologically for possible air inclusions. Exclusion criteria were air inclusions or deviations from the required geometry. As described in the ISO, the unground bottom surface was used as the tensile face during the four-point bending test. The samples of the revision bone cement were examined with a scanning electron microscope (SEM, LEO 440 with EDS detector Oxford X-Max 80, Leo, Oberkochen, Germany) at a magnification ×250 to evaluate the fracture surface between the two cement layers.

2.3. Bending Strength

The bending strength was determined using a four-point bending test as described in ISO 5833:2002-05 and in ISO 16402:2008-05 [17,19]. The sample dimensions were measured before testing. Each measurement was performed three times with an accuracy of ± 0.1 mm, and an average value was calculated for the respective sample geometry. The four-point bending tests were carried out with a material testing machine (Zwick/Roell Z005, Ulm, Germany) and a cross-head speed of 5 mm/min (Figure 2). The force on the central loading points was increased, starting from zero until the specimen broke. The deflection of the specimen was recorded as a function of the applied force. For each tested specimen, the bending strength was calculated using the following equation: $B = \frac{3Fa}{bh^2}$. Where F is the force at break (in N), b is the average measured width of the specimen (in mm), h is the average thickness of specimen (in mm), and a is the distance between the inner and outer loading points. According to the ISO 5833:2002-05, the distance between the outer and inner loading points was 20 mm [17].

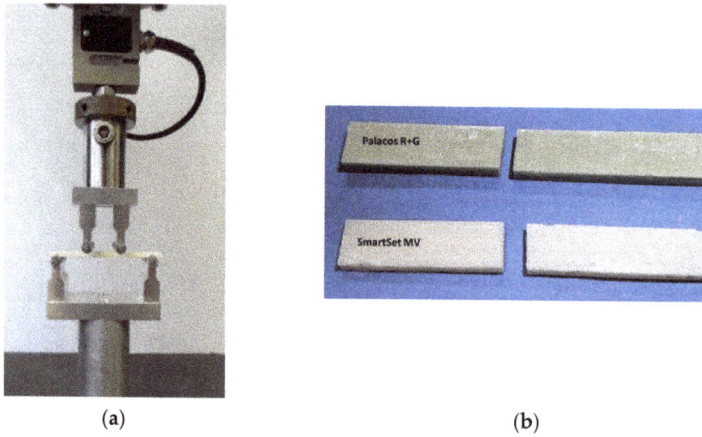

(a) (b)

Figure 2. (a) Four-point bending test with integrated cement specimen; (b) specimen after the testing.

2.4. Statistical Analysis

For statistical analysis, the software SPSS 25 (IBM Inc., Armonk, New York, NY, USA) was used. A descriptive analysis (arithmetic mean, standard deviation, minimum, and maximum) was performed. With the Shapiro–Wilk test, the normal distribution of the data was confirmed. Therefore, a repeated-measures ANOVA of independent variables was applied. To compare the groups, an ANOVA with a Bonferroni correction was used. A p-value of <0.05 was considered significant.

3. Results

A repeated-measures ANOVA showed that there is a statistically significant difference between the four groups, $F(3, 12) = 34.315$, $p < 0.001$. Additionally, a repeated-measures ANOVA determined that the aging of bone cement showed a statistically significant difference between testing points, $F(3, 36) = 17.589$, $p < 0.001$ (Figure 3).

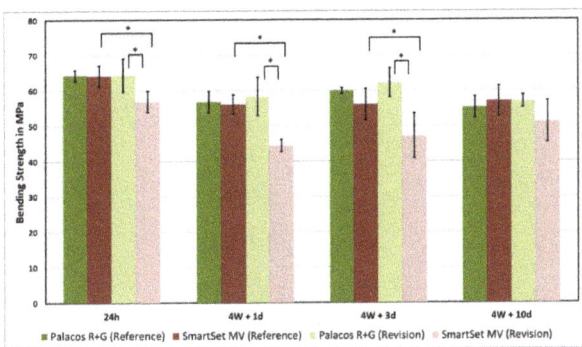

Figure 3. The results of the Bending Strength in MPa. * symbolizes the statistically significant difference between groups ($p < 0.05$).

3.1. Palacos R+G (Reference–Revision)

A Bonferroni post hoc analysis revealed no significant difference ($p = 1.000$) between the bending strength of the reference and revision groups of Palacos R+G at any testing time (Table 2).

Table 2. Comparison of the bending strength of the Palacos R+G groups. Mean (SD) in MPa.

	Palacos R+G		
	Reference	Revision	p-Value
24 h	64.2 (1.6)	64.4 (4.7)	1.000
4W + 1d	56.7 (3.0)	58.3 (5.4)	1.000
4W + 3d	59.9 (0.9)	62.2 (4.2)	1.000
4W + 10d	55.2 (3.0)	56.8 (1.8)	1.000

3.2. SmartSet MV (Reference–Revision)

The SmartSet MV bone cement showed in a Bonferroni post hoc analysis a statistically significant difference at all testing times except after 4 weeks plus 10 days of aging ($p = 0.239$). Compared to the reference group, the revision group had a lower bending strength (Table 3).

Table 3. Comparison of the bending strength of the SmartSet MV groups. Mean (SD) in MPa.

	SmartSet MV		
	Reference	Revision	p-Value
24 h	64.1 (2.9)	56.9 (3.0)	0.043
4W + 1d	56.1 (2.6)	44.4 (1.7)	<0.001
4W + 3d	56.1 (4.4)	47.1 (5.9)	0.023
4W + 10d	56.9 (4.2)	51.2 (5.8)	0.239

3.3. Reference/Revision (Palacos R+G–SmartSet MV)

While comparing the two different types of bone cement, the two reference groups showed no significant difference at any time of testing ($p > 0.8$).

However, the revision samples of SmartSet MV showed a significantly lower bending strength compared to Palacos R+G except at the testing time of 4 weeks plus 10 days (24 h $p = 0.008$; 4W + 1d $p < 0.001$; 4W + 3d $p < 0.001$; and 4W + 10d $p = 0.221$).

The adhesion between the two cement layers of the revision samples is seen in Figure 4. While SmartSet MV showed two layers of bone cement, the Palacos R+G bone cement had no visibly separated layers of old and new cement at the fractured surface after 4 weeks plus

3 days and 4 weeks plus 10 days. For both types of cement, the fractures occurred in the middle of the sample, and no delamination was observed at the cement–cement interface.

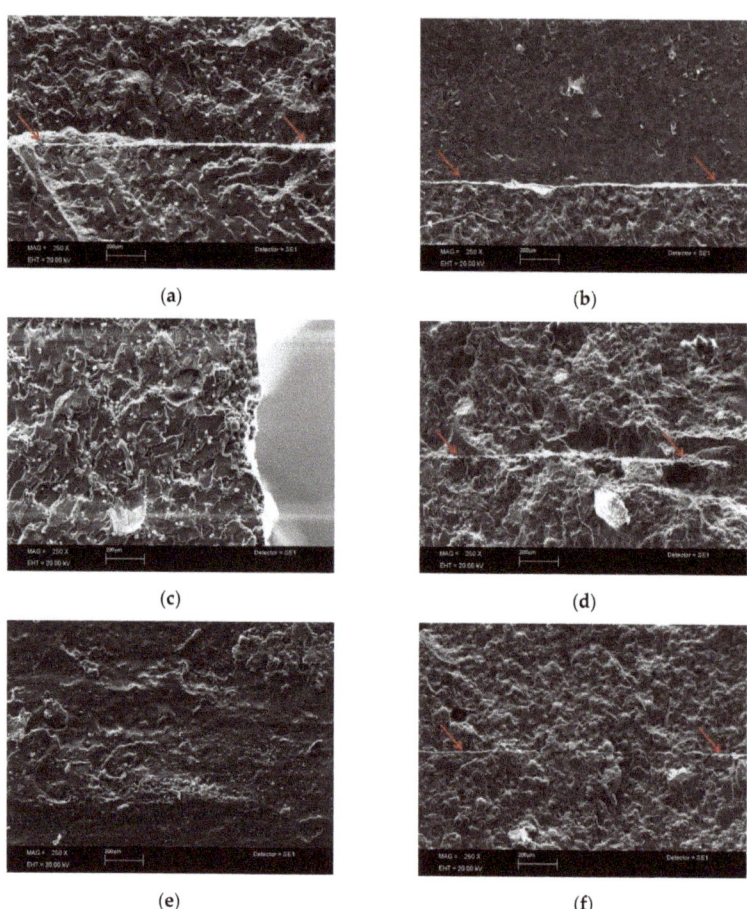

Figure 4. Images of the fractured surface with the scanning electron microscope (SEM); Palacos R+G revision at 4W + 1d (**a**), 4W + 3d (**c**), and 4W + 10d (**e**); (**b**) SmartSet MV revision at 4W + 1d (**b**), 4W + 3d (**d**), and 4W + 10d (**f**), red arrows show the line between the two layers.

4. Discussion

The arthroplasty registries show an increase in joint arthroplasties. Related to this, the incidences of revisions are increasing too, while the aseptic loosening of the endoprosthesis is still the main cause [1]. Despite the positive long-term prognosis of cemented endoprostheses, a revision is a challenging task. Due to the previous implant, in revisions, the loss of bone is already processed. To avoid or at least minimize possible complications, the cement-in-cement technique can be an alternative for hip or knee revision surgery.

In our experimental in vitro study, the bone cement Palacos R+G showed no significant difference between the reference group and the revision group at any testing time. The mean value of the reference and revision groups with Palacos R+G bone cement also had a bending strength of more than 50 MPa, which is recommended by ISO 5833:2002-05 [17]. A revision with the cement-in-cement technique and the bone cement Palacos R+G appears to be comparable to a standard cement layer under standardized conditions without the contamination of blood and lipids.

The SmartSet MV bone cement showed a different result between the reference and the revision groups. After only 4 weeks plus 10 days of aging, the bending strength did not differ significantly between the two groups. All aging points before showed that the revision group had a significantly decreased bending strength. Especially at the testing times of 4 weeks plus 1 day and 4 weeks plus 3 days, the mean value of the revision group was below the recommended 50 MPa.

While comparing the two kinds of cement, the references of the Palacos R+G and the SmartSet MV had similar values of bending strength. Therefore, there were no significant differences between the two reference groups at any testing time.

The SmartSet MV bone cement sample had a significantly lower performance than the Palacos R+G sample with the revision technique. The aging of a revision construct influenced the bending strength of the SmartSet MV more than Palacos R+G. Ayre et al. also showed that PMMA bone cements had a decrease in bending strength over the aging time [18]. If the bone cement gets in contact with blood or lipids, it can further decrease the bending strength [20,21]. Further investigations have to be conducted.

In recent years, the use of the cement-in-cement technique has increased more and more. It showed promising clinical results. Quinlan et al. had an excellent outcome using the cement-in-cement technique [22]. Other studies also showed results with the new technique and a decrease in complications due to the revision [5,13,23,24]. Sandiford et al. also investigated the cement-in-cement technique in multiple revised total hip replacements. Even though the results were less promising than other studies investigating the cement-in-cement technique, the outcome was still acceptable, especially for patients with a background with more comorbidity [12]. A systematic review of Xará-Leite et al. in 2020 showed that the cement-in-cement technique is a useful option to minimize intraoperative complications and immediate postoperative morbidity, and the rate of implant survival also remains low [10]. However, it is often unclear which cement was used in the primary arthroplasty, and therefore, different combinations of cements are possible.

Due to the time interval between the primary replacement and the revision and the possible change of hospital, the cement types may differ from each other. It is often unclear which bone cement was used in the primary replacement [11].

A further problem could be the preparation of the old cement mantle. Liddle et al. analyzed the effect on the cement-in-cement interface when the old cement is ultrasonically prepared versus a preparation with a burr or no preparation of the cement mantle at all. The shear strength was significantly decreased while using an ultrasonic device. It is possible that the generated heat produces foam on top of the surface, which can lead to a weaker connection between the two bonding cement layers. [16]

Dang et al. also investigated the strength between the connection of the old cement and the new cement [15]. The question in their study was if there is an impact from combining two different kinds of cement and if the interface between the aged cement and the new one is the weakest point of this construct. However, the type of cement was not a significant factor for the flexural strength. Additionally, they found that the cement–cement interface is not the primary weakness in this study.

Even though the method of Dang et al. had similarities to our study, there is a relevant difference between them. The samples for the four-point bending test had a different layout than ours. They put the aged cement next to the new cement, instead of on top of each other. Both cement layers were aged the same time. In our study, we aged one layer 4 weeks and the new layer from an additional day to up to 10 days.

The bending strength of aged bone cement was also studied by Oonishi et al. [25]. They performed a three-point bending test on in vivo-aged bone cement. As a result, there was a correlation between the time in situ and the bending strength. However, the impact of porosity and density should be considered. Our study showed that the time of aged cement has a significant impact on the bending strength.

This study also has limitations. Even though we used two different kinds of bone cement that are commonly used, it only represents these cements and cannot be replicated on all bone cements that are used for joint arthroplasties. For other bone cements, the process of polymerization can be different. Further investigations have to be conducted. The possible contamination of the cement with blood and bone marrow in vivo was not considered. The negative effect of contamination on stability is proven [20,21]. Contamination can reduce the bond stability by 99% [26]. However, our study was performed under laboratory conditions. Further, it was found that if the bone cement is applied early onto the implant, the interface stability is increased by 72%, and a late application increases failure by 73% [26].

5. Conclusions

In conclusion, our experimental in vitro study showed that the aging of a revision construct had a significant difference between the two analyzed bone cements. There were no significant differences between the primary-aged bone cements. However, in the revision groups, there was a significant difference between the SmartSet MV and the Palacos R+G. Further investigations are required to invest the clinical impact of the bending strength under the recommended 50 MPa of the SmartSet MV bone cement.

Author Contributions: Conceptualization, M.S. and S.J.; Data curation, M.S. and S.J.; Formal analysis, M.S. and S.J.; Methodology, S.J.; Project administration, M.S. and S.J.; Writing—original draft, M.S. and S.J.; Writing—review and editing, M.S., T.B., K.K., T.R., L.S., and S.J. All authors have read and agreed to the published version of the manuscript.

Funding: This research received no external funding.

Conflicts of Interest: The authors declare no pertinent conflict of interest. S.J. report grants from B Braun Aesculap, Johnson & Johnson Depuy Synthes, Heraeus Medical, Waldemar Link, Peter Brehm, and Zimmer Biomet that are not related to the current study. M.S., T.B., K.K., T.R., and L.S. report no conflict of interest.

References

1. Graves, S.E.; Davidson, D.; Ingerson, L.; Ryan, P.; Griffith, E.C.; McDermott, B.F.J.; McElroy, H.J.; Pratt, N.L. Australian Orthopaedic Association National Joint Replacement Registry—Annual Report. *Med. J. Aust.* **2004**, *180*, S31–S34. [CrossRef] [PubMed]
2. National Joint Registry—17th Annual Report 2020. Available online: https://www.njrcentre.org.uk/ (accessed on 20 March 2021).
3. *Swedish Hip Arthroplasty Register—Annual Report 2018*; Department of Orthopaedics, Sahlgrenska University Hospital: Gothenburg, Sweden, 2019.
4. Kraay, M.J. Cemented Component Removal: Tricks of the Trade. *Orthop. Proc.* **2015**, *97*, 52. [CrossRef]
5. Kumar, A.; Porter, M.; Shah, N.; Gaba, C.; Siney, P. Outcomes of Cement in Cement Revision, in Revision Total Hip Arthroplasty. *Open Access Maced. J. Med. Sci.* **2019**, *7*, 4059–4065. [CrossRef]
6. Burgo, F.J.; Mengelle, D.E.; Feijoo, M.; Autorino, C.M. A minimally invasive technique to remove broken cemented stems and its reconstruction with cement-in-cement. *Hip Int. J. Clin. Exp. Res. Hip Pathol. Ther.* **2019**, *29*, Np1–Np5. [CrossRef] [PubMed]
7. Bernthal, N.M.; Hegde, V.; Zoller, S.D.; Park, H.Y.; Ghodasra, J.H.; Johansen, D.; Eilber, F.; Eilber, F.C.; Chandhanayingyong, C.; Eckardt, J.J. Long-term outcomes of cement in cement technique for revision endoprosthesis surgery. *J. Surg. Oncol.* **2018**, *117*, 443–450. [CrossRef] [PubMed]
8. Gu, A.; Wei, C.; Chen, A.Z.; Malahias, M.A.; Fassihi, S.C.; Ast, M.P.; Liu, J.; Cross, M.B.; Sculco, P.K. Operative time greater than 120 minutes is associated with increased pulmonary and thromboembolic complications following revision total hip arthroplasty. *Eur. J. Orthop. Surg. Traumatol. Orthop. Traumatol.* **2020**, *30*, 1393–1400. [CrossRef] [PubMed]
9. Greenwald, A.S.; Narten, N.C.; Wilde, A.H. Points in the technique of recementing in the revision of an implant arthroplasty. *J. Bone Jt. Surg. Br. Vol.* **1978**, *60*, 107–110. [CrossRef]
10. Xará-Leite, F.; Pereira, A.D.; Andrade, R.; Sarmento, A.; Sousa, R.; Ayeni, O.R.; Espregueira-Mendes, J.; Soares, D. The cement-in-cement technique is a reliable option in hip arthroplasty revision surgery: A systematic review. *Eur. J. Orthop. Surg. Traumatol. Orthop. Traumatol.* **2020**, *31*, 7–22. [CrossRef]
11. Duncan, W.W.; Hubble, M.J.; Howell, J.R.; Whitehouse, S.L.; Timperley, A.J.; Gie, G.A. Revision of the cemented femoral stem using a cement-in-cement technique: A five- to 15-year review. *J. Bone Jt. Surg. Br. Vol.* **2009**, *91*, 577–582. [CrossRef] [PubMed]
12. Sandiford, N.A.; Jameson, S.S.; Wilson, M.J.; Hubble, M.J.; Timperley, A.J.; Howell, J.R. Cement-in-cement femoral component revision in the multiply revised total hip arthroplasty: Results with a minimum follow-up of five years. *Bone Jt. J.* **2017**, *99*, 199–203. [CrossRef]
13. Cnudde, P.H.; Karrholm, J.; Rolfson, O.; Timperley, A.J.; Mohaddes, M. Cement-in-cement revision of the femoral stem: Analysis of 1179 first-time revisions in the Swedish Hip Arthroplasty Register. *Bone Jt. J.* **2017**, *99*, 27–32. [CrossRef]

14. te Stroet, M.A.; Moret-Wever, S.G.; de Kam, D.C.; Gardeniers, J.W.; Schreurs, B.W. Cement-in-cement femoral revisions using a specially designed polished short revision stem; 24 consecutive stems followed for five to seven years. *Hip Int. J. Clin. Exp. Res. Hip. Pathol. Ther.* **2014**, *24*, 428–433. [CrossRef]
15. Dang, K.; Pelletier, M.H.; Walsh, W.R. Factors affecting flexural strength in cement within cement revisions. *J. Arthroplast.* **2011**, *26*, 1540–1548. [CrossRef]
16. Liddle, A.; Webb, M.; Clement, N.; Green, S.; Liddle, J.; German, M.; Holland, J. Ultrasonic cement removal in cement-in-cement revision total hip arthroplasty: What is the effect on the final cement-in-cement bond? *Bone Jt. Res.* **2019**, *8*, 246–252. [CrossRef]
17. *ISO 5833:2002-05, Implants for Surgery—Acrylic Resin Cements*; ISO: Geneva, Switzerland, 2002.
18. Ayre, W.N.; Denyer, S.P.; Evans, S.L. Ageing and moisture uptake in polymethyl methacrylate (PMMA) bone cements. *J. Mech. Behav. Biomed. Mater.* **2014**, *32*, 76–88. [CrossRef]
19. *ISO 16402:2008-05, Implants for Surgery—Acrylic Resin Cement—Flexural Fatigue Testing of Acrylic Resin Cements Used in Orthopaedics*; ISO: Geneva, Switzerland, 2008.
20. Karpiński, R.; Szabelski, J.; Maksymiuk, J. Effect of Physiological Fluids Contamination on Selected Mechanical Properties of Acrylate Bone Cement. *Materials* **2019**, *12*. [CrossRef]
21. Tan, J.H.; Koh, B.T.; Ramruttun, A.K.; Wang, W. Compression and flexural strength of bone cement mixed with blood. *J. Orthop. Surg.* **2016**, *24*, 240–244. [CrossRef] [PubMed]
22. Quinlan, J.F.; O'Shea, K.; Doyle, F.; Brady, O.H. In-cement technique for revision hip arthroplasty. *J. Bone Jt. Surg. Br. Vol.* **2006**, *88*, 730–733. [CrossRef] [PubMed]
23. Mandziak, D.G.; Howie, D.W.; Neale, S.D.; McGee, M.A. Cement-within-cement stem exchange using the collarless polished double-taper stem. *J. Arthroplast.* **2007**, *22*, 1000–1006. [CrossRef] [PubMed]
24. Berg, A.J.; Hoyle, A.; Yates, E.; Chougle, A.; Mohan, R. Cement-in-cement revision with the Exeter Short Revision Stem: A review of 50 consecutive hips. *J. Clin. Orthop. Trauma* **2020**, *11*, 47–55. [CrossRef] [PubMed]
25. Oonishi, H.; Akiyama, H.; Takemoto, M.; Kawai, T.; Yamamoto, K.; Yamamuro, T.; Oonishi, H.; Nakamura, T. The long-term in vivo behavior of polymethyl methacrylate bone cement in total hip arthroplasty. *Acta Orthop.* **2011**, *82*, 553–558. [CrossRef] [PubMed]
26. Billi, F.; Kavanaugh, A.; Schmalzried, H.; Schmalzried, T.P. Techniques for improving the initial strength of the tibial tray-cement interface bond. *Bone Jt. J.* **2019**, *101*, 53–58. [CrossRef] [PubMed]

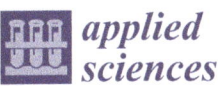

Article

Establishment of a Rolling-Sliding Test Bench to Analyze Abrasive Wear Propagation of Different Bearing Materials for Knee Implants

Jessica Hembus [1,*], Felix Ambellan [2], Stefan Zachow [2] and Rainer Bader [1]

1. Biomechanics and Implant Technology Research Laboratory, Department of Orthopaedics, University Medicine Rostock, Doberaner Str. 142, 18057 Rostock, Germany; rainer.bader@med.uni-rostock.de
2. Visual and Data-Centric Computing, Zuse Institute Berlin, Takustraße 7, 14195 Berlin, Germany; ambellan@zib.de (F.A.); zachow@zib.de (S.Z.)
* Correspondence: jessica.hembus@med.uni-rostock.de; Tel.: +49-381-494-9375

Citation: Hembus, J.; Ambellan, F.; Zachow, S.; Bader, R. Establishment of a Rolling-Sliding Test Bench to Analyze Abrasive Wear Propagation of Different Bearing Materials for Knee Implants. *Appl. Sci.* **2021**, *11*, 1886. https://doi.org/10.3390/app11041886

Academic Editor: Frank Seehaus

Received: 3 February 2021
Accepted: 18 February 2021
Published: 21 February 2021

Publisher's Note: MDPI stays neutral with regard to jurisdictional claims in published maps and institutional affiliations.

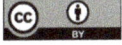

Copyright: © 2021 by the authors. Licensee MDPI, Basel, Switzerland. This article is an open access article distributed under the terms and conditions of the Creative Commons Attribution (CC BY) license (https://creativecommons.org/licenses/by/4.0/).

Abstract: Currently, new materials for knee implants need to be extensively tested but such tests are expensive in a knee wear simulator in a realized design. However, using a rolling-sliding test bench, these materials can be examined under the same test conditions, but with simplified geometries. In the present study, the test bench was optimized, and forces were adapted to the physiological contact pressure in the knee joint using the available geometric parameters. Various polymers made of polyethylene and polyurethane, articulating against test wheels made of cobalt-chromium and aluminum titanate, were tested in the test bench using adapted forces based on ISO 14243–1. Polyurethane materials showed distinctly higher wear rates than polyethylene materials and showed inadequate wear resistance for use as knee implant material. Thus, the rolling-sliding test bench is an adaptable test setup to evaluate newly developed bearing materials for knee implants. It combines the advantages of screening and simulator tests and allows for the testing of various bearing materials under physiological load and tribological conditions of the human knee joint. The wear behavior of different material compositions and the influence of surface geometry and quality can be initially investigated without the need to produce complex implant prototypes of total knee endoprosthesis or interpositional spacers.

Keywords: knee joint kinematics; wear bearing; rolling-sliding mechanism; test bench

1. Introduction

The knee is the largest synovial fluid-filled joint in the human body [1] and exhibits different articulating surfaces. The tibiofemoral joint is the weight-bearing component of the knee [1,2], consisting of two biconvex femoral condyles that articulate on a concave medial and a convex lateral plateau of the tibia. The complex structure of the native knee joint enables flexion and extension, anterior posterior (AP) translation, abduction and adduction, as well as axial rotation movements. The degree of freedom of knee movements is mainly limited by the ligaments [3]. The dominant movements are flexion and extension, where the femoral component performs a complex rolling-sliding movement on the tibial plateau. The ratio of rolling and sliding is determined by the extent of flexion [4,5]. At the beginning of the flexion movement, the rolling mechanism prevails. From approximately 20 to 30 degrees of flexion, rolling-sliding dominates until pure gliding occurs at the maximum degree of flexion movement. The extent of rolling-sliding is lower in the medial than in the lateral compartment [4–6]. The viscoelastic menisci ensures a consistent distribution of joint load [1].

Osteoarthritis is one of the most common diseases of the knee joint. Affected patients suffer from severe pain and reduced joint mobility, and are often treated with knee arthroplasty. This procedure is one of the most common surgical interventions in orthopedics [2].

However, one major problem of knee endoprostheses is their limited ability to replicate the natural rolling-sliding mechanism and wear propagation at bearing surfaces. Enhanced mechanical loading due to high physical activity influences the durability and functionality of knee implants [5,7]. One of the main causes of implant failure and revision is aseptic loosening due to the release of wear debris, accompanied by an adverse biological reaction to the particles [8,9].

Therefore, preclinical tribological and biological investigations on abrasive wear and deformation behavior are relevant for the development of suitable knee implant materials and designs. For this purpose, various wear test methods are available, which differ in complexity and testing parameters. These methods can be divided into screening and simulator studies [10]. Initial tribological screening tests mainly examine the contact surface over a short time period using simplified sample geometries and kinematics. The most commonly used test methods include pin-on-disc or cylinder-on-cylinder tests [7,10]. To simulate wear behavior under more physiological conditions, new endoprosthetic implant materials and designs need to be tested according to international testing standards, where advanced joint-specific motion sequences and load profiles are applied. However, these tests are time-consuming and the running costs for wear data acquisition are high. Furthermore, only finalized implant prototypes are tested regarding their wear behavior at articulating surfaces, which are complex to produce [7,10,11]. Before such implants are produced, a test device that enables the screening of new materials with simplified geometries under biomechanical boundary conditions, adapted to the in vivo situation, should be available. Some previous studies have introduced the concept of executing combined rolling-sliding movements while applying physiological joint forces and motions. In 2004, Citters et al. developed a rolling-sliding tribotester that was capable of generating realistic contact stresses [12]. The extent and frequency of rolling and sliding could be adjusted separately for each test station. Cylindrical samples of cobalt-chromium (CoCr) and polyethylene (PE) were tested in test fluid until macroscopic failure of the samples occurred [12,13]. However, the geometric contact conditions were simplified. Richter et al. [11] developed a test bench in which an axial load was applied statically with a cylinder made of CoCr to a horizontally moving plate made of PE, resulting in a rolling movement of the rotating cylinder on the plate. After stopping the CoCr cylinder, a sliding movement occurs due to the continuous movement of the PE plate in a tempered test fluid [11]. As this test chamber is not sealed, there is a risk of contamination by foreign particles. In another rolling-sliding test bench, an axial sinusoidal load is applied to a plate made of PE by means of a CoCr cylinder [14]. The rolling-sliding movement results from the horizontal movement of the test chamber. These test rigs represent an appropriate mixture of screening and simulator tests and are designed for wear and endurance testing. However, none of them replicate the dynamically acting load conditions in the human knee joint.

To address this, Goebel et al. developed a rolling-sliding test bench (RST) [7]. Comparable to the test benches of Wieser [14] and Richter et al. [11], the force is applied to a flat sample of PE using CoCr cylinders. The rolling-sliding movement is caused by the coupled movement of a lifting arm. With this test bench, the forces acting on the knee during normal gait can be dynamically and variably applied to the sample during the roll-slide movement [7]. Furthermore, it is possible to simulate the roll-slide movement of a femoral component made of CoCr under wear conditions that are as close as possible to physiological conditions [7]. However, this test bench has some limitations. Goebel et al. used the same force, according to ISO 14243–1 [15], that is used for the testing of total endoprostheses in knee wear simulators, although only one knee condyle was simulated on the test bench. Furthermore, the test bench had only one station, resulting in time-consuming sample screening [7].

In the present study, the test bench was optimized, and the forces were adapted to the physiological contact pressure in the knee joint using the available geometric parameters. In this study, a knee spacer, which is a unicompartmental interpositional implant, was developed with the aim to postpone the implantation of a unicondylar or bicondylar knee endoprosthesis. For this purpose, we adapted the test bench and test conditions described by Goebel et al. [7] to simulate the contact conditions of an osteoarthritic femoral condyle on the spacer material. Furthermore, a second station was added to the rolling-sliding test bench. The joint reaction force according to ISO 14243–1 [15] was adjusted to the load situation at the unicompartmental implant surface, and different bearing material pairs were compared.

2. Materials and Methods

2.1. Construction of the Rolling-Sliding Test Bench

In the test setup, the physiological rolling-sliding movement of the knee joint was transferred to a simple movement algorithm with simplified sample geometries, according to Schwittalle et al. [16]. The bearing components included a rolling cylinder, which was guided through a hole, with an additional pin to lock the rotation of the cylinder. This cylinder simulated one femoral condyle. The corresponding tibial plateau with an integrated insert was simulated by a flat polymer sample disc placed on an inclined metallic plane. The test bench applied flexion-extension movements. The application of the forces and movements of the femoral and tibial components was ensured by coupling to two electromechanical cylinders (CMS63S series; SEW-EURODRIVE GmbH and Co KG, Güstrow, Germany). The loads and movements of the cylinders could be freely adjusted using MOVITOOLS®-Motion-Studio software (SEW-EURODRIVE GmbH and Co KG, Güstrow, Germany). The test bench with the electromechanical cylinders was embedded in a frame constructed of anodized aluminum profiles. One pivoted electromechanical cylinder was used for the transmission of force (Figure 1), while the second electromechanical cylinder performed the rolling-sliding movement simultaneously in a kinematic chain.

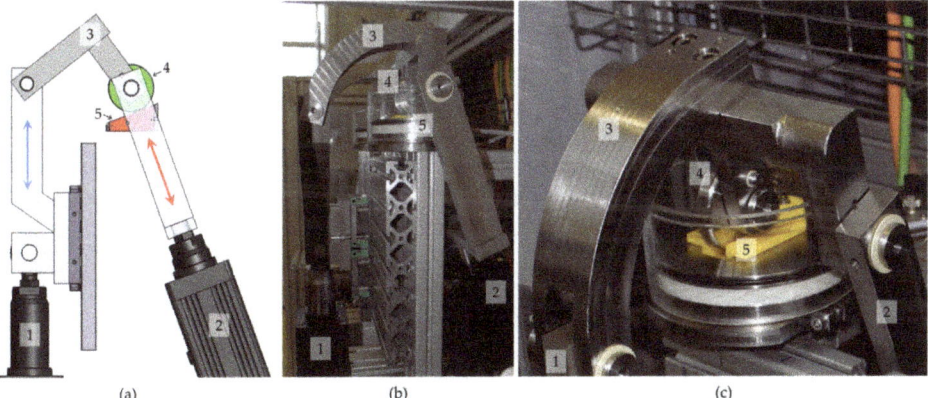

Figure 1. Rolling-sliding test bench (**a**) initially developed by Goebel et al. [7]; (**b**) enhanced with a second station and tempered testing chamber (**c**); with a lifting cylinder and linear guide (1, blue arrow indicates the direction of movement), pivoted force cylinder (2, red arrow indicates the direction of applied forces), right-angled lever (3), rolling cylinder (4, CoCr) with a rotation lock pin, and the sample on an inclined plane fixed with a yellow clamp (5).

The rolling cylinder was firmly connected to a right-angled lever, which was connected to the lifting cylinder with a linear guide (see Figure 1) driven by an electromechanical cylinder. This enabled a consistent forward movement, whereby the cylinder rolled on the inclined plane through the rotation lock (Figure 2a). From half of the stroke length at 55 mm, the cylinder was rolled to the upper point (reversal point). The coupling point with the lifting cylinder was at the level of the center of rotation of the test wheel. With further lifting of the lifting cylinder, the coupling point rose higher than the center of the rotation and the test wheel slid down the inclined plane (Figure 2b). The lifting cylinder moved upwards for 110 mm, and the test wheel stopped at the lowest position on the bearing surface (Figure 2c). According to the physiological kinematics, the rolling of the test wheel occurred approximately during the first 55% of the gait cycle (see Figure 2, left panel). Subsequently, the pure sliding movement was simulated, which appeared in the knee at approximately 30° of flexion, corresponding to about 55% of the gait cycle. The linear movement of the lifting cylinder was adjusted in such a way that the roll-slide movement was completed after 1 s, thus completing a full gait cycle. Just as in the knee joint, the rolling-sliding test bench simulates movement of the rotation axis of the knee condyle. During the downward movement of the lifting cylinder, the rolling-sliding mechanism occurred in reverse order.

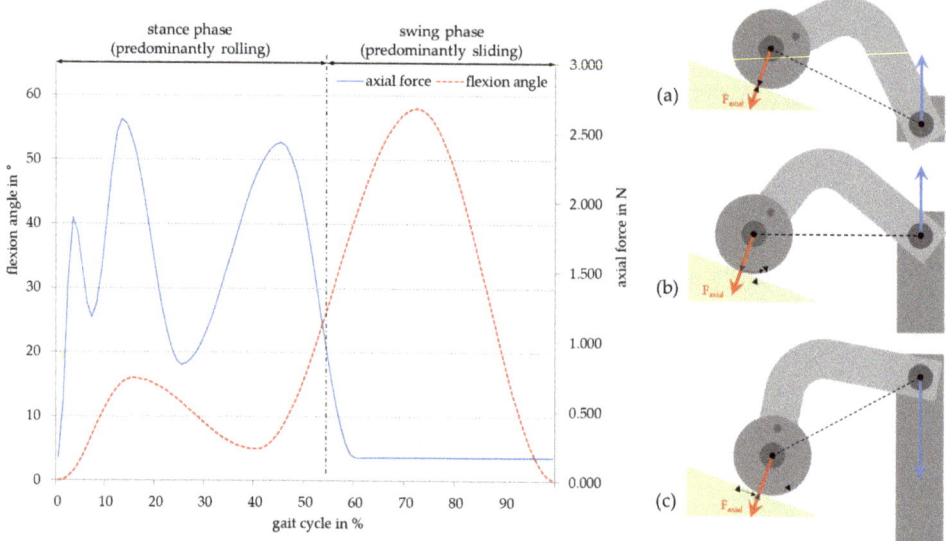

Figure 2. Motion sequence of the rolling-sliding test bench with the corresponding force according to ISO 14243–1 [15]: (**a**) Starting position of the lifting cylinder and rolling of the cylinder during lifting; (**b**) end of rolling and start of sliding down the plane; and (**c**) end of the motion sequence and start of the reverse cycle by sinking of the lifting cylinder.

The sample was loaded axially with a force cylinder, which was coupled to the axis of the test wheel (Figure 1). The application of force by the first electromechanical cylinder was synchronized with the linear lifting movement driven by the second electromechanical cylinder. The force curve was freely programmable and could therefore be applied statically, and it was also time dependent. In order to simulate a physiological joint load, the force curve of normal walking, as specified in ISO 14232–1, was applied between the test wheel and the polymer sample [15]. Thus, the applied forces were correlated to the corresponding angles of the flexion-extension movement according to the ISO standard [7,15].

In order to simulate the physiological axial joint load, the applied force based on ISO 14243–1 was adapted to the prevailing physiological contact pressure of the condyles in the following section (see Section 2.3).

Goebel et al. [7] initially included one station in the test bench. In the present study, a second station, operating in parallel, was integrated into the test bench. For this purpose, a second force cylinder and a second pair of bearing surfaces were integrated in parallel to the first station with the same load profile. In order to apply an identical rolling-sliding movement, both stations were coupled with the lifting arm (Figure 3d).

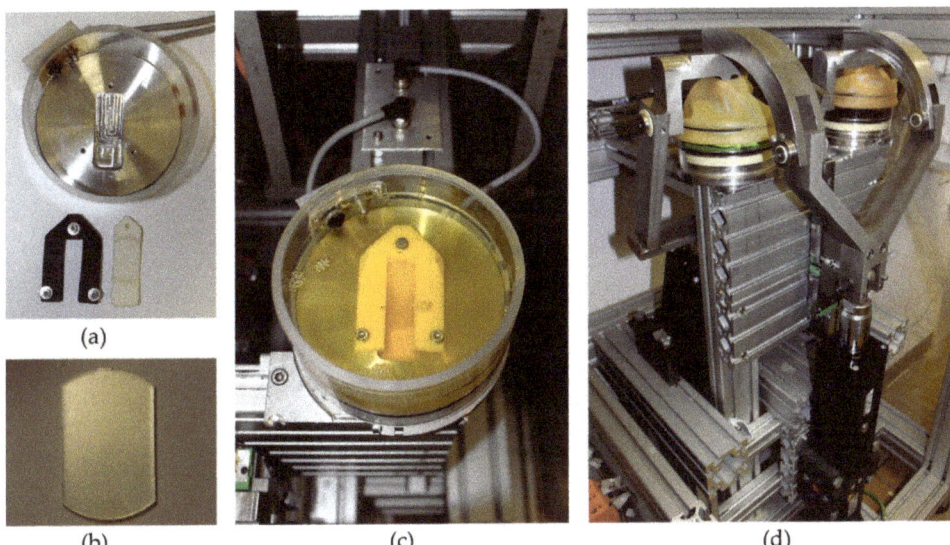

Figure 3. Setup of the rolling-sliding test bench. (**a**) Testing chamber with the sample clamp (black) and sample holder (white), (**b**) prepared polyurethane (PU) sample for testing, (**c**) tempered testing chamber with the fixed PU sample (yellow clamp) in test fluid, and (**d**) rolling-sliding test bench with two testing stations.

To ensure that the polymer specimens were loaded identically and would not slip out of the holder during dynamic loading, they were fixed with a clamp (Figure 3a,c). This also prevented high backside abrasive wear. The bearing partners were loaded according to ISO 14243–1 at 1 ± 0.1 Hz at 37 ± 2 °C in 150 mL bovine serum with a protein content of 20 g/L [15]. These parameters were intended to simulate the environment of the human knee joint. Integrated level and temperature sensors allowed for long-term automated and controlled operation of the test bench. The test bench was made of stainless steel to prevent corrosion as well as third body wear through the chamber. The setup of the rolling-sliding test bench is shown in Figure 3. To ensure a load frequency of 1 ± 0.1 Hz, the feed force of the lifting cylinder must be adapted to the increased weight by coupling of the second station.

In the present study, interpositional implant samples made of polyurethane (PU), which should imitate cartilage and articulate against a simulated subchondral bone, were tested as an example. For this purpose, test wheels made of aluminum titanate (Alutit T; CeramTec GmbH, Plochingen, Germany) were used. This ceramic material has a similar Young's modulus (17,000 MPa) to that of cortical bone. Furthermore, the bearing combination of a cobalt-chromium test wheel articulating against ultra-high-molecular-weight polyethylene was analyzed in the test bench with adapted contact forces.

2.2. Test Samples

The test samples (disks with a height of 3.5 mm, diameter of 40 mm, and cut to a width of 24 mm; see Figure 3b) were made of polyurethane and polyethylene. The test wheels (cylinders with a width of 12 mm and diameter of 60 mm) consisted of Alutit and CoCr. The samples were dynamically loaded in the test bench according to ISO 14243–1 [15]. For each sample material, one sample was loaded statically as a reference for fluid absorption [15]. As knee spacer materials, two thermoplastic polycarbonate urethane (TPCU) materials provided by the University of Applied Sciences, Reutlingen, were tested [17,18]. These polyurethane materials were tested using a ceramic test wheel made of thermal shock-optimized Alutit T.

To facilitate comparison to abrasion data from the knee simulator, a conventional ultra-high-molecular-weight polyethylene (GUR1050) sample was articulated against Alutit T and CoCr test wheels under the same conditions.

2.3. Adjustment of Load Pattern

According to ISO 14243–1 [15], forces between 0.17 and 2.6 kN occur in the human knee during the normal gait cycle. In the rolling-sliding test bench, tests were carried out with a cylindrical test wheel, which is considerably narrower than a knee condyle. Therefore, in order to achieve a roll-slide movement under physiological forces, the force specified by the ISO standard needed to be reduced. In addition to the different geometries, the differences in material properties, such as the elasticity of the bearing partners, also needed to be taken into account. Furthermore, it is important to consider that only one knee condyle is represented in the roll-sliding test bench. According to Hella et al., 70% of the axial force is transmitted with the medial condyle and 30% with the lateral condyle [19]. Hence, the spacer material was tested by simulating loading at the medial condyle.

In order to determine the force to be transferred between the two articulating surfaces, A and B, taking into account the geometry and material properties, the formula for the contact pressure according to Hertz (Equation (1)) was chosen, with consideration of the material parameters (Equation (2)) for the case of a cylinder (A) on a plane (B):

$$p_H = \sqrt{\frac{F}{2\pi r l} \times \frac{E}{1-v^2}} \quad (1)$$

$$\frac{E}{1-v^2} = \left(\frac{1-v_A^2}{E_A} + \frac{1-v_B^2}{E_B}\right)^{-1} \quad (2)$$

To calculate the forces for the roll-slide test rig, the physiological contact pressure in the human knee joint must first be determined. Therefore, the maximum axial force from ISO 14243–1 was considered. For the medial condyle, a maximum force of 2.6 kN resulted in an axial maximum force F_{medial} of 1.82 kN. The knee spacer material tested in this study was developed for the treatment of knee joints with progressive osteoarthritis. Patients often suffer from a severe lesion of the femur cartilage down to the surface of the subchondral bone. Therefore, the contact model of cortical bone (femoral site) on cartilage (tibial site) was chosen for the determination of the contact pressure. The Young's modulus and Poisson's ratio of cortical bone, which were articulated against cartilage, were chosen as parameters to test the material properties of the bearing materials. Hayes and Mockros determined variable properties for long- and short-term loaded cartilage [20]. To ensure that the worst-case scenario is covered, we used the higher value for the short-term loaded cartilage to calculate the contact pressure on the articulating surface. Since progressive osteoarthritis often results in a joint space narrowing accompanied by meniscal extrusion, the meniscus was not taken into account for the calculation of the contact pressure [21]. To determine the radius and width of the medial condyle, it is necessary to ascertain the flexion axis according to the ISO norm. Since the knee does not have a fixed center of rotation and the flexion axis shifts to anterior with increasing flexion, this axis needs to be approximated for the determination. For an accurate determination, both parameters were measured at maximum force. According to ISO 14243–1, this occurs at 15.32° of flexion [15].

2.4. Shape Analysis for Parameter Detection

In order to measure parameters, we performed 3D surface reconstruction from magnetic resonance imaging (MRI) scans of 261 female femoral surfaces based on quality assured manual segmentations of the distal femur bone. The segmentations were part of the previously published OAI–ZIB dataset [22]. For further technical details, we refer the reader to that publication. We calculated the point-wise mean shape, a standard procedure in statistical shape modeling [23], and performed an error-minimizing cylinder fit to the condyle region with respect to the contact points obtained by virtually mimicking the flexion-rolling of the distal femur bone (see Figure 4a,b). The radius of the determined cylinder serves as parameter r_{medial}. Taking the center line of the fitted cylinder as the (flexion) axis, we intersected the medial condyle region with a plane deflected by 15.32° and adapted the resulting intersection curve to the load-bearing cartilage interface by restriction to the segment connecting the two points of maximal curvature. The parameter l_{medial} could then be defined as the Euclidean distance between these points (see Figure 4c). In contrast to most studies in which the condylar radius is determined by considering the condyles as independent spheres [24,25], this study fitted a cylinder around the flexion axis of both condyles. This approach was chosen because ISO 14243–1:2009 also takes the flexion axis into account when both condyles contact the tibial plateau. Furthermore, in the study by Howel et al. [24], only very small differences between the radii of the medial and lateral condyles of a human knee joint were determined (on average 0.1 to 0.2 mm, accompanied with high standard deviations), although the condyles were considered individually as spheres. As these are very small differences, we assume that the use of a cylinder in the determination of the radius is suitable.

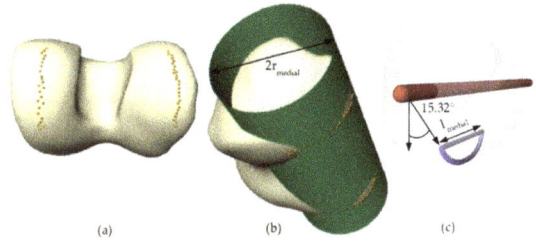

Figure 4. Algorithmic estimation of condyle radius and width. (**a**) Contact points of simulated flexion movement on the distal femur; (**b**) optimal cylinder fitted to the contact points; and (**c**) curve along and through the medial condyle approximating the describing contact for a flexion angle of 15.32°.

The parameters used are summarized in Table 1.

Table 1. Parameters used to determine the physiological contact pressure in the medial knee joint.

Parameter	Value	Meaning
F	0.17 to 2.6 kN	Axial force according to ISO 14243–1 [15]
F_{medial}	0.12 to 1.82 kN	Axial force that is transmitted via the medial condyle (F_{medial} = 70% F [19])
r_{medial}	20.584 mm	Cylinder radius/radius of the condyle
l_{medial}	25.29 mm	Length of contact of the cylinder with the plane/cartilage surface
$E_A = E_{cortical\ bone}$	17,000 N/mm²	Young's modulus of cortical bone [26]
$v_A = v_{cortical\ bone}$	0.3	Poisson's ratio of cortical bone [26]
$E_B = E_{cartilage}$	12 N/mm²	Young's modulus of cartilage [20]
$v_B = v_{cartilage}$	0.42	Poisson's ratio of cartilage [20]

This resulted in a constant value of $E/(1 - v^2) = 14.56$ N/mm² for the bearing materials cortical bone on cartilage with the material parameters after insertion in Equation (2). This resulted in the following equation for the physiological contact pressure:

$$p_H = \sqrt{\frac{F_{medial} \times 14.56\ N/mm^2}{2\pi \times 20.58\ mm \times 25.29\ mm}} \quad (3)$$

In order to determine the force for the rolling-sliding test bench, Equation (1) had to be modified according to the force and the determined natural contact pressure with the geometric data and the material data of the samples to be tested. The geometric parameters used in the calculation were the radius (r_{RST} = 30 mm) and width (l_{RST} = 12 mm) of the rolling cylinder. The parameters of the bearing materials investigated in this study are summarized in Table 2.

$$F_{RST} = \frac{p_H^2 \, 2\pi \, r_{RST} \, l_{RST}}{E/(1-v^2)} = \frac{p_H^2 \, 2\pi \times 30 \, mm \times 12 \, mm}{E/(1-v^2)} \quad (4)$$

with

$$\frac{E}{1-v^2} = \left(\frac{1-v_{cylinder}^2}{E_{cylinder}} + \frac{1-v_{plane}^2}{E_{plane}} \right)^{-1} \quad (5)$$

Table 2. Parameters used to determine the axial load curves in the rolling-sliding test bench.

Parameter	Bearing Material Pair 1		Bearing Material Pair 2		Bearing Material Pair 3	
	Alutit T [1]	PU	CoCr [27]	PE [28,29]	Alutit T	PE
$E_{cylinder}$ in N/mm²	17,000	-	230,000	-	17,000	-
$v_{cylinder}$	0.22	-	0.3	-	0.22	-
E_{plane} in N/mm²	-	18.9	-	945	-	945
v_{plane}	-	0.4	-	0.45	-	0.45

[1] Specified by the manufacturer.

A material constant of $E/(1-v^2)$ = 22.47 N/mm² was determined for the bearing material pair Alutit against PU, which resulted in a maximum force of 815.43 N. For CoCr against PE, a maximum force of 15.5 N was calculated with $E/(1-v^2)$ = 1179.42 N/mm². For bearing material pair 3, Alutit against PE, a maximal force of 16.5 N was calculated with $E/(1-v^2)$ = 1111.24 N/mm². For programming the rolling-sliding test bench, an adapted load curve was calculated using the force curve from ISO 14243–1. The computerized force curve for the two bearing materials, PU against Alutit, is shown in Figure 5.

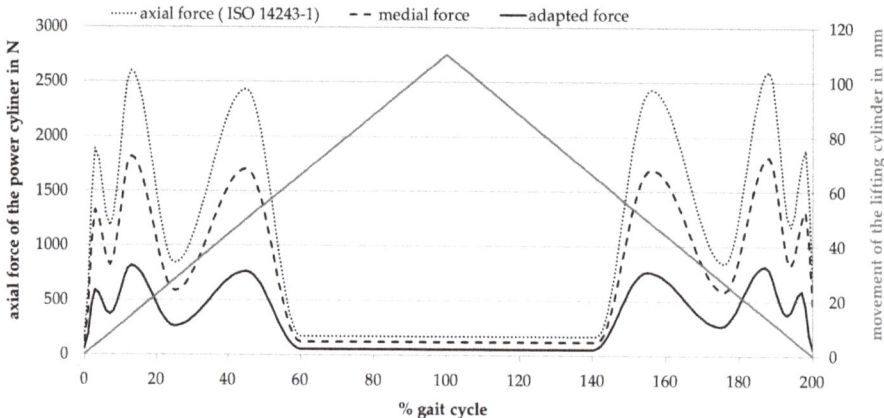

Figure 5. Adapted load curve in the rolling-sliding test bench and corresponding movement of the lifting cylinder.

2.5. Abrasive Wear Measurement

Similar to standard knee wear simulator tests, three samples of each pair of bearing materials were tested in the rolling-sliding test bench under dynamic loading, as well as an additional soak control. Before loading, the polymer samples were saturated in the test medium in accordance with ISO 14243–2 [30]. As the test fluid, bovine serum (protein content 20 g/L; Biochrom GmbH, Berlin, Germany), ethylene diamine tetra acetic acid (EDTA) and sodium azide (NaN$_3$) were used. Deviating from the ISO standard, the load was applied with an adapted force profile in the rolling-sliding test bench with two stations over a million cycles in total, as the PU materials had already been subjected to severe wear during this period. To validate the fluid absorption of the inserts, the soak control was only loaded with the axial force. For this purpose, the rolling-sliding movement was inhibited by decoupling of the lifting cylinder so that no wear was generated in the soak control sample. To validate the progress of sample saturation and the measurement before loading, the weight of the samples was measured gravimetrically after 0.5 million and 1 million cycles using a high precision balance (Sartorius ME235S; Sartorius AG, Göttingen, Germany; sensitivity 0.01 mg, uncertainty 0.03 mg) with an accuracy of 0.1 mg, according to ISO 14243–2. The wear of the samples was determined, taking the fluid absorption of the soak control into account. Before the gravimetric measurement, the samples were cleaned and dried in accordance with ISO 14243–2 [30]. To avoid damaging the PU samples, they were not treated with propanol. To ensure an identical load of all samples and to avoid station-related influences, the samples were exchanged between the two stations every 0.5 million cycles. In addition, the medium was replaced, and the test chambers were cleaned. The serum was stored for further examination [15,30].

2.6. Surface Analysis and Roughness Measurement

After completion of the wear measurement analysis, optical surface analysis was carried out using a laser scanning microscope (LSM; VHX–900F; Keyence, Osaka, Japan). This was used to characterize the surface roughness and the patterns of wear that occurred. Measurements were made in the articulated area, in the area of clamping and in the unloaded area of the plane. The arithmetical mean height (Sa) and the maximum height (Sz) were determined according to DIN EN ISO 4288:1998 and DIN EN ISO 3274:1998 [31,32]. The wear patterns and roughness values were compared to the images and values of unloaded samples.

3. Results
3.1. Amount of Wear

Four different bearing pairs were tested on the rolling-sliding test bench over one million cycles under standard conditions. We were unable to detect any signs of wear on the PE inserts articulated against the CoCr and Alutit test wheels after loading with 15.5 N (PE–CoCr) or 16.5 N (PE-Alutit); therefore, the PE inserts were also loaded with the higher force (815.43 N) from the pairing of Alutit against PU. The wear rates of the three test specimens were calculated for each pairing considering the material saturation with the test fluid (soak control). The worn running surface of the PU materials was about 35 mm, while the worn surface of the PE samples was distinctly flatter and shorter (20 mm). This is also reflected in the wear data presented in Figure 6. The mean gravimetric wear of the PU materials after one million cycles amounted to 1223.46 ± 87.02 mg for PU1 and 466.92 ± 69.44 mg for PU2. The PE material articulated against Alutit showed an average wear of $7.9 \times 10^{-3} \pm 2.0 \times 10^{-4}$ mg after one million cycles. The wear rates of the PE samples articulated against CoCr were the lowest, with a rate of $2.5 \times 10^{-4} \pm 3.4 \times 10^{-4}$ mg. All PU and PE samples showed significant backside wear respective to the measured amount of wear (Figure 7). The gravimetric wear after 0.5 million cycles was also included in the calculation of wear rates (Figure 6). All curves showed a linear wear behavior.

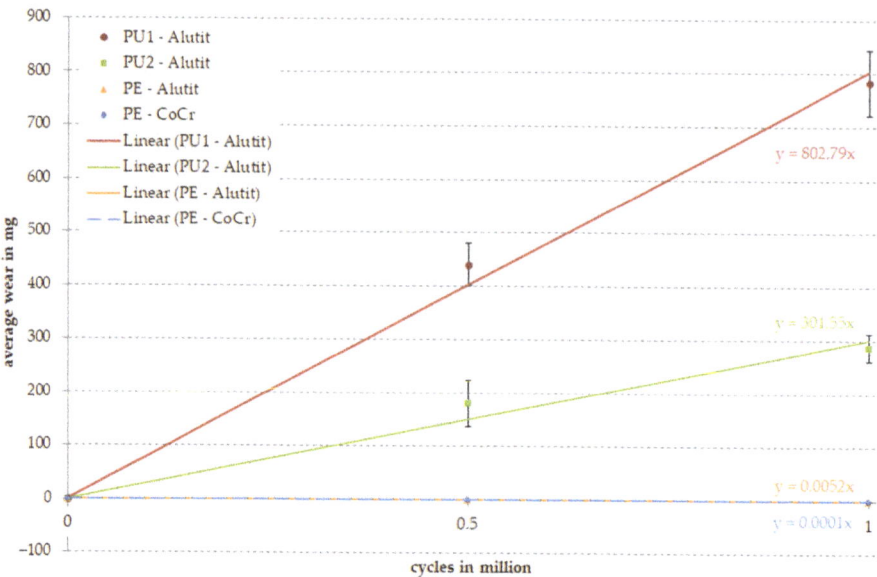

Figure 6. Overall wear of samples after loading in the rolling-sliding test bench. The straight line results from linear regression of the data for estimating the abrasion after 1 million cycles. Different to ISO 14243–1, the zero time point is used in this calculation.

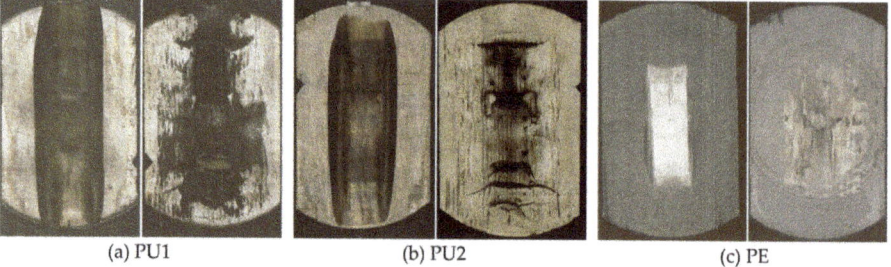

Figure 7. Worn surfaces (each left) and backsides (each right) of the three tested materials: (**a**) PU1, (**b**) PU2, and (**c**) PE.

3.2. Surface Analysis and Roughness Measurement

After loading in the rolling-sliding test bench and the gravimetric measurement, the running surfaces of all samples were examined by LSM and compared to the initial state. The PU samples showed a higher penetration depth of the test wheel into the material (see Figure 7). All samples showed slight scratches and ruts along the direction of movement, as well as scattered pitting. The PU samples also showed partial delamination of the surface. Furthermore, partial smoothing of manufacturing marks could be found on the running surface of the PE samples. Pronounced backside wear was observed, particularly for the PU samples (Figure 7). The extent of the running surface and the strength of the backside wear were consistent with the wear rates.

To measure surface roughness, the parameters Sa and Sz were recorded. The measured roughness values are shown in Figure 8. The dynamically tested PU samples showed increased surface roughness of the running surface. The arithmetical mean height of the PE samples decreased while the maximum height stayed consistent, which was due to smoothing of the manufacturing marks. The PU1 material showed the highest roughness values. The soak control samples showed polished contact surfaces, and thus, reduced roughness compared to the initial state.

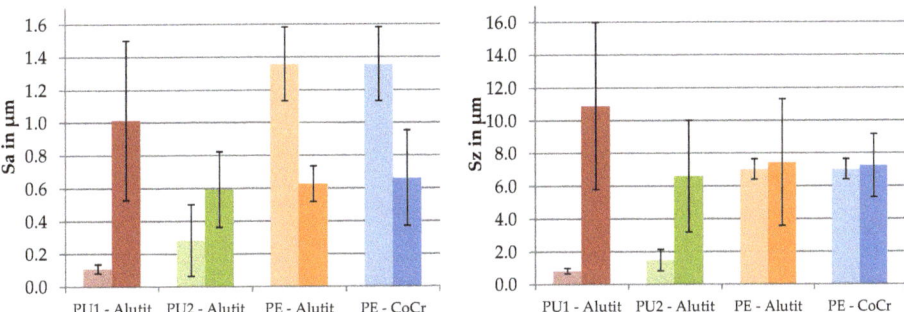

Figure 8. Surface roughness of the running surfaces of the tested samples before (left bars) and after (right bars) the wear test.

4. Discussion

Using the rolling-slide test bench described here, different knee implant materials with simple geometries can be tested under the physiological loading conditions of the knee joint. The applied force was adjusted in the test bench so that different tribological pairings could be tested at the same physiological contact pressure. Nevertheless, some limitations must be considered when using the test bench. The simplified geometries offer the advantage that new materials can initially be screened with an affordable cost and little effort. For further investigations, long-term tests in a wear simulator are required, which take into account realistic implant geometries. A further limitation is related to the simplification of the geometries, since there is a lack of anterior-posterior translation and rotational movements. Hence, no transverse motions can be generated, which are considered important for PE wear propagation [33,34]. However, because flexion and extension are the main directions of movement in the knee [3], this is only a minor limitation. In order to ensure consistent loading on the tested samples, both test chambers with samples have to be perfectly aligned under the test wheels of each station. Otherwise, station-related differences in the wear patterns may appear. Since congruent worn surfaces of the polymer samples could be observed in both stations after loading, an adequate alignment of both test chambers can be assumed. Likewise, during articulation, approximately one-third of the testing wheel surface was in contact with the running surface of the polymer samples in the two stations.

To prevent the results from being influenced by friction-related sample heating, various tribological situations (loading in a dry test chamber, loading in medium, static and dynamic loading, and loading at room temperature and with connected heating) were investigated in preliminary tests using a thermal imaging camera and temperature sensors. A maximum warming of 4 °C was detected only in the dry running test. Since no temperature differences of the PU sample were detected under lubricated test conditions with medium, the influence of friction on the temperature was considered to have a negligible effect. Temperature-dependent changes in sample volume during wear testing could be excluded. Furthermore, the rolling-sliding test bench allows only minor changes in the volume of samples.

Force curves according to ISO 14243–1 were adapted to the tested bearing material to simulate the same surface pressure that is present in the natural knee joint. In addition, load curves other than those from the ISO 14243–1 can be created, and, if necessary, they can be adapted to specific material and load cases. Higher loading or other gait patterns, such as stair climbs, can be implemented in the rolling-sliding test bench based on data derived from biomechanical studies [35]. Since native cartilage is a material with nonlinear behavior, the use of the Hertzian contact model as a contact model for the transmission of the physiologically acting contact pressure represents a limitation of our test bench. Since samples with linear material behavior are tested in this study and a complete simulation of the conditions in the native knee joint is not possible, we assume this simplification is suitable for the present study. Madeti et al. [36] has also used a Hertzian contact model to determine physiological surface pressure. An even more accurate determination of the surface contact pressure could be achieved using multibody models [37,38]. Hence, nonlinear material models for cartilage or acting muscle forces may be considered in future studies.

Since the developed soft PU materials showed high abrasive wear during preliminary tests, the PU samples were only tested over 1 million cycles instead of 5 million cycles, as recommended in ISO 14243–1. A high amount of wear is also reflected in the increased surface roughness of the PU samples. To exclude the influence of laser scanning on the sample material during the surface analysis, this was carried out only after wear testing of the samples was complete.

Since PE is an established bearing material in total knee arthroplasty, it was used as the reference material. In contrast to PU, no significant abrasive wear could be detected when the PE samples were loaded with 15.5 N or 16.5 N. To ensure comparability between PE and PU, the same force curve was used for all materials tested. Therefore, for the algorithmic estimation of condyle radius and contact length, we examined three datasets consisting of only female, only male, or both male and female data. We found that the radius and contact lengths for females are smaller than males by a few millimeters (radius ~2.5 mm, contact length ~4 mm). Hence, we considered only female data for the final evaluation because a lower radius and contact lengths, together with constant force, as specified by ISO 14243–1, result in a higher surface contact pressure (cf. Equation (1)). Implant materials should be designed not only for an average load situation, but also for severe conditions. Thus, by selecting appropriate datasets, the adjustment of applied forces to specific patient groups (for example, by age or sex) can be easily accomplished.

ISO 14243–1 specifies that the samples should be subjected to a load of more than 5 million cycles. Furthermore, due to running-in behavior, the abrasion rate should only be determined after 0.5 million cycles. The high wear rates of PU samples in the current study suggest that this material is not suitable as a direct bearing partner for a unicompartmental interpositional knee implant. Since no comparable wear studies on PU in the knee joint using physiological rolling-sliding movements have been carried out to date, it is not possible to classify the abrasive wear rates of PU materials. Our results were not consistent with the findings of Schwartz et al. [39], who showed lower wear rates for PU than for PE materials. However, a direct comparison of both studies is not possible due to non-comparable methods. We assume that the high wear rates of PU materials observed in the current study are related to the different properties of the material, and not the geometry of the test bench. The observed high wear rates were partly caused by pronounced backside wear of the PU materials. The wear patterns of the surface and backside of the samples correspond to the determined wear rates of the samples. On the PE samples, only polishing and smoothing of the manufactured surface was observed. The test wheels were able to sink much deeper into the PU samples during loading, which led to massive ruts in the direction of movement. Partial delamination of the PU surface was observed. However, we cannot conclude that the high backside wear and the high wear rates of the PU materials are caused only by abrasive wear and not adhesive wear. Nevertheless, PU could potentially be used in other human joints with reduced loading and friction, such as finger joints.

The rolling-sliding test bench was successfully established as a tribological testing method. In order to test even more samples in parallel, it would be useful to expand this test bench with additional stations. In contrast to a knee wear simulator according to ISO 14243–1, simplified implant geometries can be used in the rolling-sliding test bench. Hence, the effort required to produce test prototypes of new implant materials for the first abrasive wear screening is reduced. Due to the simplified implant geometry and design of the test bench, reduced lubricant volumes are required when compared to knee wear simulator tests. The reduction of the amount of lubricating fluid leads to additional cost savings. The wear data of the PU materials can be classified due to the direct comparison of their wear rates with a clinically established PE material. A comparative study using same bearing materials to compare our rolling-sliding test bench with the standard knee wear simulator should be carried out in further validation studies. Compared to other screening tests, such as those that use a tribometer, the rolling-sliding test bench allows testing under conditions that are more similar to physiological conditions. Further, the material of the sample and the material of the test wheel as well as the lubricating medium can be varied. For the rolling-sliding test bench, wear particles released from the material sample during testing can be isolated from the lubricant and analyzed according to ISO 14243–1.

5. Conclusions

The rolling-sliding test bench was successfully established through the application of load profiles adjusted to realistic contact pressures. The rolling-sliding test bench combines the advantages of screening and simulator tests, allowing for the testing of various bearing materials under physiological load and tribological conditions of the human knee joint. Therefore, both the wear behavior of different materials and the influence of the surface geometry and quality can be further investigated without the need to produce complex implant prototypes of total knee endoprosthesis or interpositional spacers. Hence, the test bench allows the suitability of new implant materials as bearing materials to be checked prior to further testing, where promising materials and surface modifications are subjected to advanced testing in a knee wear simulator in their final implant design.

Author Contributions: Conceptualization, J.H., F.A., S.Z. and R.B.; methodology, J.H. and F.A.; software, F.A.; validation, J.H.; formal analysis, J.H. and F.A.; investigation, J.H.; resources, S.Z. and R.B.; data curation, J.H. and F.A.; writing—original draft preparation, J.H. and F.A.; writing—review and editing, J.H., F.A., S.Z. and R.B.; visualization, J.H. and F.A.; supervision, S.Z. and R.B.; project administration, S.Z. and R.B.; funding acquisition, R.B. All authors have read and agreed to the published version of the manuscript.

Funding: This research was funded by the German Federal Ministry of Education and Research within the project TOKMIS (grant numbers 01EC1406F and 01EC1406E). This research did not receive any specific grant from commercial or not-for-profit sectors.

Institutional Review Board Statement: Not applicable.

Informed Consent Statement: Not applicable.

Data Availability Statement: Data is contained within the article.

Acknowledgments: We would like to thank the German Federal Ministry of Education and Research (BMBF) for facilitating the implementation of the TOKMIS project (grant numbers 01EC1406F and 01EC1406E) in addition to our project partners at the University of Applied Sciences, Reutlingen, for provision of the test samples. The authors thank the mechanical workshop of the Institute of Physics, University of Rostock, for manufacturing the components for the test bench and Mario Jackszis for his support with the installation and alignment of the test bench.

Conflicts of Interest: The authors declare no conflict of interest.

References

1. Drake, R.L.; Vogl, W.; Mitchell, A.W.M. *Drake, Gray's Anatomie SC*; Elsevier, Urban&FischerVerlag: Munich, Germany, 2007; ISBN 978-3-437-41231-8.
2. Krukemeyer, M.G.; Möllenhoff, G. *Endoprothetik: Ein Leitfaden für den Praktiker*, 3rd ed.; De Gruyter: Berlin, Germany, 2013; ISBN 978-3-11-028261-0.
3. Faller, A.; Schünke, M. *Der Körper des Menschen: Einführung in Bau und Funktion*; Georg Thieme Verlag: Stuttgart, Germany, 2016; ISBN 978-3-13-151957-3.
4. Nägerl, H.; Frosch, K.H.; Wachowski, M.M.; Dumont, C.; Abicht, C.; Adam, P.; Kubein-Meesenburg, D. A novel total knee replacement by rolling articulating surfaces. In vivo functional measurements and tests. *Acta Bioeng. Biomech.* **2008**, *10*, 55–60.
5. Abicht, C. *Artifical Knee Joints Following the Principle of a Four-Bar Linkage—Concept, Design and Tribological Properties of a New Natural Shaped Knee Endoprothesis*; Ernst-Moritz-Arndt-Universität, Medizinische Fakultät: Greifswald, Germany, 2006.

6. Kapandji, I.A.; Koebke, J. *Funktionelle Anatomie der Gelenke: Obere Extremität—Untere Extremität—Rumpf und Wirbelsäule*, 5th ed.; Georg Thieme Verlag: Stuttgart, Germany, 2009; ISBN 978-3-13-142215-6.
7. Goebel, P.; Zietz, C.; Bieck, R.; Kluess, D.; Bader, R. A novel method for tribological evaluation of bearing materials in total knee replacements. *Biomed. Tech. Eng.* **2012**, *57*. [CrossRef]
8. Robertsson, O.; Lidgren, L.; Sundberg, M.; W-Dahl, A. *The Swedish Knee Arthroplasty Register—Annual Report 2018*; Lund University Department of Clinical Sciences, Orthopedics Skåne University Hospital: Holmgrens, Malmö, Sweden, 2019.
9. Abu-Amer, Y.; Darwech, I.; Clohisy, J.C. Aseptic loosening of total joint replacements: Mechanisms underlying osteolysis and potential therapies. *Arthritis Res. Ther.* **2007**, *9*, S6. [CrossRef]
10. Kretzer, J.; Zietz, C.; Schröder, C.; Reinders, J.; Middelborg, L.; Paulus, A.; Sonntag, R.; Bader, R.; Utzschneider, S. Grundlagen zur tribologischen Analyse von Endoprothesen. *Der Orthopäde* **2012**, *41*, 844–852. [CrossRef]
11. I Richter, B.; Ostermeier, S.; Turger, A.; Denkena, B.; Hurschler, C. A rolling-gliding wear simulator for the investigation of tribological material pairings for application in total knee arthroplasty. *Biomed. Eng. Online* **2010**, *9*, 24. [CrossRef]
12. Van Citters, D.W.; Kennedy, F.E.; Currier, J.H.; Collier, J.P.; Nichols, T.D. A Multi-Station Rolling/Sliding Tribotester for Knee Bearing Materials. *J. Tribol.* **2004**, *126*, 380–385. [CrossRef]
13. Van Citters, D.W.; Kennedy, F.E.; Collier, J.P. Rolling sliding wear of UHMWPE for knee bearing applications. *Wear* **2007**, *263*, 1087–1094. [CrossRef]
14. Wieser, J. Testung Unterschiedlicher Polyethylene im Roll-Gleit-Prüfstand. Text. Ph.D. Thesis, Ludwig-Maximilians-Universität München, Munich, Germany, 2014.
15. ISO 14243-1:2009 Implants for Surgery—Wear of Total Knee-Joint Prostheses—Part 1: Loading and Displacement Parameters for Wear-Testing Machines with Load Control and Corresponding Environmental Conditions for Test. Available online: https://www.iso.org/cms/render/live/en/sites/isoorg/contents/data/standard/04/42/44262.html (accessed on 18 June 2020).
16. Schwitalle, M.; Just, A.; Mark, T.; Bodem, F.; Schwitalle, E.; Koller, S. Kinematische Analyse vor und nach bikondylaerem Oberflaechenersatz des Kniegelenks. *Der Orthopäde* **2003**, *32*, 266–273. [CrossRef]
17. Kutuzova, L.; Athanasopulu, K.; Schneider, M.; Kandelbauer, A.; Lorenz, G.; Kemkemer, R. In vitro bio-stability screening of novel implantable polyurethane elastomers. *Curr. Dir. Biomed. Eng.* **2018**, *4*, 535–538. [CrossRef]
18. Athanasopulu, K.; Kutuzova, L.; Thiel, J.; Lorenz, G.; Kemkemer, R. Enhancing the biocompatibility of siliconepolycarbonate urethane based implant materials. *Curr. Dir. Biomed. Eng.* **2019**, *5*, 453–455. [CrossRef]
19. Heller, M.O.; Taylor, W.R.; Perka, C.; Duda, G.N. The influence of alignment on the musculo-skeletal loading conditions at the knee. *Langenbeck's Arch. Surg.* **2003**, *388*, 291–297. [CrossRef] [PubMed]
20. Hayes, W.C.; Mockros, L.F. Viscoelastic properties of human articular cartilage. *J. Appl. Physiol.* **1971**, *31*, 562–568. [CrossRef]
21. Adams, J.; McAlindon, T.; Dimasi, M.; Carey, J.; Eustace, S. Contribution of meniscal extrusion and cartilage loss to joint space narrowing in osteoarthritis. *Clin. Radiol.* **1999**, *54*, 502–506. [CrossRef]
22. Ambellan, F.; Tack, A.; Ehlke, M.; Zachow, S. Automated segmentation of knee bone and cartilage combining statistical shape knowledge and convolutional neural networks: Data from the Osteoarthritis Initiative. *Med Image Anal.* **2019**, *52*, 109–118. [CrossRef] [PubMed]
23. Ambellan, F.; Lamecker, H.; Von Tycowicz, C.; Zachow, S. Statistical Shape Models: Understanding and Mastering Variation in Anatomy. In *Advances in Experimental Medicine and Biology*; Springer International Publishing: Basel, Switzerland, 2019; Volume 1156, pp. 67–84.
24. Howell, S.M.; Howell, S.J.; Hull, M.L. Assessment of the Radii of the Medial and Lateral Femoral Condyles in Varus and Valgus Knees with Osteoarthritis. *J. Bone Jt. Surg.-Am. Vol.* **2010**, *92*, 98–104. [CrossRef] [PubMed]
25. Sancisi, N.; Parenti-Castelli, V. A sequentially-defined stiffness model of the knee. *Mech. Mach. Theory* **2011**, *46*, 1920–1928. [CrossRef]
26. Schultze, C.; Klüss, D.; Martin, H.; Hingst, V.; Mittelmeier, W.; Schmitz, K.-P.; Bader, R. Finite-Elemente-Analyse einer zementierten, keramischen Femurkomponente unter Berücksichtigung der Einbausituation bei künstlichem Kniegelenksersatz/Finite element analysis of a cemented ceramic femoral component for the assembly situation in total knee arthroplasty. *Biomed. Tech. Eng.* **2007**, *52*, 301–307. [CrossRef]
27. Mattei, L.; Di Puccio, F.; Piccigallo, B.; Ciulli, E. Lubrication and wear modelling of artificial hip joints: A review. *Tribol. Int.* **2011**, *44*, 532–549. [CrossRef]
28. Kluess, D.; Martin, H.; Mittelmeier, W.; Schmitz, K.-P.; Bader, R. Influence of femoral head size on impingement, dislocation and stress distribution in total hip replacement. *Med Eng. Phys.* **2007**, *29*, 465–471. [CrossRef]
29. Eichmiller, F.; Tesk, J.A.; Croarkin, C.M. Mechanical Properties of Ultra High Molecular Weight Polyethylene NIST Reference Material RM 8456. *Soc. Biomater.* **2001**, *22*, 6.
30. ISO 14243-2:2009 Implants for Surgery—Wear of Total Knee-Joint Prostheses—Part 2: Methods of Measurement. Available online: https://www.iso.org/standard/69851.html (accessed on 18 June 2020).
31. DIN EN ISO 4288:1998 Geometrische Produktspezifikation (GPS)—Oberflächenbeschaffenheit: Tastschnittverfahren—Regeln und Verfahren für die Beurteilung der Oberflächenbeschaffenheit (ISO 4288:1996); Beuth Verlag: Berlin, Germany, 1998. [CrossRef]
32. DIN EN ISO 3274:1998 Geometrische Produktspezifikationen (GPS)—Oberflächenbeschaffenheit: Tastschnittverfahren—Nenneigenschaften von Tastschnittgeräten (ISO 3274:1996); Beuth Verlag: Berlin, Germany, 1998. [CrossRef]

33. Jin, Z.; Fisher, J. Tribology in joint replacement*Note: This chapter is an updated version of Chapter 2, from the first edition of Joint replacement technology, edited by P. A. Revell and published by Woodhead Publishing, 2008*. *Jt. Replace. Technol.* **2014**, 31–61. [CrossRef]
34. Sivananthan, S.; Goodman, S.; Burke, M. Failure mechanisms in joint replacement**Note: This chapter is an updated version of Chapter 12, from the first edition of Joint replacement technology, edited by P. A. Revell and published by Woodhead Publishing, 2008. *Jt. Replace. Technol.* **2014**, 370–400. [CrossRef]
35. Taylor, W.R.; Heller, M.O.; Bergmann, G.; Duda, G.N. Tibio-femoral loading during human gait and stair climbing. *J. Orthop. Res.* **2004**, *22*, 625–632. [CrossRef] [PubMed]
36. Madeti, B.K.; Rao, C.S.; Rao, B.S.S. Failure analysis of ACL and Hertz contact stress in human knee. *Int. J. Biomed. Eng. Technol.* **2014**, *16*, 317. [CrossRef]
37. Machado, M.; Flores, P.; Claro, J.C.P.; Ambrósio, J.; Silva, M.; Completo, A.; Lankarani, H.M. Development of a planar multibody model of the human knee joint. *Nonlinear Dyn.* **2010**, *60*, 459–478. [CrossRef]
38. Khoshgoftar, M.; Vrancken, A.; Van Tienen, T.; Buma, P.; Janssen, D.; Verdonschot, N. The sensitivity of cartilage contact pressures in the knee joint to the size and shape of an anatomically shaped meniscal implant. *J. Biomech.* **2015**, *48*, 1427–1435. [CrossRef]
39. Schwartz, C.J.; Bahadur, S. Development and testing of a novel joint wear simulator and investigation of the viability of an elastomeric polyurethane for total-joint arthroplasty devices. *Wear* **2007**, *262*, 331–339. [CrossRef]

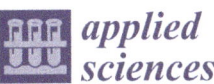

Article

Partial Threading of Pedicle Screws in a Standard Construct Increases Fatigue Life: A Biomechanical Analysis

Fon-Yih Tsuang [1], Chia-Hsien Chen [2,3], Lien-Chen Wu [2,3], Yi-Jie Kuo [4,5], Yueh-Ying Hsieh [2,5] and Chang-Jung Chiang [2,5,*]

[1] Department of Surgery, Division of Neurosurgery, National Taiwan University Hospital, Taipei City 10022, Taiwan; tsuangfy@ntu.edu.tw
[2] Department of Orthopedics, Shuang Ho Hospital, Taipei Medical University, New Taipei City 23561, Taiwan; chiaxian@tmu.edu.tw (C.-H.C.); d98548019@tmu.edu.tw (L.-C.W.); 11154@s.tmu.edu.tw (Y.-Y.H.)
[3] Graduate Institute of Biomedical Materials and Tissue Engineering, College of Biomedical Engineering, Taipei Medical University, Taipei City 11031, Taiwan
[4] Department of Orthopedic Surgery, Taipei Municipal Wanfang Hospital, Taipei Medical University, Taipei City 116, Taiwan; benkuo5@tmu.edu.tw
[5] Department of Orthopedic Surgery, School of Medicine, College of Medicine, Taipei Medical University, Taipei City 110, Taiwan
* Correspondence: cjchiang@s.tmu.edu.tw

Abstract: This study proposed a pedicle screw design where the proximal 1/3 of the screw is unthreaded to improve fixation in posterior spinal surgery. This design was also expected to reduce the incidence of mechanical failure often observed when an unsupported screw length is exposed outside the vertebra in deformed or degenerated segments. The aim of this study was to evaluate the fatigue life of the novel pedicle screw design using finite element analysis and mechanical testing in a synthetic spinal construct in accordance with American Society for Testing and Materials (ASTM) F1717. The following setups were evaluated: (i) pedicle screw fully inserted into the test block (EXP-FT-01 and EXP-PU-01; full thread (FT), proximal unthread (PU)) and (ii) pedicle screw inserted but leaving an exposed shaft length of 7.6 mm (EXP-FT-02 and EXP-PU-02). Corresponding finite element models FEM-FT-01, FEM-FT-02, FEM-PU-01, and FEM-PU-02 were also constructed and subjected to the same loading conditions as the experimental groups. The results showed that under a 220 N axial load, the EXP-PU-01 group survived the full 5 million cycles, the EXP-PU-02 group failed at 4.4 million cycles on average, and both EXP-FT-01 and EXP-FT-02 groups failed after less than 1.0 million cycles on average, while the fatigue strength of the EXP-FT-02 group was the lowest at 170 N. The EXP-FT-01 and EXP-FT-02 constructs failed through fracture of the pedicle screw, but a rod fractured in the EXP-PU-02 group. In comparison to the FEM-FT-01 model, the maximum von Mises stress on the pedicle screw in the FEM-PU-01 and FEM-PU-02 models decreased by −43% and −27%, respectively. In conclusion, this study showed that having the proximal 1/3 of the pedicle screw unthreaded can reduce the risk of screw fatigue failure when used in deformed or degenerated segments.

Keywords: pedicle screws; partial threading; fatigue life; biomechanical analysis; spinal fixation

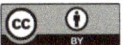

1. Introduction

The primary function of pedicle screw systems is to maintain spinal stability while fusion occurs. However, in weakened or osteoporotic bone, the bone–screw interface is often poor and prone to failure, resulting in screw loosening or back-out after surgery. Transpedicular instrumentation in patients with osteoporosis is difficult because of the challenge in achieving sufficient fixation strength. In addition, biomechanical studies have shown a reduction in the pull-out strength of pedicle screws in osteoporotic bone, which can ultimately lead to failure of internal fixation [1–3]. As such, fixation problems are common in patients suffering from osteoporosis, and gaining sufficient pedicle screw fixation is a major challenge for spinal surgeons. Loosening of pedicle screws is a leading cause of non-union, pseudarthrosis, and back pain after surgery.

One method to improve the interface strength between pedicle screws and surrounding bone in osteoporotic patients is to use a bone-cement-augmented pedicle screw, which has been shown to increase the pull-out strength [4–6]. However, complications such as cement leakage outside the vertebral body and difficulty in removing the fixed screw have been reported. Symptomatic cement leakage with augmented screws has been reported at up to 17% [7,8], while Mueller et al. indicated that periverterbral cement leakage occurs in 73.3% of cases, but most are clinically asymptomatic [9]. Besides cement augmentation, changing the screw design, including diameter, length, and thread design, may be used to improve fixation [10–13]. Because the holding power of the bone–screw interface is poor in osteoporosis, increasing the diameter of the screw may improve fixation and stability [14]. However, the maximum diameter of the screw is limited by the anatomical shape of the pedicle, and so the viable size range for the screw is limited.

A previous study by the authors demonstrated that having the proximal 1/3 of the pedicle screw left unthreaded significantly improves the pull-out strength and withdrawal force in comparison to a fully threaded screw [15]. The authors considered that this novel screw design could also improve the fatigue life of the pedicle screw in cases where only partial screw insertion is required [16]. Hence, this study aimed to evaluate the fatigue life and stress distribution of proximally unthreaded screws in accordance with American Society for Testing and Materials (ASTM) F1717 [17] and using finite element analysis. The results were compared with those obtained from fully threaded pedicle screws.

2. Materials and Methods

2.1. Mechanical Fatigue Testing

The test constructs were subjected to fatigue testing through dynamic bending in accordance with ASTM F1717. As shown in Figure 1a, each construct consisted of four pedicle screws (Ti-6Al-4V, 4.0 mm diameter, 30 mm length) and two titanium rods (Ti-6Al-4V, 5.5 mm diameter, 120 mm length) inserted into ultra-high molecular weight polyethylene (UHMWPE) test blocks to simulate a vertebrectomy. Both fully threaded (FT) and partially unthreaded (PU) pedicle screws were tested, and the screws and rods had been pre-treated by sandblasting and anodization. For the fatigue test, the UWMWPE blocks were clamped in an MTS 370 machine (MTS Systems Corporation, Eden Prairie, MN, USA) and a compressive force applied.

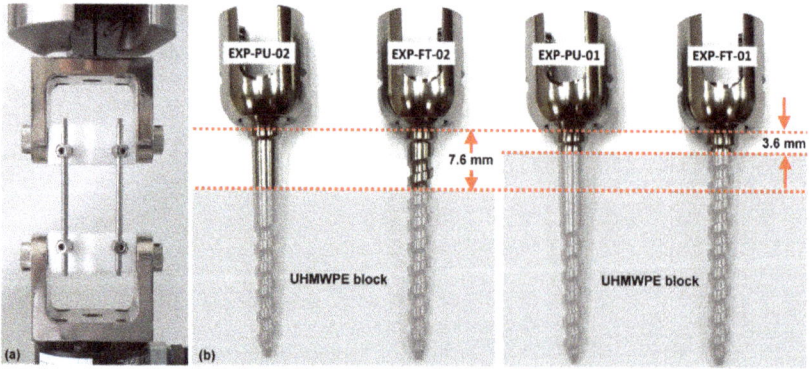

Figure 1. (a) American Society for Testing and Materials (ASTM) F1717 standard configuration. (b) Two different setups were evaluated: (i) pedicle screw fully inserted into the test block with an exposed length of 3.6 mm (EXP-FT-01 and EXP-PU-01) and (ii) pedicle screw inserted leaving 7.6 mm of the screw shaft exposed (EXP-FT-02 and EXP-PU-02).

A previous study by our institute [16] determined the critical condition for pedicle screw insertion as having the threaded portion exposed by 1 or 2 threads to accommodate rod placement and ensure alignment between the tulip of the screw and the rod. Two different setups were evaluated (Figure 1b): (i) pedicle screw fully inserted into the test block with an exposed length of 3.6 mm [16] (EXP-FT-01 and EXP-PU-01) and (ii) pedicle screw inserted leaving 7.6 mm [16] of the screw shaft exposed (EXP-FT-02 and EXP-PU-02).

Loading was applied in a cyclic sine wave at a frequency of 5 Hz with a load ratio of 0.1 (minimum load divided by maximum load). Static testing was first used to determine the ultimate load for the EXP-FT-01 model as 340 N [16]. In accordance with ASTM F1717, loading for fatigue testing should begin at 50% of the ultimate load, which is 170 N for the EXP-FT-01 construct. Therefore, for all test setups (Figure 1b), loading began at 170 N and was incrementally increased after every third sample (170 N to 190 N to 220 N) until either the construct underwent permanent deformation or failed or the number of cycles reached 5,000,000 cycles. Otherwise, the load level was decreased every 3 samples until sample run-out. The maximum and minimum loads and the number of cycles sustained were used to calculate the fatigue strength for each test setup.

2.2. Finite Element Models

Four finite element models (FEM-FT-01, FEM-FT-02, FEM-PU-01, and FEM-PU-02) were created using the same boundary and loading conditions as the experimental fatigue test setup detailed above (Figure 2a,b). A vertical load was applied to the analytically rigid surface, which was inserted within the horizontal hole of the UHMWPE test block; the lower rigid surface was fixed [16]. These two rigid surfaces were assumed to have a frictionless contact with the test block. The contact interface between the screws and rods was bonded [18,19]. All meshing and simulations were conducted using ANSYS 16.0 (ANSYS Inc., Park City, UT, USA). The pedicle screws, support rods, and UHMWPE test blocks were modeled as linearly elastic materials with the properties detailed in Table 1 [16]. The rods were meshed using eight-node hexahedral elements, and the screws used four-node tetrahedral elements. A mesh sensitivity study was performed to ensure the convergence of the mesh solution. The final model had 72,471 elements in each rod, 38,541 elements in each fully threaded polyaxial screw (8582 and 30,059 for the head and body, respectively), and 36,437 elements in each proximally unthreaded polyaxial screw (8582 and 27,855 for the head and body, respectively). The UHMWPE block in the FEM-FT-01 and FEM-PU-01 models had 61,059 elements, and in the FEM-FT-02 and FEM-PU-02 models had 55,832 elements (Table 2). When placed under a 170 N vertical load, the mesh was assumed to converge when the change in von Mises stress on the screws and rods was less than 2%.

Table 1. Material properties of finite element models.

	Modulus (MPa)	v
Ultra-high molecular weight polyethylene (UHMWPE) blocks [16]	1050	0.4
Titanium rods [16]	110,000	0.3
Titanium pedicle screws [16]	110,000	0.3

The FEM-FT-01 model was validated by demonstrating that the stiffness of the entire model (43.18 N/mm) was within the range of experimental data (42.78–43.72 N/mm), as shown in Figure 2c.

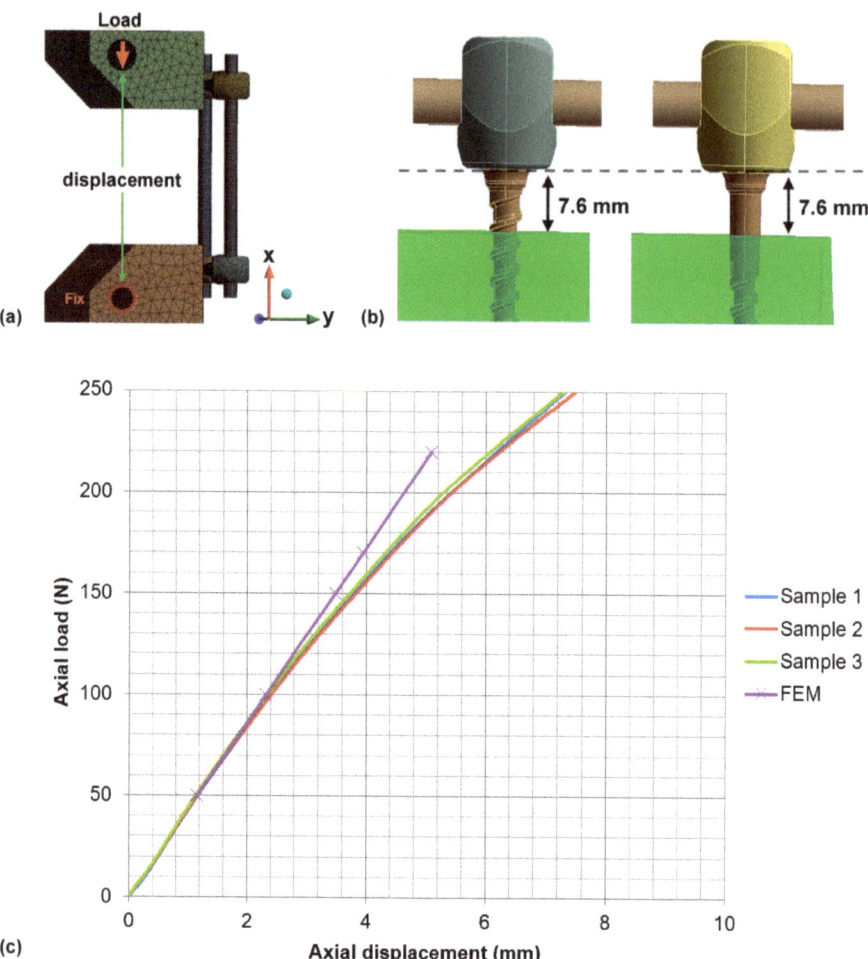

Figure 2. (**a**) Finite element model in accordance with ASTM F1717 standard configuration. (**b**) Pedicle screw inserted leaving 7.6 mm unsupported length (FEM-FT-02 and FEM-PU-02). (**c**) The axial displacement and load curve of experimental data of EXP-FT-01 and finite element model FEM-FT-01.

Table 2. Type of elements, number of elements, and nodes in each part of the finite element models.

	Fully Threaded Polyaxial Screw (Head/Body)	Proximally Unthreaded Polyaxial Screw (Head/Body)	UHMWPE Block of FEM-FT-01 and FEM-PU-01	UHMWPE Block of FEM-FT-02 and FEM-PU-02	Rod
Type of elements	4-node tetrahedral				8-node hexahedron
Number of elements	8582/30,059	8582/27,855	61,059	55,832	72,471
Number of nodes	15,448/54,407	15,448/49,582	109,296	99,381	289,878

3. Results

3.1. Dynamic Compression Bending Test

Table 3 details the results of the dynamic bending compression test. The EXP-PU-01 construct was found to have the greatest fatigue strength of 220 N, while both the EXP-FT-01 and EXP-PU-02 groups had a lower fatigue strength of 190 N. In the fully threaded (FT) groups, the screw failed where it inserted into the UHMWPE block, whereas it was the rod that failed in the proximally unthreaded (PU) groups (Figure 3). Under a maximum load of 190 N, one sample from the EXP-PU-02 group survived to run-out (>5,000,000 cycles), which was superior to the EXP-FT-02 group, which had an average cycle count of 1,116,787 cycles.

Table 3. Results of the dynamic compression bending test.

Min. and Max. of Axial Force	17–170 (N)		19–190 (N)		22–220 (N)	
Group	No. of samples	Cycles	No. of samples	Cycles	No. of samples	cycles
EXP-FT-01	1	Run-out	4	Run-out	7	719,021 *
	2	Run-out	5	Run-out	8	791,733 *
	3	Run-out	6	Run-out	9	736,885 *
EXP-FT-02	10	Run-out	13	1,361,467 *	16	18,209 *
	11	Run-out	14	971,656 *	17	21,779 *
	12	Run-out	15	1,017,237 *	18	7562 *
EXP-PU-01	19	Run-out	22	Run-out	25	Run-out
	20	Run-out	23	Run-out	26	Run-out
	21	Run-out	24	Run-out	27	Run-out
EXP-PU-02	28	Run-out	31	Run-out	34	4,152,887 **
	29	Run-out	32	Run-out	35	4,001,455 **
	30	Run-out	33	Run-out	36	Run-out

* Pedicle screw fracture; ** rod fracture; run-out: run out at 5 million cycles.

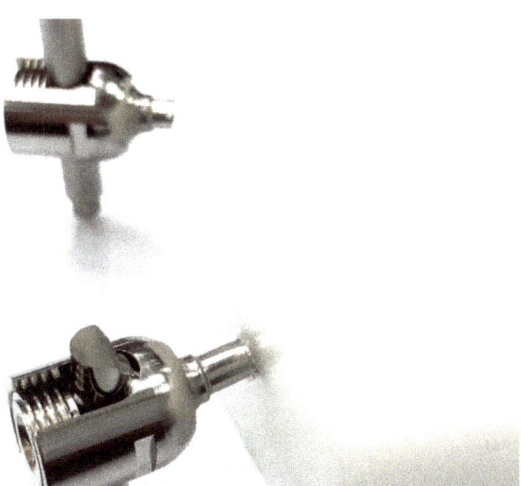

Figure 3. Rod failed in the proximally unthreaded (PU) groups in the dynamic compression bending test.

3.2. Maximum Von Mises Stress on Pedicle Screw and Rod

The maximum von Mises stress on the screws in the computational models appeared at the region where the screws entered the UHMWPE blocks (Figure 4a). The von Mises stress on the pedicle screws was recorded as 677.23 MPa, 1070.91 MPa, 385.809 MPa, and 491.50 MPa in the FEM-FT-01, FEM-FT-02, FEM-PU-01, and FEM-PU-02 models, respectively, when placed under an axial force of 170 N. When the load was increased to 220 N, the FEM-FT-02 model showed the highest von Mises stress on the pedicle screws (Table 4). For the rod component in the FEM-FT-01, FEM-FT-02, FEM-PU-01, and FEM-PU-02 models, the maximum von Mises stress was 341.66 MPa, 369.67 MPa, 361.36 MPa, and 362.24 MPa, respectively, under a 170 N axial load, and the maximum value occurred at the interface between screw and rod. When the load was increased to 220 N, the FEM-FT-02 model showed the highest von Mises stress on the rods (Figure 4b and Table 5). The maximum von Mises stress on the pedicle screws in the FEM-PU-01 and FEM-PU-02 models was 43% and 54% less than that in the FEM-FT-01 and FEM-FT-02 models, respectively, while the maximum von Mises stress on the rod component decreased by 1.4% in both models. The stiffness of the FEM-PU-01 (45.09 N/mm) and FEM-PU-02 (30.09 N/mm) models increased by 4.4% and 14.2%, respectively, in comparison to the FEM-FT-01 (43.18 N/mm) and FEM-FT-02 (26.34 N/mm) models. The stiffness of all FEM models was found to be similar to the results from the mechanical fatigue test (EXP-FT-01: 42.48 ± 0.42 N/mm; EXP-FT-02: 26.69 ± 0.63 N/mm; EXP-PU-01: 44.96 ± 0.71 N/mm; EXP-PU-02: 29.52 ± 0.93 N/mm).

Table 4. Maximum von Mises stress on pedicle screws.

Axial Force (N)	170	220
Screw of FEM-FT-01 (MPa)	677.23	875.23
Screw of FEM-FT-02 (MPa)	1070.91	1384.01
Screw of FEM-PU-01 (MPa)	385.89	498.71
Screw of FEM-PU-02 (MPa)	491.5	635.20

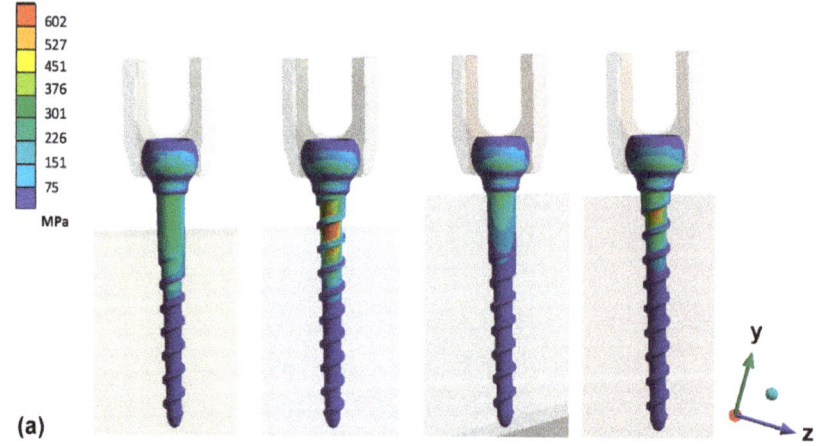

(a)

Figure 4. Cont.

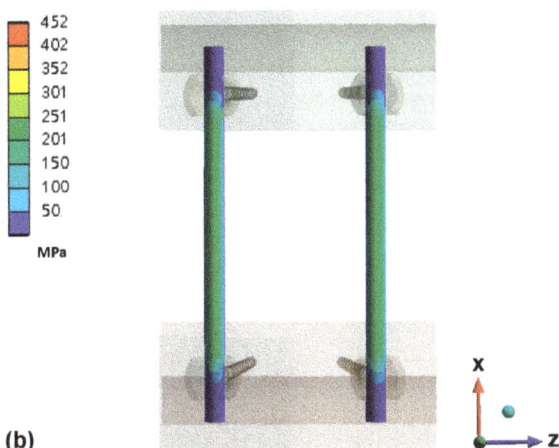

Figure 4. The distribution of the maximum von Mises stress on (**a**) pedicle screws of four models and (**b**) rods of the FEM-FT-01 model under 170 N axial loading.

Table 5. Maximum von Mises stress on rods.

Axial Force (N)	170	220
Rod of FEM-FT-01 (MPa)	341.66	440.12
Rod of FEM-FT-02 (MPa)	369.67	475.36
Rod of FEM-PU-01 (MPa)	361.36	465.49
Rod of FEM-PU-02 (MPa)	362.24	468.78

4. Discussion

Fracture of pedicle screws can lead to considerable complications in the spine, such as loss of curvature and symptomatic pseudarthrosis, which often requires reoperation. Screw fracture mostly occurs following high-energy impact injuries or metal fatigue from repetitive stress. Chu et al. [16] demonstrated a reduction in the fatigue life and strength of pedicle screws when a portion of the screw threads was left exposed outside of the bone. This is echoed in the results of this study, where the EXP-FT-02 construct clearly had the lowest fatigue strength of all groups. However, Table 3 also shows that by omitting threads from the exposed portion of the screw (1/3 proximally unthreaded), the fatigue strength increased in comparison to a fully threaded screw.

It is worth noting that the fatigue life of EXP-PU-02 was higher than EXP-FT-01, signifying that the fatigue strength of the proximally unthreaded (PU) screw when not fully inserted is higher than the fully threaded (FT) screw when fully inserted into the test block. In addition, whereas the construct with fully threaded screws failed through screw fracture, the construct with PU screws failed by fracture of the rods. This shows that the unthreaded portion (shank) of the PU screw plays an important role in the fatigue life and supports the hypothesis of this study that the fatigue strength would be superior to a fully threaded screw. A possible contributing factor to the greater fatigue strength is the diameter of the screw. The smooth shank on the PU screw had a diameter of 4.0 mm, whereas the inner/minor diameter of the fully threaded screw was 3.0 mm. The second axial moment of area of the PU screw was greater than the fully threaded screw at the point where the screws entered the test block. This might contribute to the better fatigue bending strength.

According to Chen et al. [20], the most stressed site on a pedicle screw is the junction between the shank and threads, and the threads at the screw–bone interface tend to be less stressed than threads outside the interface. This is consistent with the findings of this study. Whether considering the FT or PU screw, the major stress occurred on the proximal part of screw, and the maximum von Mises stress occurred at the interface between the screw and the block. In all of the FT screw groups, the maximum von Mises stress on the screw exceeded that on the rod. Previous studies [20–22] have demonstrated an increase in stress at the screw head and a loss in fatigue strength with increasing unsupported screw length, which is consistent with the findings of this study. The FE model demonstrated that in comparison to the FT screw, the PU screw design produced a lower maximum von Mises stress on the screw and provided superior fatigue strength when partially inserted. This was supported by the fact that it was the rod rather than the screw that fractured during the dynamical compression test.

Despite the clearly superior results obtained from the proximally unthreaded screw in this study, there are some limitations to the methods used. (i) The vertebrectomy model was developed in compliance with ASTM F1717, which is the correct approach to use for this form of study [22–24]. However, the simplifications incorporated into any such model cannot truly represent the multidirectional loading conditions in a normal human spine. (ii) Similarly, the finite element models were subjected to a single vertical load on a specific point on the test block to validate the models, but again this is a gross simplification against in vivo conditions in the spine. Future studies may consider incorporating a wider range of forces. The computational model was also simplified to assign all constructs with linearly elastic homogeneous isotropic properties with all contact interfaces bonded. These assumptions are simplifications of the real situation, where the insertion of the pedicle screw within the UHMWPE block would produce an initial residual stress/damage on the surrounding of the UHMWPE block (plastic deformed) [23], which increased the displacement in the experiments and showed non-linear behavior (Figure 2c). These assumptions also result in a stiffer construct and linear behavior of load displacement in the finite element model, as shown in Figure 2c. (iii) Different screw sizes or thread designs were also not considered in this study because the primary goal was to analyze how incomplete insertion of the proximally unthreaded pedicle screw compared to a standard fully threaded pedicle screw in terms of stress and fatigue life.

5. Conclusions

The results of this study show that the 1/3 proximally unthreaded (PU) pedicle screw design offers superior fatigue strength and fatigue life over a traditional fully threaded pedicle screw during both partial and full insertion. The PU pedicle screw can not only reduce the risk of screw fatigue failure but also increase implant survival when used in deformed or degenerated segments where the pedicle screws need to be exposed by one or multiple threads to accommodate rod placement.

Author Contributions: Conceptualization, F.-Y.T., C.-H.C. and C.-J.C.; methodology, F.-Y.T., Y.-J.K. and Y.-Y.H.; project administration, C.-H.C. and C.-J.C.; resources, C.-H.C. and L.-C.W.; software, F.-Y.T. and L.-C.W.; validation, F.-Y.T., C.-H.C., Y.-J.K. and C.-J.C.; writing—original draft, F.-Y.T.; writing—review and editing, F.-Y.T., Y.-J.K. and C.-J.C. All authors have read and agreed to the published version of the manuscript.

Funding: This research received no external funding.

Institutional Review Board Statement: Not applicable.

Informed Consent Statement: Not applicable.

Data Availability Statement: All relevant data are within the manuscript.

Acknowledgments: Not applicable.

Conflicts of Interest: The authors declare no conflict of interest.

References

1. Dvorak, M.F.; Pitzen, T.; Zhu, Q.; Gordon, J.D.; Fisher, C.G.; Oxland, T.R. Anterior cervicalplate fixation: A biomechanical study to evaluate the effects of plate design, endplate preparation, and bone mineral density. *Spine* **2005**, *30*, 294–301. [CrossRef]
2. Ramaswamy, R.; Evans, S.; Kosashvili, Y. Holding power of variable pitch screws inosteoporotic, osteopenic and normal bone: Are all screws created equal? *Injury* **2010**, *41*, 179–183. [CrossRef]
3. Halvorson, T.L.; Kelley, L.A.; Thomas, K.A.; Whitecloud, T.S., III; Cook, S.D. Effects of bone mineral density on pedicle screw fixation. *Spine* **1994**, *19*, 2415–2420. [CrossRef]
4. Lattig, F. Bone cement augmentation in the prevention of adjacent segment failure after multilevel adult deformity fusion. *J. Spinal Disord. Tech.* **2009**, *22*, 439–443. [CrossRef] [PubMed]
5. Par'e, P.E.; Chappuis, J.L.; Rampersaud, R.; Agarwala, A.O.; Perra, J.H.; Erkan, S.; Wu, C. Biomechanical evaluation of a novel fenestrated pedicle screw augmented with bone cement in osteoporotic spines. *Spine* **2011**, *36*, E1210–E1214. [CrossRef]
6. Kayanja, M.; Evans, K.; Milks, R.; Lieberman, I.H. The mechanics of polymethyl-methacrylate augmentation. *Clin. Orthop. Relat. Res.* **2006**, *443*, 124–130. [CrossRef]
7. Chen, L.-H.; Tai, C.-L.; Lai, P.-L.; Lee, D.-M.; Tsai, T.-T.; Fu, T.-S.; Niu, C.-C.; Chen, W.-J. Pullout strength for cannulated pedicle screws with bone cement augmentation in severely osteoporotic bone: Influences of radial hole and pilot hole tapping. *Clin. Biomech.* **2009**, *24*, 613–618. [CrossRef]
8. Klingler, J.-H.; Scholz, C.; Kogias, E.; Sircar, R.; Krüger, M.T.; Volz, F.; Scheiwe, C.; Hubbe, U. Minimally Invasive Technique for PMMA Augmentation of Fenestrated Screws. *Sci. World J.* **2015**, *2015*, 1–7. [CrossRef] [PubMed]
9. Mueller, J.U.; Baldauf, J.; Marx, S.; Kirsch, M.; Schroeder, H.W.; Pillich, D.T. Cement leakage in pedicle screw augmentation: A pro-spective analysis of 98 patients and 474 augmented pedicle screws. *J. Neurosurg. Spine* **2016**, *25*, 103–109. [CrossRef] [PubMed]
10. Patel, P.S.; Shepherd, D.E.; Hukins, D.W. The effect of screw insertion angle and thread type on the pullout strength of bone screws in normal and osteoporotic cancellous bone models. *Med. Eng. Phys.* **2010**, *32*, 822–828. [CrossRef] [PubMed]
11. Zindrick, M.R.; Wiltse, L.L.; Widell, E.H.; Thomas, J.C.; Holland, W.R.; Field, B.T.; Spencer, C.W. A biomechanical study of intrapeduncular screw fixation in the lumbosacral spine. *Clin. Orthop. Relat. Res.* **1986**, *203*, 99–112. [CrossRef]
12. Weinstein, J.N.; Rydevik, B.L.; Rauschning, W. Anatomic and technical considerations of pedicle screw fixation. *Clin. Orthop. Relat. Res.* **1992**, *284*, 34–46. [CrossRef]
13. Krenn, M.H.; Piotrowski, W.P.; Penzkofer, R.; Augat, P. Influence of thread design on pedicle screwfixation: Laboratory investigation. *J. Neurosurg. Spine* **2008**, *9*, 90–95. [CrossRef]
14. Varghese, V.; Krishnan, V.; Kumar, G.S. Comparison of pullout strength of pedicle screws following revision using larger di-ameter screws. *Med. Eng. Phys.* **2019**, *74*, 180–185. [CrossRef] [PubMed]
15. Tsuang, F.-Y.; Chen, C.-H.; Wu, L.-C.; Kuo, Y.-J.; Lin, S.-C.; Chiang, C.-J. Biomechanical arrangement of threaded and unthreaded portions providing holding power of transpedicular screw fixation. *Clin. Biomech.* **2016**, *39*, 71–76. [CrossRef] [PubMed]
16. Chu, Y.L.; Chen, C.H.; Tsuang, F.Y.; Chiang, C.J.; Wu, Y.; Kuo, Y.J. Incomplete insertion of pedicle screws in a standard construct re-duces the fatigue life: A biomechanical analysis. *PLoS ONE* **2019**, *14*, e0224699. [CrossRef] [PubMed]
17. ASTM F1717-18. Standard Test Methods for Spinal Implant Constructs in a Vertebrectomy Model. ASTM Int West Con-Shohocken, PA [Internet], 2018; pp. 1–16. Available online: https://www.astm.org/Standards/F1717.htm (accessed on 11 March 2019).
18. Galbusera, F.; Schmidt, H.; Wilke, H.-J. Lumbar interbody fusion: A parametric investigation of a novel cage design with and without posterior instrumentation. *Eur. Spine J.* **2011**, *21*, 455–462. [CrossRef]
19. Schmidt, H.; Heuer, F.; Wilke, H.-J. Which axial and bending stiffnesses of posterior implants are required to design a flexible lumbar stabilization system? *J. Biomech.* **2009**, *42*, 48–54. [CrossRef] [PubMed]
20. Chen, C.-S.; Chen, W.-J.; Cheng, C.-K.; Jao, S.-H.E.; Chueh, S.-C.; Wang, C.-C. Failure analysis of broken pedicle screws on spinal in-strumentation. *Med. Eng. Phys.* **2005**, *27*, 487–496. Available online: http://www.ncbi.nlm.nih.gov/pubmed/15990065 (accessed on 28 March 2019). [CrossRef]
21. La Barbera, L.; Galbusera, F.; Wilke, H.-J.; Villa, T. Preclinical evaluation of posterior spine stabilization devices: Can we compare in vitro and in vivo loads on the instrumentation? *Eur. Spine J.* **2016**, *26*, 200–209. [CrossRef]
22. La Barbera, L.; Galbusera, F.; Wilke, H.-J.; Villa, T. Preclinical evaluation of posterior spine stabilization devices: Can the current standards represent basic everyday life activities? *Eur. Spine J.* **2016**, *25*, 2909–2918. Available online: http://www.ncbi.nlm.nih.gov/pubmed/27236658 (accessed on 10 April 2019). [CrossRef] [PubMed]
23. La Barbera, L.; Galbusera, F.; Villa, T.; Costa, F.; Wilke, H.-J. ASTM F1717 standard for the preclinical evaluation of posterior spi-nal fixators: Can we improve it? *Proc. Inst. Mech. Eng. Part H J. Eng. Med.* **2014**, *228*, 1014–1026. Available online: http://www.ncbi.nlm.nih.gov/pubmed/25319550 (accessed on 16 March 2019). [CrossRef] [PubMed]
24. Stanford, R.E.; Loefler, A.H.; Stanford, P.M.; Walsh, W.R. Multiaxial Pedicle Screw Designs: Static and Dynamic Mechanical Testing. *Spine* **2004**, *29*, 367–375. [CrossRef] [PubMed]

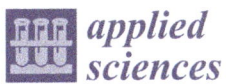

Article

Correlation of Biomechanical Alterations under Gonarthritis between Overlying Menisci and Articular Cartilage

Johannes Pordzik [1,*], Anke Bernstein [1], Julius Watrinet [1], Hermann O. Mayr [1,2], Sergio H. Latorre [1], Hagen Schmal [1] and Michael Seidenstuecker [1,*]

1. G.E.R.N. Tissue Replacement, Regeneration & Neogenesis, Department of Orthopedics and Trauma Surgery, Medical Center—Albert-Ludwigs-University of Freiburg, Faculty of Medicine, Albert-Ludwigs-University of Freiburg, Hugstetter Straße 55, 79106 Freiburg, Germany; anke.bernstein@uniklinik-freiburg.de (A.B.); julius@watrinet.net (J.W.); hermann.mayr@uniklinik-freiburg.de (H.O.M.); Sergio.Hernandez-Latorre@dzne.de (S.H.L.); hagen.schmal@uniklinik-freiburg.de (H.S.)
2. Schoen Clinic Munich Harlaching, Teaching Hospital of Paracelsus Medical University, 5026 Salzburg, Austria
* Correspondence: johannes.prodzik@t-online.de (J.P.); michael.seidenstuecker@uniklinik-freiburg.de (M.S.)

Received: 30 October 2020; Accepted: 2 December 2020; Published: 4 December 2020

Abstract: Just like menisci, articular cartilage is exposed to constant and varying stresses. Injuries to the meniscus are associated with the development of gonarthritis. Both the articular cartilage and the menisci are subject to structural changes under gonarthritis. The aim of this study was to investigate biomechanical alterations in articular cartilage and the menisci under gonarthritis by applying an indentation method. The study assessed 11 menisci from body donors as controls and 21 menisci from patients with severe gonarthritis. For the simultaneous examination of the articular cartilage and the menisci, we only tested the joint surfaces of the tibial plateau covered by the corresponding menisci. Over the posterior horn of the meniscus, the maximum applied load—the highest load registered by the load cell—of the arthritic samples of 0.02 ± 0.02 N was significantly greater ($p = 0.04$) than the maximum applied load of the arthritis-free samples of 0.01 ± 0.01 N. The instantaneous modulus (IM) at the center of the arthritic cartilage covered by the meniscus with 3.5 ± 2.02 MPa was significantly smaller than the IM of the arthritis-free samples with 5.17 ± 1.88 MPa ($p = 0.04$). No significant difference was found in the thickness of the meniscus-covered articular cartilage between the arthritic and arthritis-free samples. Significant correlations between the articular cartilage and the corresponding menisci were not observed at any point. In this study, the biomechanical changes associated with gonarthritis affected the posterior horn of the meniscus and the mid region of the meniscus-covered articular cartilage. The assessment of cartilage thickness as a structural characteristic of osteoarthritis may be misleading with regard to the interpretation of articular cartilage's biomechanical properties.

Keywords: gonarthritis; meniscus; articular cartilage; biomechanical testing; mapping; indentation; instantaneous modulus; tissue biomechanics

1. Introduction

Arthritis is the most common joint disease, with the knee joint being one of the most frequently affected joints [1]. Constantly changing multidirectional and dynamic forces stress the knee joint daily [2]. One of the structural characteristics of arthritis is the loss of articular cartilage [3]. Degenerative changes are manifested in a softening and continuous thinning of the joint cartilage, potentially leading to the complete loss of cartilage [4].

The meniscus improves weight distribution in the knee joint by increasing the contact surface between the femoral condyles and the tibial plateau [5], serving as shock absorption [5,6] and protecting the joint cartilage beneath it [7]. Consequently, meniscus displacement or meniscus extrusion is a strong predictive factor for the loss of cartilage tissue, indicating that the biomechanical properties of the meniscus have failed [8,9]. This results in the current approaches that aim to preserve as much meniscus tissue as possible [10].

There exist a variety of forms of meniscus replacement, such as autogenous replacement, but also artificial implants. However, in contrast to articular cartilage replacement [11], a widely applicable meniscus replacement with clear scientifically proven efficacy is not yet available [12]. Given this gap in research, a deeper understanding of the biomechanical behavior of meniscus and cartilage tissue appears vital.

Thus far, for both menisci and joint cartilage, animal samples have predominantly been studied [13–18]. Previous biomechanical examination of the articular cartilage, as well as for the meniscus, included both unconfined compression tests [16,19,20] and confined compression tests [21,22]. However, a complete mapping of the biomechanical properties of the tissue with a large number of measurement points was only possible to a limited extent [23,24], with exception of Seidenstuecker et al. [25], who examined the articular cartilage with a complete mapping of biomechanical properties. This was possible by using an indentation test. The main objective of the indentation test is to determine the instantaneous modulus (IM) and hardness of a sample. IM thus describes the ability of an elastic material to resist deformation under applied mechanical stress. The work from Sim et al. [26,27] and Seidenstuecker et al. [25] showed that automatic mapping of articular cartilage with Biomomentum Inc. technology (Montreal, QC, Canada) is possible.

Studies on human menisci and their corresponding articular cartilage concerning the difference between arthritic and arthritis-free samples are missing thus far.

The aim of this study was therefore to investigate the relationship between the biomechanical properties of the meniscus-covered cartilage and the corresponding menisci in the pathogenesis of osteoarthritis (OA) to better understand the role of the meniscus in the protection of the articular cartilage and contribute to the development of meniscus scaffolds.

2. Materials and Methods

A total of 32 menisci and the underlying articular cartilage were used for the measurements: 21 arthritic menisci and 11 arthritis-free samples.

The arthritic menisci were removed from the arthritic tibial plateau and the tissues were frozen within 24 h after surgery for total knee replacement (TKR) due to severe osteoarthritis [25].

The average age of the patients was 71.76 ± 7.23 years. Of the patients, 15 were female and 6 were male.

The arthritis-free samples originated from fresh frozen knees of body donors [25]. OA was excluded by specialists in orthopaedics and trauma surgery at the investigating hospital. During preparation of the arthritis-free samples by specialists in orthopaedics and trauma surgery, degenerative changes of the cartilage due to the patients age were observed. This includes softening and swelling as well as fibrillation of the cartilage surface in little areas. A further assessment including a grading system of these macroscopic changes has not been performed.

All arthritic samples were handled according to approved institutional ethics committee certificates (ethics vote 305/10 of the ethics commission of the Freiburg University Medical Center).

2.1. Indentation Testings

The description of the biomechanical measurement methods concerning the articular cartilage is based on Seidenstuecker et al. [25]. The indentation test (DIN EN ISO 14577) was carried out first, followed by thickness measurement using the needle measuring method [28].

Biomechanical testing of the menisci and cartilage was carried out by means of indentation tests (DIN EN ISO 14577-1:2015) [29] (see Figure 1). A Mach-1 Model V500css test machine (Biomomentum Inc., Laval, Canada), a multiaxial load cell with 17 N MA 233 (ATI industrial Automation, Apex, NC, USA) for the menisci and a multiaxial load cell with 70 N Model FTIFPS1 (ATI industrial Automation, Apex, NC, USA) for the articular cartilage [25], and a Newport Motion Controller ESP 301 (Newport, Irvine, CA, USA) were used. These materials allow for the examination of soft tissue as well as the complete mapping of the tissue [25,26,30]. The menisci were fixed to the MA646 specimen holder (Biomomentum Inc., Laval, QC, Canada) by Loctide (Henkel AG and CoAG KGaA, Düsseldorf-Holthausen, Germany) according to physiological conditions and were then anchored in the testing device. For biomechanical testing of the articular cartilage of the tibial plateau, we first marked the meniscus-covered areas with tissue markers [25]. The samples were then fixed in the testing machine.

After that, the measuring points had to be determined. For this purpose, the glued menisci and tibial plateaus were recorded with a camera. In the Mach-1 Analysis Software Version 4.1.0.17 (Biomomentum, Montreal, QC, Canada), a position grid could then be projected on these images with which the measurements were taken [25].

The position grid was created mechanically for the arthritis-free meniscus and all tibial plateaus and manually adapted to the shape and size of the arthritic meniscus. The indentation test (DIN EN ISO 14577) was then carried out using a spherical indenter MA680 (Biomomentum Inc., Laval, QC, Canada) with a diameter of 1 mm [25]. In this way, the entire tissue can be tested. The maximum applied load was defined as the highest load registered by the load cell per measuring point. An average of 45 measuring points was distributed over the meniscus. When the articular cartilage was tested in the same way as the meniscus, an average of 35 measuring points was distributed over the entire tibial plateau.

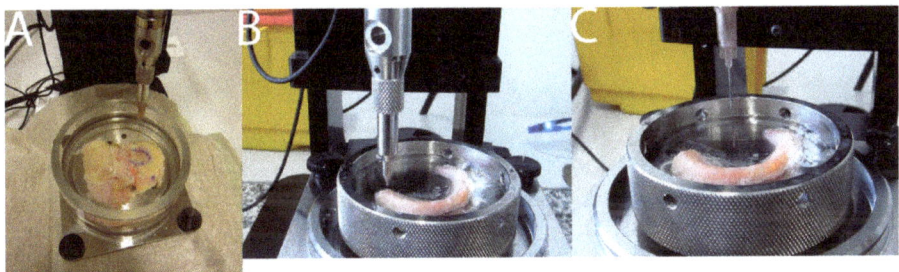

Figure 1. (**A**) Mach-1 thickness measurement by needle method (joint cartilage); (**B**) Mach-1 Indentation (meniscus); (**C**) Mach-1 thickness measurement by needle method (meniscus).

Since meniscus and articular cartilage differ in their biomechanical properties, the testing criteria differ. The testing criteria chosen are in the range of previous studies [25,26]. The meniscus is less stiff than the cartilage. Therefore, a 0.1 mm/s faster indentation speed was chosen in comparison to the indentation speed of the cartilage [25]. The articular cartilage lies flat on the subchondral bone. Therefore a 0.1 mm higher indentation depth was chosen. Since the meniscus was glued on the metal, we selected a smaller depth. Otherwise, the indenter could touch the metal before reaching the predefined indentation depth. Thus, following testing criteria were used:

The following criteria were used to test the meniscus: Poisson ratio: 0.5, contact criterion: 0.1 N, predefined indentation amplitude: 0.2 mm, indentation speed: 0.2 mm/s, and relaxation time: 10 s.

The following criteria were used to test the joint cartilage [25]: Poisson ratio: 0.5 contact criterion: 0.1 N, predefined indentation amplitude: 0.3 mm, indentation velocity: 0.1 mm/s, and relaxation time: 10 s.

In order to prevent dehydration of the tissue, we added NaCl 0.9% to the tissue repeatedly using a disposable pipette during the measurement.

2.2. Thickness Measurement

The indentation test was followed by a thickness measurement. The indenter for measuring the meniscus was replaced with a size 18 cannula (B. Braun, Melsungen, Germany). The following criteria were selected: stop criterion: 5 N, and speed: 0.5 mm/s. The cannula was perpendicular to the samples and moved in the direction of the samples at a constant speed. This movement was stopped as soon as the cannula reached the metal below the meniscus. To prevent damage of the load cell, we stopped the cannula at a maximum axial load of 5 N.

The needle technique was also used to measure the thickness of the articular cartilage [28]. The indenter was replaced with a 27G × $\frac{3}{4}$ intradermal cannula (B. Braun, Melsungen, Germany). The following criteria were used to measure the thickness of the joint cartilage [25]: stop criterion: 7 N, and speed 0.5 mm/s. The cannula was perpendicular to the sample and moved at a constant speed until it reached the subchondral bone and the stop criterion was met [25,26].

The thickness mapping used the same measuring grid as the automated indentation mapping in order to get the thickness information on the exact same positions [25].

2.3. Evaluation of Biomechanical Results

The findings were analyzed using the software Mach-1 Analysis Version 4.1.0.17 (Biomomentum, Montreal, Canada) and SPSS 25 (IBM, Armonk, NY, USA). The collected data were evaluated according to Sim et al. [26] and Seidenstuecker et al. [25]. The thickness of both the menisci and the articular cartilage was evaluated in the same way. The thickness was calculated as the difference between the first point of contact of the cannula with the tissue, where the load cell registers a load, and the point of transition, where the load cell perceives a load against the stop criterion. The IM was then evaluated at each measuring position using the following formula [31]:

$$IM = \frac{P}{H} \cdot \frac{1 - v^2}{2ak \cdot \left(\frac{a}{h}, v\right)}$$

where IM is instantaneous modulus, P is load, H is indentation depth, a is radius of the contact region, v is Poisson's ratio, k is correction factor dependent on a/h and v (values of k were chosen automatically by the software Mach-1 Analysis Version 4.1.0.17 (Biomomentum, Montreal, Canada) according to values determined by Hayes et al. [31] depending on a/h and v), and h is specimen thickness.

2.4. Statistics

The data were evaluated using Mach-1 Analysis Software Version 4.1.0.17 (Biomomentum, Montreal, QC, Canada), Origin 2018 Professional (Origin Lab, Northampton, MA, USA), SPSS 25 (IBM, Armonk, NY, USA) and Excel 2016 (Microsoft Corporation, Redmond, WA, USA). The menisci were divided into thirds. The mean value of each third was calculated with Excel 2016 (Microsoft Corporation, Redmond, WA, USA). The mean value of the entire meniscus was calculated as well. Like the meniscus, the meniscus-covered area of the tibial plateau was also divided into thirds. Mean values were then calculated the same way. All biomechanical results were expressed as mean values with a standard deviation. Statistical analysis was conducted with SPSS 25 (IBM, Armonk, NY, USA). Samples were compared using the Mann–Whitney U test. Samples were correlated according to Spearman's rank correlation coefficient. Results with $p < 0.05$ were considered statistically significant.

After pre-tests of the meniscus, mean values for the maximum applied load of 0.01 N for arthritis-free samples and 0.03 N for arthritic samples were expected. The SD was hypothesized as 0.01. To reach an alpha error level of 1%, at least 11 samples of each (specimen and control) were necessary. The online sample size and power calculator www.dssresearch.com were used. The calculated power for 2 different samples and two-tailed test with a difference of maximum applied load with 0.02 N, 21 samples and 11 controls, SD of 0.01 each, and alpha error level of 1% was calculated to be 99.7%.

After pre-tests of the cartilage, mean values for the IM of 5 MPa for arthritis-free samples and 3 MPa for arthritic samples were expected. The SD was hypothesized as 1. To reach an alpha error level of 1%, at least 11 samples of each (specimen and control) were necessary. The online sample size and power calculator www.dssresearch.com were used. The calculated power for 2 different samples and two-tailed test with a difference of IM with 2 MPa, 21 samples and 11 controls, SD of 1 MPa each, and alpha error level of 1% was calculated to be 99.7%.

3. Results

3.1. Biomechanical Results of the Meniscus

Over the posterior horn, the maximum applied load of the arthritic samples of 0.02 ± 0.02 N was significantly greater ($p = 0.04$) than the maximum applied load of the arthritis-free samples of 0.01 ± 0.01 N (see Figure 2).

Over the posterior horn, the IM of the arthritic samples of 0.18 ± 0.1 MPa was not significantly greater ($p = 0.17$) than the IM of the arthritis-free samples of 0.13 ± 0.07 (see Figure 2).

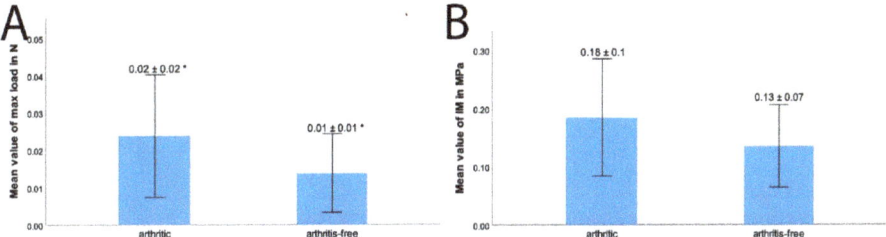

Figure 2. (A) Differences in the maximum applied load in N over the posterior horn of the meniscus ($p = 0.03$): arthritic: 0.02 ± 0.02 N (error bar: ± 1 SD); arthritis-free: 0.01 ± 0.01 N (error bar: ± 1 SD). (B) Differences in instantaneous modulus (IM) in MPa over the posterior horn of the meniscus: arthritic: 0.18 ± 0.1 MPa (error bar: ± 1 SD); arthritis-free: 0.13 ± 0.07 MPa (error bar: ± 1 SD); * = statistically significant with $p < 0.05$.

3.2. Biomechanical Results of the Meniscus-Covered Cartilage Tissue

Significant differences were found in both the IM and the maximum applied load (see Figure 3) between arthritic and arthritis-free samples at the center of the meniscus-covered articular cartilage. The IM of the arthritic samples with 3.5 ± 2.02 MPa was significantly smaller than the IM of the arthritis-free samples with 5.17 ± 1.88 MPa ($p = 0.04$). The maximum applied load of the arthritic samples with 1.04 ± 0.63 N was significantly smaller than the maximum applied load of the arthritis-free samples with 1.51 ± 0.47 N ($p = 0.03$).

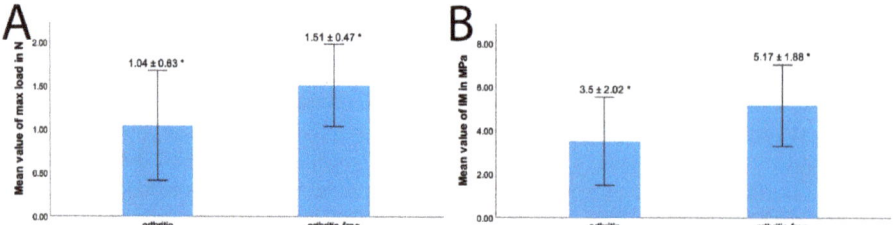

Figure 3. (**A**): Differences in maximum applied load in N over the mid part of the meniscus-covered cartilage ($p = 0.04$): arthritic: 1.04 ± 0.63 N (error bar: 1 SD); arthritis-free: 1.51 ± 0.47 N (error bar: 1 SD). (**B**) Differences in IM in MPa over the mid part of the meniscus-covered cartilage tissue ($p = 0.03$): arthritic: 3.5 ± 2.02 MPa (error bar: 1 SD); arthritis-free: 5.17 ± 1.88 MPa; * = statistically significant with $p < 0.05$.

The maximum applied load over the entire meniscus-covered articular cartilage with 1.06 ± 0.67 N was also significantly smaller for the arthritic samples compared to the arthritis-free samples with 1.55 ± 0.58 N ($p = 0.04$) (see Figure 4).

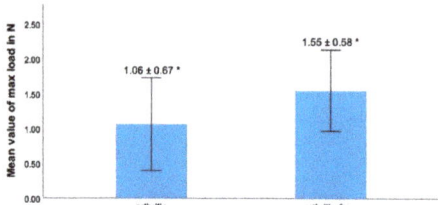

Figure 4. Differences in maximum applied load in N over the entire meniscus-covered cartilage tissue ($p = 0.04$): arthritic: 1.06 ± 0.67 N (error bar: 1 SD); arthritis-free: 1.55 ± 0.58 N (error bar: 1 SD); * = statistically significant with $p < 0.05$.

Over the entire meniscus-covered cartilage, the thickness of the arthritic articular cartilage with 2.11 ± 0.58 mm was not significantly smaller ($p = 0.76$) compared to the arthritis-free samples with 2.13 ± 0.42 mm (see Figure 5). At the mid region of the meniscus-covered cartilage, the thickness of the arthritic cartilage with 2.17 ± 0.71 mm was not significantly smaller than the thickness of the arthritis-free cartilage with 2.17 ± 0.5 mm ($p = 0.82$).

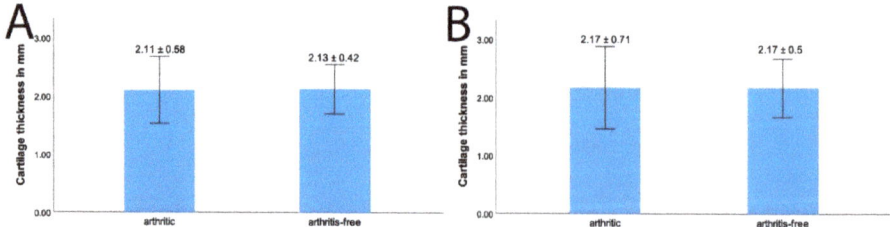

Figure 5. (**A**) Differences in entire meniscus-covered cartilage thickness in mm: arthritic: 2.11 ± 0.58 mm; arthritis-free: 2.13 ± 0.42 mm (error bar: 1 SD). (**B**) Differences in meniscus-covered cartilage thickness in the mid part in mm: arthritic: 2.17 ± 0.71 mm; arthritis-free: 2.17 ± 0.5 mm (error bar: 1 SD).

3.3. Correlation Between the Results of the Meniscus-Covered Cartilage Tissue and the Meniscus

Only the menisci and their corresponding tibial plateaus were correlated (see Figure 6). Significant correlations were not observed at any point. Neither the maximum applied load nor the IM between the articular cartilage and the corresponding meniscus correlated significantly.

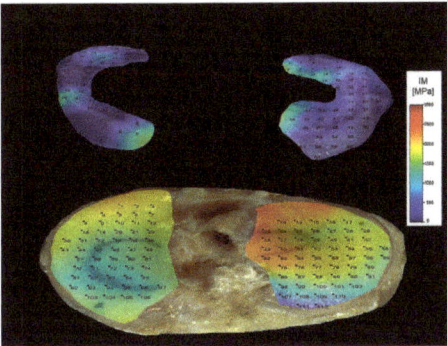

Figure 6. Combined mapping of IM of joint cartilage and associated menisci.

4. Discussion

4.1. Biomechanics of the Meniscus

The present study showed that the posterior horn is affected in cases of OA. In this study, the maximum applied load on the posterior horn of the arthritic menisci was twice as high as that of the menisci in arthritis-free knees. This means that over the posterior horn, the stiffness of the meniscus increases under arthritis. In relation to the arthritis-free samples, a 100% higher force was required to indent the arthritic samples to an equal depth (200 µm). This can be explained by the special type of rolling–sliding movement in the knee joint [32]. The finding that the posterior horn of the meniscus was affected in knee arthritis is consistent with previous studies. A medial meniscus study showed that the posterior horn carried the highest percentage of shear stress [33]. Warnecke et al. [34] showed by examining degenerative lateral menisci that the highest values for the respective hydraulic permeability "k" were in the posterior region of the meniscus, indicating that degenerative processes initially occur at the posterior horn. Under increased load, stiffness seems to increase in the particularly stressed regions of the meniscus, i.e., the posterior horn.

4.2. Biomechanics of the Articular Cartilage

Both the IM and the maximum applied load at the center region of the articular cartilage covered by the meniscus significantly decreased in arthritis. Degenerative changes are manifested in softening and continuous thinning of the articular cartilage to complete bone baldness [4]. In particular, the central part of the articular cartilage, where local loads are greatest [35] is affected by arthritis [36]. This concerns in particular the uncovered cartilage but also the meniscus-covered regions [36]. With 2.11 ± 0.58 mm for arthritic articular cartilage and 2.13 ± 0.42 mm for arthritis-free articular cartilage, the cartilage thicknesses were very similar. The values measured for human cartilage tissue of the tibial plateau correspond to the values described in literature on human cartilage tissue of the tibial plateau. Thambyah et al. [37] reported cartilage thicknesses between 3.2 and 3.9 mm for the meniscus-uncovered parts and between 1.7 and 2.1 mm for the meniscus-covered areas. Bohringer et al. [38] found a clear difference in cartilage thickness between the different stages of osteoarthritis—cartilage thickness was greatly reduced in severe osteoarthritis. Seidenstuecker et al. [25] found a statistically significant ($p < 0.001$) difference in cartilage thickness between arthritic articular cartilage of the tibial plateau with 2.25 ± 0.11 mm and arthritis-free articular cartilage of the tibial plateau with 2.0 ± 0.07 mm. In this study, there was no significant difference in cartilage thickness between arthritic samples and arthritis-free samples. An important task of the meniscus is the protection of the articular cartilage beneath [5,7,39]. Due to this protection, the articular cartilage may not have been reduced in the meniscus-covered area even under arthritic conditions. The biomechanical properties of the meniscus-covered articular cartilage decrease under arthritis significantly, although there is no relevant loss of articular cartilage. This means that the cartilage thickness as a structural characteristic of osteoarthritis may be misleading with regard to the interpretation of the biomechanical properties. Previous studies have shown that early stage OA processes occur without macroscopic changes in the cartilage morphology [40,41]. Sim et al. [26] showed that visual and thickness assessments are much less sensitive in distinguishing early degenerated cartilage than mechanical assessments where the functional and structural properties of cartilage play important roles. There are existing non-invasive and non-contact methods to test the biomechanical properties by using ultrasound imaging technologies [42]. Both ultrasound elasticity (UEI) and ultrasound shear wave elasticity imaging (USWEI) have limitations [42]. Therefore, minimally invasive indentation tests could better provide intraoperative information about the severity of joint damage and thus contribute to the decision between joint replacement and joint-preserving therapy.

4.3. Correlation between the Results of the Meniscus-Covered Cartilage Tissue and the Meniscus

The IM of the meniscus-covered cartilage tissue was higher for the arthritis-free samples than for the arthritic samples. These observations are consistent with the current literature [25]. For the menisci, the opposite was observed. Both observations can be explained with the changes in the proteoglycan content. In arthritic articular cartilage, proteoglycan synthesis is inhibited in particular by Interleukin-1β [43], whereas more proteoglycan is present in arthritis-free tissue. Proteoglycans bind water and thus stiffen the tissue [44]. In the meniscus, this is the opposite—degenerative or arthritic altered menisci have a higher content of proteoglycan [45,46]. In meniscus tissue, an increased glycosaminoglycan content correlates with an increased compression modulus [47]. In addition, the articular cartilage was most affected by arthritis in the central part in contrast to the meniscus, where the posterior horn was mainly affected by arthritis. The finding that the biomechanical results of the articular cartilage did not correlate with those of the meniscus and vice versa appears to be imperative to the background research described above.

4.4. Weaknesses of This Study

The arthritis-free samples are a population from the Pathological Institute. The age of the arthritis-free samples is not known. However, it can be assumed that the age is advanced. Degenerative changes occurred. Age-related degenerative changes influence the biomechanical properties of the meniscus and of the articular cartilage. Tsujii et al. [48] showed that age-related compositional changes, such as advanced glycation end-products, largely contribute to tissue stiffness. For the meniscus, age-related changes are at least in tendency comparable to changes caused by osteoarthritis. This also applies to the joint cartilage. Hudelmaier et al. [49] showed that knee cartilage thickness becomes thinner with age. Pataki et al. [50] showed that age leads to impaired synthesis of proteoglycans as well as osteoarthritis. Therefore, the age-related changes and osteoarthritis-related changes are comparable. This reinforces the assumption that osteoarthritis leads to an even greater change in biomechanical properties compared to a healthy young control group than observed in this study. Due to the limited and different number of samples from the arthritic group and the arthritis-free group, further investigations are necessary to determine if the assessment of cartilage thickness as a structural characteristic of osteoarthritis is misleading with regard to the interpretation of articular cartilage's biomechanical properties. Laboratory studies are not fully comparable with in vivo conditions.

5. Conclusions

This study is the first to establish a direct connection between biomechanical alterations of the meniscus and the articular cartilage beneath the meniscus under OA by applying an indentation method that allows for the examination of the entire tissue. It could be shown that biomechanical changes mainly affect the posterior horn of the meniscus and the middle part of the meniscus-covered joint cartilage. During OA, the stiffness of the meniscus increased while the stiffness of articular cartilage increased. Despite the change in the biomechanical properties of the articular cartilage, no significant difference was found in the thickness of articular cartilage between arthritic and arthritis-free samples. Therefore, the cartilage thickness as a landmark of osteoarthritis may be misleading with regard to the interpretation of the biomechanical properties. Indentation tests may help us to better understand the biomechanical behavior of the meniscus and thus contribute to the further development of meniscus grafts. In addition, minimally invasive indentation tests could provide intraoperative information about the severity of joint damage and thus contribute to the decision between joint replacement and joint-preserving therapy.

Author Contributions: H.O.M., M.S., H.S., and A.B. conceived and designed the experiments; J.P., M.S., S.H.L., and J.W. performed the experiments; J.P. and M.S. analyzed the data; A.B., H.S., and H.O.M. contributed reagents/materials/analysis tools; J.P. and M.S. wrote the paper. All authors have read and agreed to the published version of the manuscript.

Funding: The project was financially supported by Alwin Jäger Foundation. The article processing charge was funded by the Baden-Wuerttemberg Ministry of Science, Research and Art and the University of Freiburg in the funding program Open Access Publishing.

Acknowledgments: The authors would like to thank Arthrex for providing the controls and Melanie L. Hart for proofreading.

Conflicts of Interest: The authors declare no conflict of interest.

References

1. Heijink, A.; Gomoll, A.H.; Madry, H.; Drobnic, M.; Filardo, G.; Espregueira-Mendes, J.; van Dijk, C.N. Biomechanical considerations in the pathogenesis of osteoarthritis of the knee. *Knee Surg. Sports Traumatol. Arthrosc.* **2012**, *20*, 423–435. [CrossRef] [PubMed]
2. Gilbert, S.; Chen, T.; Hutchinson, I.D.; Choi, D.; Voigt, C.; Warren, R.F.; Maher, S.A. Dynamic contact mechanics on the tibial plateau of the human knee during activities of daily living. *J. Biomech.* **2014**, *47*, 2006–2012. [CrossRef] [PubMed]
3. Kellgren, J.H.; Lawrence, J.S. Radiological assessment of osteo-arthrosis. *Ann. Rheum. Dis.* **1957**, *16*, 494–502. [CrossRef] [PubMed]
4. Bailey, A.J.; Mansell, J.P.; Sims, T.J.; Banse, X. Biochemical and mechanical properties of subchondral bone in osteoarthritis. *Biorheology* **2004**, *41*, 349–358.
5. Seedhom, B.B.; Dowson, D.; Wright, V. Proceedings: Functions of the menisci. A preliminary study. *Ann. Rheum. Dis.* **1974**, *33*, 111. [CrossRef]
6. Rath, E.; Richmond, J.C. The menisci: Basic science and advances in treatment. *Br. J. Sports Med.* **2000**, *34*, 252–257. [CrossRef]
7. Mow, V.C.; Arnoczky, S.P.; Jackson, D.W. *Knee Meniscus Basic and Clinical Foundations*; Raven Press: New York, NY, USA, 1992; Volume xi, 190p.
8. Berthiaume, M.J.; Raynauld, J.P.; Martel-Pelletier, J.; Labonte, F.; Beaudoin, G.; Bloch, D.A.; Choquette, D.; Haraoui, B.; Altman, R.D.; Hochberg, M.; et al. Meniscal tear and extrusion are strongly associated with progression of symptomatic knee osteoarthritis as assessed by quantitative magnetic resonance imaging. *Ann. Rheum. Dis.* **2005**, *64*, 556–563. [CrossRef]
9. Hunter, D.J.; Zhang, Y.Q.; Niu, J.B.; Tu, X.; Amin, S.; Clancy, M.; Guermazi, A.; Grigorian, M.; Gale, D.; Felson, D.T. The association of meniscal pathologic changes with cartilage loss in symptomatic knee osteoarthritis. *Arthritis Rheum.* **2006**, *54*, 795–801. [CrossRef]
10. Noyes, F.R.; Barber-Westin, S.D. Repair of complex and avascular meniscal tears and meniscal transplantation. *J. Bone Jt. Surg. Am.* **2010**, *92*, 1012–1029.
11. Brittberg, M.; Lindahl, A.; Nilsson, A.; Ohlsson, C.; Isaksson, O.; Peterson, L. Treatment of deep cartilage defects in the knee with autologous chondrocyte transplantation. *N. Engl. J. Med.* **1994**, *331*, 889–895. [CrossRef]

12. Starke, C.; Kopf, S.; Becker, R. Indication and limitations of meniscus replacement. *Der Orthopade* **2017**, *46*, 831–838. [PubMed]
13. Joshi, M.D.; Suh, J.K.; Marui, T.; Woo, S.L. Interspecies variation of compressive biomechanical properties of the meniscus. *J. Biomed. Mater. Res.* **1995**, *29*, 823–828. [CrossRef] [PubMed]
14. Fithian, D.C.; Kelly, M.A.; Mow, V.C. Material properties and structure-function relationships in the menisci. *Clin. Orthop. Relat. Res.* **1990**, *252*, 19–31. [CrossRef]
15. Proctor, C.S.; Schmidt, M.B.; Whipple, R.R.; Kelly, M.A.; Mow, V.C. Material properties of the normal medial bovine meniscus. *J. Orthop. Res.* **1989**, *7*, 771–782. [CrossRef] [PubMed]
16. Sweigart, M.A.; Zhu, C.F.; Burt, D.M.; DeHoll, P.D.; Agrawal, C.M.; Clanton, T.O.; Athanasiou, K.A. Intraspecies and interspecies comparison of the compressive properties of the medial meniscus. *Ann. Biomed. Eng.* **2004**, *32*, 1569–1579. [CrossRef] [PubMed]
17. Chen, A.C.; Bae, W.C.; Schinagl, R.M.; Sah, R.L. Depth- and strain-dependent mechanical and electromechanical properties of full-thickness bovine articular cartilage in confined compression. *J. Biomech.* **2001**, *34*, 1–12. [CrossRef]
18. Franke, O.; Durst, K.; Maier, V.; Goken, M.; Birkholz, T.; Schneider, H.; Hennig, F.; Gelse, K. Mechanical properties of hyaline and repair cartilage studied by nanoindentation. *Acta Biomater.* **2007**, *3*, 873–881. [CrossRef]
19. Boschetti, F.; Peretti, G.M. Tensile and compressive properties of healthy and osteoarthritic human articular cartilage. *Biorheology* **2008**, *45*, 337–344. [CrossRef]
20. Pereira, H.; Caridade, S.G.; Frias, A.M.; Silva-Correia, J.; Pereira, D.R.; Cengiz, I.F.; Mano, J.F.; Oliveira, J.M.; Espregueira-Mendes, J.; Reis, R.L. Biomechanical and cellular segmental characterization of human meniscus: Building the basis for tissue engineering therapies. *Osteoarthr. Cartil.* **2014**, *22*, 1271–1281. [CrossRef]
21. Martin Seitz, A.; Galbusera, F.; Krais, C.; Ignatius, A.; Durselen, L. Stress-relaxation response of human menisci under confined compression conditions. *J. Mech. Behav. Biomed. Mater.* **2013**, *26*, 68–80. [CrossRef]
22. Alexopoulos, L.G.; Williams, G.M.; Upton, M.L.; Setton, L.A.; Guilak, F. Osteoarthritic changes in the biphasic mechanical properties of the chondrocyte pericellular matrix in articular cartilage. *J. Biomech.* **2005**, *38*, 509–517. [CrossRef] [PubMed]
23. Deneweth, J.M.; Newman, K.E.; Sylvia, S.M.; McLean, S.G.; Arruda, E.M. Heterogeneity of tibial plateau cartilage in response to a physiological compressive strain rate. *J. Orthop. Res.* **2013**, *31*, 370–375. [CrossRef] [PubMed]
24. Danso, E.K.; Oinas, J.M.T.; Saarakkala, S.; Mikkonen, S.; Toyras, J.; Korhonen, R.K. Structure-function relationships of human meniscus. *J. Mech. Behav. Biomed. Mater.* **2017**, *67*, 51–60. [CrossRef] [PubMed]
25. Seidenstuecker, M.; Watrinet, J.; Bernstein, A.; Suedkamp, N.P.; Latorre, S.H.; Maks, A.; Mayr, H.O. Viscoelasticity and histology of the human cartilage in healthy and degenerated conditions of the knee. *J. Orthop. Surg. Res.* **2019**, *14*, 256. [CrossRef]
26. Sim, S.; Chevrier, A.; Garon, M.; Quenneville, E.; Lavigne, P.; Yaroshinsky, A.; Hoemann, C.D.; Buschmann, M.D. Electromechanical probe and automated indentation maps are sensitive techniques in assessing early degenerated human articular cartilage. *J. Orthop. Surg. Res.* **2017**, *35*, 858–867. [CrossRef]
27. Sim, S.; Hadjab, I.; Garon, M.; Quenneville, E.; Lavigne, P.; Buschmann, M.D. Development of an electromechanical grade to assess human knee articular cartilage quality. *Ann. Biomed. Eng.* **2017**, *45*, 2410–2421. [CrossRef]
28. Jurvelin, J.S.; Räsänen, T.; Kolmonens, P.; Lyyra, T. Comparison of optical, needle probe and ultrasonic techniques for the measurement of articular cartilage thickness. *J. Biomech.* **1995**, *28*, 231–235. [CrossRef]
29. ISO. *14577-1 Metallic Materials-Instrumented Indentation Test for Hardness and Materials Parameters—Part 1: Test Method*; ISO: Geneva, Switzerland, 2015.
30. Zhou, Y.; Tang, Y.; Hoff, T.; Garon, M.; Zhao, F.Y. The verification of the mechanical properties of binder jetting manufactured parts by instrumented indentation testing. *Procedia Manuf.* **2015**, *1*, 327–342. [CrossRef]
31. Hayes, W.C.; Keer, L.M.; Herrmann, G.; Mockros, L.F. A mathematical analysis for indentation tests of articular cartilage. *J. Biomech.* **1972**, *5*, 541–551. [CrossRef]
32. Kummer, B. *Biomechanik: Form und Funktion des Bewegungsapparates Mit 3 Tabellen*; Dt. Ärzte-Verl.: Köln, Germany, 2005; Volume XV, p. 604 S.
33. Walker, P.S.; Arno, S.; Bell, C.; Salvadore, G.; Borukhov, I.; Oh, C. Function of the medial meniscus in force transmission and stability. *J. Biomech.* **2015**, *48*, 1383–1388. [CrossRef]

34. Warnecke, D.; Balko, J.; Haas, J.; Bieger, R.; Leucht, F.; Wolf, N.; Schild, N.; Stein, S.; Seitz, A.; Ignatius, A.; et al. Degeneration alters the biomechanical properties and structural composition of lateral human menisci. *Osteoarthr. Cartil.* **2020**, *28*, 1482–1491. [CrossRef] [PubMed]
35. Bae, J.Y.; Park, K.S.; Seon, J.K.; Kwak, D.S.; Jeon, I.; Song, E.K. Biomechanical analysis of the effects of medial meniscectomy on degenerative osteoarthritis. *Med. Biol. Eng. Comput.* **2012**, *50*, 53–60. [CrossRef] [PubMed]
36. Pelletier, J.P.; Raynauld, J.P.; Berthiaume, M.J.; Abram, F.; Choquette, D.; Haraoui, B.; Beary, J.F.; Cline, G.A.; Meyer, J.M.; Martel-Pelletier, J. Risk factors associated with the loss of cartilage volume on weight-bearing areas in knee osteoarthritis patients assessed by quantitative magnetic resonance imaging: A longitudinal study. *Arthritis Res. Ther.* **2007**, *9*, R74. [CrossRef] [PubMed]
37. Thambyah, A.; Nather, A.; Goh, J. Mechanical properties of articular cartilage covered by the meniscus. *Osteoarthr. Cartil.* **2006**, *14*, 580–588. [CrossRef]
38. Bohringer, M.E.; Beyer, W.F.; Weseloh, G. Comparative histomorphometry of subchondral bone density and articular cartilage thickness in the tibial head in early human arthritis. *Z. Orthop. Ihre Grenzgeb.* **1995**, *133*, 291–302.
39. Fischenich, K.M.; Lewis, J.; Kindsfater, K.A.; Bailey, T.S.; Haut Donahue, T.L. Effects of degeneration on the compressive and tensile properties of human meniscus. *J. Biomech.* **2015**, *48*, 1407–1411. [CrossRef]
40. Burstein, D.; Gray, M.; Mosher, T.; Dardzinski, B. Measures of molecular composition and structure in osteoarthritis. *Radiol. Clin. N. Am.* **2009**, *47*, 675–686. [CrossRef]
41. Crema, M.D.; Roemer, F.W.; Marra, M.D.; Burstein, D.; Gold, G.E.; Eckstein, F.; Baum, T.; Mosher, T.J.; Carrino, J.A.; Guermazi, A. Articular cartilage in the knee: Current mr imaging techniques and applications in clinical practice and research. *Radiographics* **2011**, *31*, 37–61. [CrossRef]
42. Kim, K.; Wagner, W.R. Non-invasive and non-destructive characterization of tissue engineered constructs using ultrasound imaging technologies: A review. *Ann. Biomed. Eng.* **2016**, *44*, 621–635. [CrossRef]
43. Evans, C.H.; Robbins, P.D. Potential treatment of osteoarthritis by gene therapy. *Rheum. Dis. Clin. N. Am.* **1999**, *25*, 333–344. [CrossRef]
44. Lüllmann-Rauch, R. *Taschenbuch Histologie 5*; vollst. überarb. Auflage ed. 5; Thieme: Stuttgart u.a, Germany, 2015; Volume XVIII, p. 726 S.
45. Sun, Y.; Mauerhan, D.R.; Kneisl, J.S.; James Norton, H.; Zinchenko, N.; Ingram, J.; Hanley, E.N., Jr.; Gruber, H.E. Histological examination of collagen and proteoglycan changes in osteoarthritic menisci. *Open Rheumatol. J.* **2012**, *6*, 24–32. [CrossRef] [PubMed]
46. Herwig, J.; Egner, E.; Buddecke, E. Chemical changes of human knee joint menisci in various stages of degeneration. *Ann. Rheum. Dis.* **1984**, *43*, 635–640. [CrossRef] [PubMed]
47. Bursac, P.; Arnoczky, S.; York, A. Dynamic compressive behavior of human meniscus correlates with its extra-cellular matrix composition. *Biorheology* **2009**, *46*, 227–237. [CrossRef] [PubMed]
48. Tsujii, A.; Nakamura, N.; Horibe, S. Age-related changes in the knee meniscus. *Knee* **2017**, *24*, 1262–1270. [CrossRef]
49. Hudelmaier, M.; Glaser, C.; Hohe, J.; Englmeier, K.H.; Reiser, M.; Putz, R.; Eckstein, F. Age-related changes in the morphology and deformational behavior of knee joint cartilage. *Arthritis Rheumatol.* **2001**, *44*, 2556–2561. [CrossRef]
50. Pataki, A.; Ruttner, J.R.; Abt, K. Age-related histochemical and histological changes in the knee-joint cartilage of c57b1 mice and their significance for the pathogenesis of osteoarthrosis. I. Oxidative enzymes. *Exp. Cell Biol.* **1980**, *48*, 329–348. [CrossRef]

Publisher's Note: MDPI stays neutral with regard to jurisdictional claims in published maps and institutional affiliations.

© 2020 by the authors. Licensee MDPI, Basel, Switzerland. This article is an open access article distributed under the terms and conditions of the Creative Commons Attribution (CC BY) license (http://creativecommons.org/licenses/by/4.0/).

Article

Model-Based Roentgen Stereophotogrammetric Analysis Using Elementary Geometrical Shape Models: Reliability of Migration Measurements for an Anatomically Shaped Femoral Stem Component

Jing Xu [1,*], Han Cao [1,2], Stefan Sesselmann [3], Dominic Taylor [1], Raimund Forst [1] and Frank Seehaus [1]

1. Department of Orthopaedic Surgery, Friedrich-Alexander-Universität Erlangen-Nürnberg, 91054 Erlangen, Germany; han.cao@fau.de (H.C.); dominictaylor2000@yahoo.com (D.T.); raimund.forst@fau.de (R.F.); frank.seehaus@fau.de (F.S.)
2. Department of Orthopaedic Surgery, Taizhou Second People's Hospital, Taizhou 225599, China
3. Institute for Medical Engineering, Ostbayerische Technische Hochschule Amberg-Weiden, 92637 Weiden, Germany; s.sesselmann@oth-aw.de
* Correspondence: jing.xu@fau.de

Received: 24 September 2020; Accepted: 26 November 2020; Published: 28 November 2020

Featured Application: This study validated the application of Elementary Geometrical Shape (EGS) models for in vivo migration measurements of Total Hip Arthroplasty. Using EGS models for migration detection presenting an alternative to surface models resulting out of computer aided design and reverse engineering technology.

Abstract: Elementary Geometrical Shape (EGS) models present an alternative approach to detect in vivo migration of total hip arthroplasty using model-based Roentgen Stereophotogrammetric Analysis (mbRSA). However, its applicability for an irregular-shaped femoral stem and the reliability of this mbRSA approach has not been proven so far. The aim of this study is to assess the effect of multi-rater and an anatomically shaped femoral stem design onto resulting implant to bone migration results. The retrospective analysis included 18 clinical cases of anatomically shaped stem with 10-year RSA follow-ups. Three raters repeatedly measured all RSA follow-ups for evaluating the rater equivalence and intra-rater reliability. The results proved the equivalence between different raters for mbRSA using EGS models (mbRSA-EGS), hence it simplified the investigation of rater reliability to intra-rater reliability. In all in-plane migration measurements, mbRSA-EGS shows good intra-rater reliability and small intra-rater variability (translation: <0.15 mm; rotation: <0.18 deg). However, the reliability is worse in the out-of-plane measurements, especially the cranial-caudal rotation (intra-rater variability: 0.99–1.81 deg). Overall, mbRSA-EGS can be an alternative approach next to surface models while the in-plane migration of femoral stem (e.g., the implant subsidence for loosening prediction) have more research interested than other directions.

Keywords: reliability; model-based RSA; elementary geometrical shape models; accuracy; hip arthroplasty; migration

1. Introduction

Total Hip Arthroplasty (THA) is considered an effective treatment to improve the function of hip joint failure caused by: arthritis [1] (including osteoarthritis, rheumatoid arthritis, traumatic arthritis, and arthritis caused by other reasons, e.g., the microbleeds in joint capsule of congenital afibrinogenemia patients [2]), fractures [3], malignant bone tumors [4], and so on. However, the main complication of

THA, aseptic loosening [5], has plagued both patients and clinicians for many years. Next to aseptic loosening, periprosthetic infection and the subsequent biofilm formation presented a common reason for revision of THA [6,7]. The antibacterial potential of different implant materials and the strategy to avoid infection is discussed within literature [8,9]. At present, the implant to bone micromotion is considered the most important mechanical factors of aseptic loosening which represents one of the top five reasons for revision surgery [10]. The current gold standard to assess the implant to bone migration in vivo is Roentgen Stereophotogrammetric Analysis (RSA) [11,12]. The RSA method calculates implant to bone migration using rigid body kinematics. To define a rigid body of the implants surrounding bone, at least three tantalum markers must be intraoperatively injected into cancellous bone. To define the implant component as a rigid body, available RSA methods use specific approaches. (i) Marker-based RSA uses additional attached tantalum markers to the implant; model-based RSA uses on the one hand (ii) surface models of the implant, resulting out of Reverse Engineering (RE), or Computer Aided Design (CAD), or (iii) Elementary Geometrical Shape (EGS) models on the other hand [11,13]. The continuous development of the methodology should allow a more extensive application of it.

The introduction of model-based RSA (mbRSA) replaced the additionally attached implant markers of marker-based RSA method by matching a three dimensional (3D) surface implant model to implants projection contour on X-ray films [13]. By using mbRSA, the possibility of an implant marker occlusion could be avoided, and more complex designs, for which additional implant marking presents a challenge, could be overcome. Interchangeable applicability between the gold standard marker-based RSA and mbRSA approach was proved in experimental and clinical settings for surface models [14,15] as well as for EGS approach [13,16,17]. The models required for mbRSA can be derived from RE, CAD, or EGS. Both RE and CAD model have the characteristic that they are highly close to the actual shape of an implant, so that they can be easily matched up with the implant contour on X-ray images. An EGS model uses 3D geometric shapes, likewise spheres, cones, etc., to represent the implant, which will then be partially matched to the implant contours (Figure 1). For example, the femoral ball head component can be matched with a sphere and the distal part of hip stem component can be matched with a cone. mbRSA-EGS uses three virtual markers calculated from the hip stem geometry to represent the rigid body of stem component [13]. The first virtual marker is allocated to the center of femoral ball head, which is represented by the sphere. The second virtual marker represents the femoral stem tip, located at the projection of the lowest tip point on the longitudinal axis of applied EGS cone model. The projection of the first maker (origin center first virtual marker; center of the ball head) on the longitudinal axis of cone model defined the third virtual marker. Remember, this determination of the femoral stem as a rigid body (by three virtual markers) using EGS models requires a stable head-taper connection [17]. Migrations of the stem component relative to femur bone (represented by maker model) were calculated using rigid body kinematics.

This EGS approach enables us to create an individual model with each applied implant size for migration detection within a clinical study. In comparison to the mbRSA approach using CAD/RE models, for each implant size and design variation, one CAD/RE model is required as it is matched with the actual implant shape [18]. Exceptions exist, if, for a design variation, a reduced contour selection is possible [19]. For instance, a THA system with seven different sizes and three variations of caput-collum-diaphyseal (CCD) angle means 21 RE models in total. If each RE model costs approximately EUR 200–250, the total costs of RE models will amount to EUR 4200–5250. In contrast, the application of EGS model can save this cost, as it only demands the corresponding geometry of implants. The generality of EGS model enables the wide application to various types and sizes of implants [20].

At present, EGS model is mostly applied to regular-shaped femoral stems (with conical shaped distal part) [13,16]. However, an irregular-shaped design has been introduced into a large number of femoral stem designs for different reasons [21]: rectangular cross-sectional design for strong rotational stability, conical design with multiple splines for primary fixation, anatomical design to achieve maximum contact, short stem design without a long distal part to preserve bony tissue. However, the application of EGS model on those irregular-shaped femoral stems has not been proven. The development of computer assisted RSA approaches has turned most of the cumbersome manual procedures into automation, thereby reducing unnecessary sources of error from most of manual procedures [22]. Migration analysis using RSA software still contains some user interactions (Figure 2).

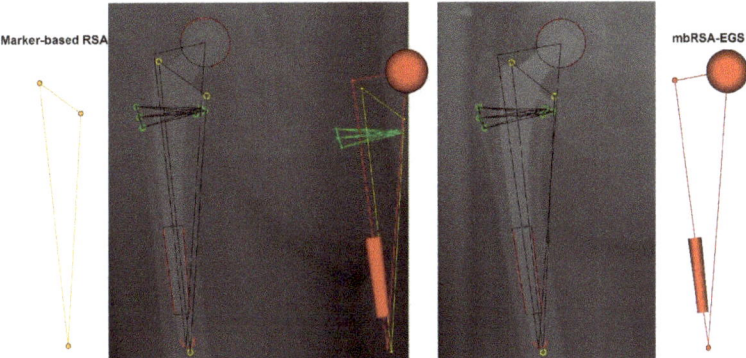

Figure 1. Investigated femoral stem component. RSA analyses by marker-based RSA and mbRSA-EGS illustrated on the same set of RSA radiographs. Bone markers: Green; Implant markers: Yellow; EGS model and projection contour: Red.

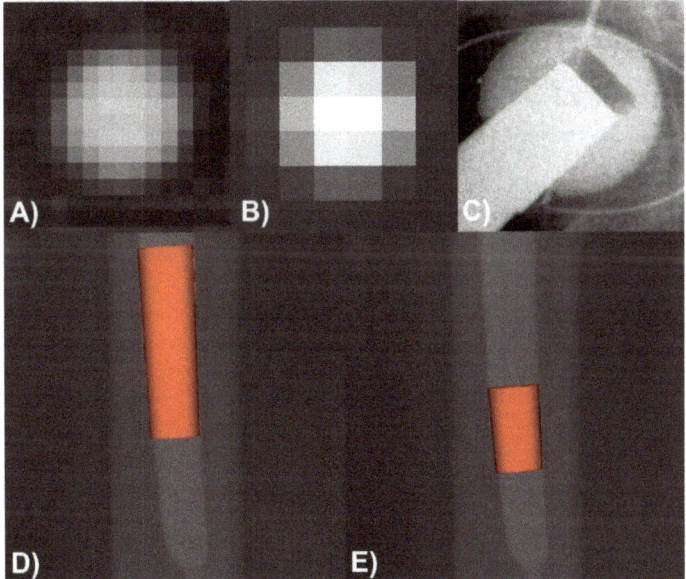

Figure 2. Potential user interactions during RSA image analyses. (**A,B**): poor image quality can lead to variations in the choosing marker center. (**C**): the blurry projection contour of a ceramic femoral head. (**D,E**): choosing two conical-shaped parts when applying EGS models to the irregular-shaped femoral stem. Variations existed in both the length and position of the cone model.

An example for user interactions presents the implant contour detection, which required the rater to select the correct contour. However, not all the implant contours can be clearly displayed on the

X-ray image. The clarity of the implant contour can be affected by the image quality, thickness of soft tissue, density of implant material, etc. For instance, the contour of ceramic femoral head is more blurred compared to metal implants (Figure 2c). In addition to the selection of implant contour, the rater needs to decide which part of distal stem is the required conical shape when applying EGS model to irregular-shaped femoral stems. The current RSA approach and available software-package for analysis is not able to standardize this procedure, considering that those user interactions may affect the resulting implant or bone rigid body definition, thereby influencing the reliability of migration measurement. Information of RSA methodology reliability is lacking. There is a need for this kind of analysis, whilst keeping in mind, that user interactions may affect migration results. Therefore, a rater reliability RSA study was designed to investigate whether the EGS model can be reliably applied to one kind of the irregularly shaped designs: an anatomically shaped stem.

The aim of this study is to answer the two following questions by investigating the rater reliability: (i) which directions of migration measurements have acceptable reliability by applying mbRSA using EGS model; (ii) the reliability of which direction of measurements may be greatly affected. This was demonstrated by the following steps:

1. Rater equivalence: the equivalence between raters was evaluated firstly, which was obtained when the inter-rater difference was so small that measurements from different raters were considered to be equivalent to the rater's own repeated measurements.
2. Intra-rater reliability: if the rater equivalence is acceptable, the investigating of rater reliability can be reduced to the evaluation of intra-rater reliability (as the definition of rater equivalence above).

- Intra-rater reliability of marker-based RSA and mbRSA-EGS
- Whether the intra-rater variability of mbRSA-EGS can be accepted compared with marker-based RSA and the upper limits of RSA accuracy.

2. Materials and Methods

RSA data of primary THA was retrospectively analysed and taken out of a previous study (ethical registration number: 1.077) [23]. Available data offers the opportunity to analyse long-term implant migration by both marker-based RSA and mbRSA-EGS method, respectively.

2.1. Image Acqusition and Analysis

RSA examinations were performed within a uniplanar RSA set up. Patients were positioned in supine position within the both X-ray sources, focused at the hip joint from above with an intersection angle of approximately 40 deg. A calibration box (RSA BioMedical Innovations AB, Umeå, Sweden) was placed under the X-ray table with a vertical distance of 140 cm from the X-ray source. Patients underwent the first reference RSA examination within the first postoperative week, and received RSA follow-ups at 3 months, 6 months, 1 year, 2 years, 5 years, and 10 years.

2.2. Patient Cohort—Inclusion Criteria

The patient cohort received a cemented THA system, consisting of an anatomically shaped femoral stem (Lubinus SP II, Waldemar Link GmbH, Hamburg, Germany) with three visible additional attached tantalum markers which was combined with a ceramic ball head (BIOLOX®forte, Ceram Tec GmbH, Plochingen, Germany) with a diameter of 28 mm. All available cases of this previous study were reviewed. Only cases with a cemented polyethylene acetabular cup (LINK® IP Acetabular Cup, Waldemar Link GmbH, Hamburg, Germany), and a complete follow-up series of RSA images and cases which were able to carry out by both marker-based RSA and mbRSA-EGS methods, were included. Exclusion criteria were: cases with the marker occlusion problem, unacceptable conditions, and cases with a metal acetabular cup component (this means that the femoral head projection can be occluded by metal cup and it resulted in an impossibility to analyze with EGS models). Finally, n = 18 cases were included.

2.3. Measurement and Analysis Protocol

RSA analyses of femoral stem components were performed with a commercially available software package (MBRSA 4.1, RSA Core, Leiden, The Netherlands). During the analysis with standard thresholds, condition number (≤100) and rigid body error (≤0.35 mm), were continuously monitored according to the recommended RSA Guidelines for producing standardized analysis procedure [11,24]. Migration was calculated based on a reference point, which represents the center of gravity of a rigid body. After aligned the reference rigid body (e.g., bone rigid body), translation could be calculated based on the difference of the migration rigid body location (e.g., location of the reference point of implant) between two follow-up time points, rotation could be calculated based on the difference of the migration rigid body orientation between two follow-up time points. The rigid body orientation can be estimated by several shape matching methods in case of using RE/CAD model [12] or EGS model [13]. To verify the quality of the image calibration procedure, standard thresholds for calibration errors (translation ≤0.05 mm, focus error ≤0.5 mm) were used for image analysis [24]. Migration of about 6 degrees of freedom using rigid body kinematics were calculated with respect to a global coordinate system. Application of a calibration box defined translation along the medial-lateral (x) and cranial-caudal (y) axes as in-plane motion, and translation along the anterior-posterior axis (z) as out-of-plane implant to bone motion (migration). Rotation around the anterior-posterior axis (Rz) described in-plane motion and around the medial-lateral (Rx) and cranial-caudal (Ry) axes, out-of-plane implant to bone motion, respectively.

Three independent raters participated in this study, two of which have 2 years' experience in RSA project (rater 1 and rater 3), one has half year experience in RSA analysis (rater 2). Each rater carried out RSA analyses with the marker-based RSA and mbRSA-EGS methods according to the standard analysis protocol in the user manual (MBRSA 4.1, RSA Core, Leiden, The Netherlands). When applying mbRSA-EGS, the raters themselves chose which conical portion of the contour of the distal stem to analyse. After all RSA radiographs were analyzed once by both methods, the raters took a one-week break. This process was repeated until each pair of RSA radiographs was analyzed three times by each rater (Figure 3). Once achieved, for an individual rater, calibration of RSA radiographic image pairs was kept unchanged for the remainder of the analysis sequence of each image pair for both RSA methods (marker-based RSA and mbRSA-EGS). However, for repeated analysis (three times with the same images) by different raters, each time the calibration and analysis were done repeatedly. During the analyses, raters were allowed to revise the analyses when any procedure went against the defined analysis protocol. However, they were not allowed to revise the analyses based only on suspicion of migration. Before all analyses were accomplished, raters had no information of the migration data from previous studies or any other source.

2.4. Statistics

The coefficient of individual agreement (CIA) was used to assess rater equivalence [25], which was adapted from the coefficient for assessing individual bioequivalence criteria (IBC) by Food and Drug Administration (FDA) guideline 2001 [26]. CIA was obtained when the inter-rater difference was so small that measurements from different raters were considered to be equivalent to the rater's own repeated measurements. The threshold of CIA was adapted from the bound of IBC recommended by FDA, 2.495, which corresponds to 0.445 of CIA [25]. Equivalence was considered acceptable if CIA greater than 0.445. The 95% confidence interval was estimated with bootstrapping method [25]. Intraclass correlation coefficient (ICC) was used to assess the intra-rater reliability. An ICC less than 0.40 was considered to be "poorly" agreement, from 0.40 to 0.59 was considered to be "acceptable", from 0.60 to 0.74 was considered to be "good", and 0.75 to 1.00 was considered to be "excellent" [27]. The intra-rater variability was calculated as within-group mean square (WMS) [28]. F-test was used to determine the significance of the intra-rater variability of mbRSA-EGS compared with the corresponding of marker-based RSA (normality was tested by Kolmogorov–Smirnov test). Chi-square test for the variance was used to determine whether intra-rater variability was significantly less than the upper limit of RSA measurement accuracy. Consistent with previous studies [29,30], the upper limit of RSA accuracy (0.5 mm for translation, 1.15 deg for rotation) was used as the threshold. In addition, implants with translation more than 0.15 mm within two years was considered to have higher risk of loosening according to a previous literature [31]. Therefore, 0.15 mm was used as an additional threshold for the intra-rater variability considering the ability of mbRSA-EGS to predict the loosening of the femoral stem. The significance level of 0.05 was considered in all the tests mentioned above. All statistical analyses were performed by R (R Foundation, Vienna, Austria) [32].

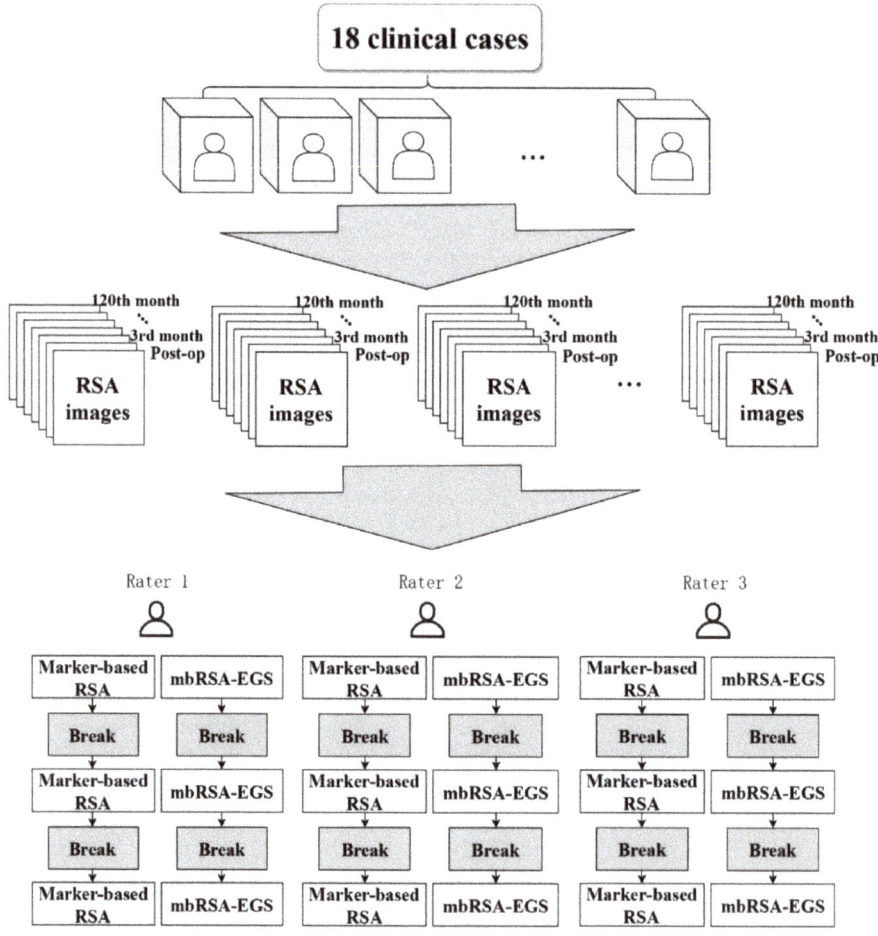

Figure 3. The flow diagram showing details of the study design. Each RSA follow-up was analyzed by 3 raters with both methods and repeated 3 times.

3. Results

The migration results of each of three raters showed similar migration patterns for the investigated femoral stem. On the cranial-caudal translation, the femoral stem showed a clear trend of subsidence within the first two years post-operation (mean migration: 0.05 mm/year), and then become stabilized from the second year to the 10th year (mean migration: 3.28×10^{-5} mm/year).

All migration measurements of mbRSA-EGS showed significant rater equivalence (all six measurements have left-sided confidence interval greater than 0.445). For marker-based RSA, four of all six measurements were found to have rater equivalence with three of them showing significant equivalence (Table 1). None of the measurements had significant inequivalence (with right-sided confidence interval lower than 0.445).

Table 1. Rater equivalence estimated by CIA and its left sided 95% confidence interval.

	Translation			Rotation		
	m.l.[1]	c.c.[2]	a.p.[3]	m.l.[1]	c.c.[2]	a.p.[3]
RSA-marker[4]	0.42 (> 0.27)	0.58 (> 0.44)	0.81 (> 0.72)	0.80 (> 0.70)	0.83 (> 0.75)	0.37 (> 0.22)
mbRSA-EGS	0.71 (> 0.55)	0.64 (> 0.48)	0.77 (> 0.69)	0.76 (> 0.69)	0.81 (> 0.74)	0.65 (> 0.52)

[1] Medial-Lateral; [2] Cranial-Caudal; [3] Anterior-Posterior; [4] Marker-based RSA.

Better intra-rater reliability was found in all in-plane measurements, 15 measurements had ICC within the range of 0.75 to 1.00 ("excellent"), and the other three measurements were within the range of 0.60 to 0.75 ("good") (Table 2). In contrast, in all out-of-plane measurements, the worst ICC value was found in the cranial-caudal rotation measurements with mbRSA-EGS (from 0.11 to 0.30, "poorly"). Furthermore the other out-of-plane measurements showed slightly worse ICC than the in-plane measurements, five measurements within the range of 0.75 to 1.00 ("excellent"), three measurements within the range of 0.60 to 0.75 ("good"), three measurements within the range of 0.4 to 0.59 ("acceptable"), one measurement showed "poorly" result.

Table 2. Intra-rater reliability estimated by ICC.

		Translation			Rotation		
		m.l.[1]	c.c[2]	a.p.[3]	m.l.[1]	c.c.[2]	a.p.[3]
RSA-marker[4]	Rater 1	0.93	0.90	0.75	0.79	0.63	0.92
	Rater 2	0.91	0.83	0.76	0.86	0.50	0.90
	Rater 3	0.90	0.88	0.68	0.83	0.47	0.87
mbRSA-EGS	Rater 1	0.83	0.84	0.62	0.64	**0.30**	0.82
	Rater 2	0.77	0.76	0.53	0.59	**0.21**	0.76
	Rater 3	0.65	0.70	**0.32**	0.51	**0.11**	0.64

[1] Medial-Lateral; [2] Cranial-Caudal; [3] Anterior-Posterior; [4] Marker-based RSA; "poorly" reliability (ICC < 0.40) was marked in bold.

Both RSA methods showed lower intra-rater variability of the in-plane measurements (translation: 0.07–0.15 mm, rotation: 0.07–0.18 deg). Compared with marker-based RSA, the intra-rater variability of mbRSA-EGS were significantly increased (with all measurements had $p < 0.05$). However, compared with the upper limits of RSA accuracy, intra-rater variability of all in-plane measurements were significantly below the upper limits (0.5 mm, 1.15 deg). A total of five out of all six in-plane translation measurements of mbRSA-EGS showed significantly lower intra-rater variability than the threshold of 0.15 mm (Table 3).

Table 3. Intra-rater variability estimated by root of WMS.

		Translation (mm)			Rotation (deg)		
		m.l.[1]	c.c.[2]	a.p.[3]	m.l.[1]	c.c.[2]	a.p.[3]
RSA-marker[4]	Rater 1	0.07 *†	0.07 *†	0.15 *	0.19 *	0.50 *	0.07 *
	Rater 2	0.08 *†	0.09 *†	0.15 *	0.15 *	0.65 *	0.08 *
	Rater 3	0.09 *†	0.07 *†	0.18 *	0.17 *	0.69 *	0.09 *
mbRSA-EGS	Rater 1	0.09 *†	0.09 *†	0.17 *	0.28 *	0.99 *	0.11 *
	Rater 2	0.11 *†	0.11 *†	0.21 *	0.31 *	1.27	0.14 *
	Rater 3	0.15 *	0.13 *†	0.32 *	0.37 *	1.81	0.18 *

[1] Medial-Lateral; [2] Cranial-Caudal; [3] Anterior-Posterior; [4] Marker-based RSA; * Significantly less than 0.5 mm or 1.15 deg ($p < 0.05$); † Significantly less than 0.15 mm ($p < 0.05$).

For the out-of-plane measurements, the largest intra-rater variability was found in the cranial-caudal rotation measurements (0.99–1.81 deg) (Table 3). This large intra-rater variability of mbRSA even leads to clear deviations of the mean cranial-caudal rotation results between raters when compared with marker-based RSA (Figure 4). Furthermore, rater 3 was found to have larger intra-rater variability (0.181 deg) on this rotation measurement compared with other two raters (0.99 and 1.27 deg) (Figure 4b).

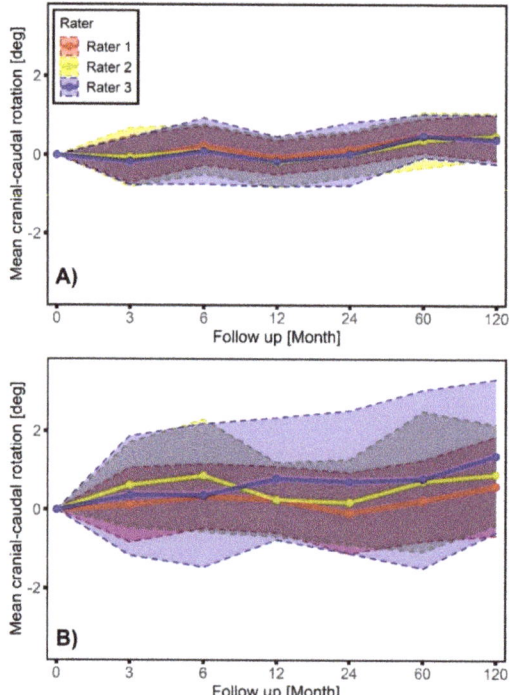

Figure 4. Mean cranial-caudal rotations of femoral stem along follow-up time analyzed by 3 raters with marker-based RSA (**A**) and mbRSA-EGS (**B**). Intra-rater variability was presented as the shaded area.

4. Discussion

Reliability of marker-based RSA and mbRSA EGS approaches and their application in the irregular-shaped femoral stem was assessed for the first time from clinical data. Results of the analyses are very encouraging, suggesting that RSA can deliver reliable and valid migration data, as confirmed within a clinical setting.

Results revealed that both marker-based RSA and mbRSA-EGS have acceptable rater equivalence for the migration measurement of the anatomically designed femoral stem (Table 1). Therefore, according to the definition of CIA, the measurements between different raters can be regarded as the repeated measurements of the same rater. Thus, the intra-rater reliability was further explored. For in-plane migration measurements, mbRSA-EGS showed as good an intra-rater reliability as the gold standard marker-based RSA, with 66.7% of the measurements having "excellent" reliability and 33.3% of the measurements having "good" reliability (Table 2). The intra-rater variability of in-plane migration of mbRSA-EGS (<0.15 mm, <0.18 deg) was much lower compared with the upper-limits of RSA accuracy (0.5 mm, 1.15 deg) (Table 3).

So far, research question (i) can be answered: the rater reliability of in-plane migration measurements by applying EGS model can be accepted. Moreover, the in-plane translation, subsidence of stem, has certain clinical value in predicting future aseptic loosening [29,33]. Systematic reviews and meta-analyses showed that femoral stem subsidence was associated with long term aseptic loosening [31]. Additionally, the results of the investigated THA design proved that the intra-rater variability of this in-plane translation measurement was significantly less than 0.15 mm (the threshold of risk implants of loosening), which means that the EGS model also has a considerable application value for predicting loosening. However, it is known that the accuracy and precision of mbRSA method in general are prosthesis design-dependent. Conclusions cannot be generally applied to each investigated THA system [18].

However, the intra-rater reliability of out-of-plane migration measurements were worse than the in-plane migration, especially in cranial-caudal rotation measurements ("poorly" reliability). The intra-rater variability of cranial-caudal rotation measurements also exceeded 1.15 deg (Table 3). One of the reasons for this large variance was considered as the limitation of its working principle using pose-estimation technique. It was demonstrated that mbRSA using CAD or RE performed less accurately than marker-based RSA on the cranial-caudal rotational measurements of femoral stem implant [14]. The implant projection contour did not change much with a slight rotation around this longitudinal axis, which provided too little information for migration measurement.

Until now, research question (ii) can be answered: the rater reliability of out-of-plane migration measurement (cranial-caudal rotation) by applying EGS model were harmed. The mismatch of EGS model and actual stem shape also played an important role on the poor reliability of this rotation measurement [16]. During the analyses, raters found that the distal part of this anatomically shaped stem was the most difficult part to determine. Rater 1 and 2 tended to choose a longer contour of the distal stem, while rater 3 chose a shorter contour. As the selection of shorter contour may provide less information about the stem axis, it led to a larger intra-rater variability as well as worse ICC of rater 3 (Figure 4), especially in the cranial-caudal rotation measurement. However, it is worth noting that the rater's choice of contour length (rater 1 ≥ rater 2 > rater 3) is not consistent with their experience of RSA analysis (rater 1 ≈ rater 3 > rater 2), as the results supported that the choice of contour length was associated with the reliability of out-of-plane migration measurement. It is recommended to clearly define the standard operating protocol for mbRSA-EGS with the region of interest (length and position) for establishing a standardized template for the contour cone segment to represent the femoral stem component. Considering that two of the three virtual markers in the EGS model depended on the position of the stem central axis, the results presupposed that the irregular-shape of investigated stems would have an impact on the reliability of mbRSA-EGS. On the other hand, these results supported that choosing a longer stem contour could help to improve the reliability harmed by the mismatch of EGS model and actual irregular stem shape of the investigated stem. Additionally, this situation can be improved when applied to stem implants which has the shape matched with available EGS models (likewise cones or cylinders). A study showed better measurement precision of mbRSA-EGS on an hip stem with a strictly conical shaped stem (precision on cranial-caudal rotation measurement: 0.614 deg) [13]. For other irregular stem designs, it could be recommended to do a proof of concept study in advance of the clinical application of mbRSA-EGS for these designs.

Therefore, these results showed that the user interaction can affect the reliability of some migration measurements, especially the choice of stem contour length when using EGS stem model. In general, the reliability of mbRSA-EGS is more sensitive to user interaction compared with marker-based RSA, which should be carefully considered before applying to clinical implant migration measurements. If considering measuring the out-of-plane migration of irregular-shaped stem with mbRSA-EGS, it is better to validate the measurement accuracy by in vitro experiments, double examination in advance, or choosing other validated methods as marker-based RSA or RSA using CAD/RE models. In addition, as the EGS stem model considers the head-stem as a rigid body compared with the CAD/RE model that considers the stem only, it can violate the definition of a rigid body when head-taper motion exists in the actual clinical situation, and consequently may cause deviations in translation measurements.

Additional attention should be paid to possible head-taper motion when applying the EGS stem model [17].

A uniplanar RSA set up was used. This presents the common set up for hip implant migration measurement [34–36]. The results of this study showed the reliability of out-of-plane migration measurements was inferior to in-plane migration measurements, which can be a common limitation of the uniplanar calibration set up [14]. However, the bi-planar set up overcomes this limitation but is rarely used for hip implant migration measurement due to its set up design. Knee and ankle implant migration measurements were much more common with the bi-planar set up [37,38].

The RSA method is in the discussion and gets an increasing importance in the approval and pre-clinical testing process of new orthopaedic implants. Pre-clinical testing is essential to assess the safety and efficacy of new implant designs, coatings, materials, etc., not only for implants in the orthopedic area but also within dentistry [39]. However, sometimes pre-clinical testing results do not correlate with the clinical results and observations (meaning laboratory environment versus real life application). Because of its high accuracy and precision, only small patient cohorts are necessary to investigate the effect of changes in implant design, new bone cements, or additional implant coating on the implant fixation [12,40]. Recently, the importance of RSA to become a tool for the pre-clinical testing and a stepwise introduction of new orthopaedic implant designs has been increasingly valued [40–42]. Therefore, it is necessary to validate the reliability of RSA methods.

Classical marker-based RSA or mbRSA approach offers the opportunities: to measure in vivo implant fixation [43,44], to investigate, e.g., new THA design or coatings, degenerative changes [45–47], joint kinematics [48] and pathomechanism [49], and bony fusion [50]. Additionally, it offers the opportunity to investigate the effect of joint material connection within total joint arthroplasty, likewise the head-taper junction [17]. The application of mbRSA eliminates the additional costs and corresponding risks caused by additional markers on the implant. The CAD/RE model can match the actual shape of implant precisely and has been proven to be as accurate as marker-based RSA [14,20]. But there are certain difficulties in obtaining CAD models. The implant manufacturer is often reluctant to share their CAD models (representing sensitive construction data files) for some commercial reasons. RE model is more convenient to be obtained compared with CAD model. However, when applying RE models to a large number of implants with different sizes or variants (which is a common situation in clinical studies), it can result in a considerable expense. EGS model is a potential alternative when CAD/RE model is not available [51].

5. Conclusions

The in-plane migration of the investigated anatomically shaped femoral stem can be reliably measured by mbRSA-EGS. Considering the loosening prediction value of the femoral stem subsidence (in-plane translation), the EGS model can be used as an alternative option when the CAD/RE model is not available. Last but not least, EGS model delivers a lower-cost alternative compared to CAD/RE model. However, it is worth noting that the mismatch between EGS model and the actual stem shape may significantly affect the reliability of out-of-plane migration measurement, the cranial-caudal rotation. The CAD/RE model presenting a better choice when the out-of-plane migration has greater research significance.

Author Contributions: Conceptualization, F.S., R.F., S.S. and J.X.; methodology, F.S. and J.X; formal analysis, J.X. and H.C.; investigation, F.S. and J.X; resources, R.F.; data curation, J.X., H.C. and F.S.; writing—original draft preparation, J.X.; writing—review and editing, F.S., R.F., S.S. and D.T.; visualization, J.X and F.S.; supervision, R.F.; project administration, F.S. All authors have read and agreed to the published version of the manuscript.

Funding: This research received no external funding.

Acknowledgments: The present work was performed in partial fulfilment of the requirements for obtaining the degree (J.X). Special thanks to D.N. for his support in performing migration analysis.

Conflicts of Interest: The authors declare no conflict of interest.

References

1. Ferguson, R.J.; Palmer, A.J.; Taylor, A.; Porter, M.L.; Malchau, H.; Glyn-Jones, S. Hip replacement. *Lancet* **2018**, *392*, 1662–1671. [CrossRef]
2. Simurda, T.; Kubisz, P.; Dobrotova, M.; Necas, L.; Stasko, J. Perioperative Coagulation Management in a Patient with Congenital Afibrinogenemia during Revision Total Hip Arthroplasty. *Semin. Thromb. Hemost.* **2016**, *42*, 689–692. [CrossRef]
3. Gautam, D.; Gupta, S.; Malhotra, R. Total hip arthroplasty in acetabular fractures. *J. Clin. Orthop. Trauma* **2020**, *11*, 1090–1098. [CrossRef] [PubMed]
4. Brown, T.S.; Salib, C.G.; Rose, P.S.; Sim, F.H.; Lewallen, D.G.; Abdel, M.P. Reconstruction of the hip after resection of periacetabular oncological lesions: A systematic review. *Bone Jt. J.* **2018**, *100*, 22–30. [CrossRef] [PubMed]
5. Goodman, S.B.; Gallo, J. Periprosthetic Osteolysis: Mechanisms, Prevention and Treatment. *J. Clin. Med.* **2019**, *8*, 2091. [CrossRef] [PubMed]
6. Dobson, P.F.; Reed, M.R. Prevention of infection in primary THA and TKA. *EFORT Open Rev.* **2020**, *5*, 604–613. [CrossRef]
7. Lenguerrand, E.; Whitehouse, M.R.; Beswick, A.D.; Kunutsor, S.K.; Foguet, P.; Porter, M.; Blom, A.W. Risk factors associated with revision for prosthetic joint infection following knee replacement: An observational cohort study from England and Wales. *Lancet Infect. Dis.* **2019**, *19*, 589–600. [CrossRef]
8. Cantore, S.; Ballini, A.; Mori, G.; Dibello, V.; Marrelli, M.; Mirgaldi, R.; De Vito, D.; Tatullo, M. Anti-plaque and antimicrobial efficiency of different oral rinses in a 3-day plaque accumulation model. *J. Biol. Regul. Homeost. Agents* **2016**, *30*, 1173–1178.
9. Czuban, M.; Kulka, M.W.; Wang, L.; Koliszak, A.; Achazi, K.; Schlaich, C.; Donskyi, I.S.; Di Luca, M.; Mejia Oneto, J.M.; Royzen, M.; et al. Titanium coating with mussel inspired polymer and bio-orthogonal chemistry enhances antimicrobial activity against Staphylococcus aureus. *Mater. Sci. Eng. C* **2020**, *116*, 111109. [CrossRef]
10. Australian Orthopaedic Association National Joint Replacement Registry (AOANJRR). *Hip, Knee & Shoulder Arthroplasty: Annual Report*; Australian Orthopaedic Association National Joint Replacement Registry: Adelaide, Australia, 2019.
11. Valstar, E.R.; Gill, R.; Ryd, L.; Flivik, G.; Borlin, N.; Karrholm, J. Guidelines for standardization of radiostereometry (RSA) of implants. *Acta Orthop.* **2005**, *76*, 563–572. [CrossRef]
12. Valstar, E.R. *Digital Roentgen Stereophotogrammetry: Development, Validation, and Clinical Application*; Leiden University: Leiden, The Netherlands, 2002.
13. Kaptein, B.L.; Valstar, E.R.; Spoor, C.W.; Stoel, B.C.; Rozing, P.M. Model-based RSA of a femoral hip stem using surface and geometrical shape models. *Clin. Orthop. Relat. Res.* **2006**, *448*, 92–97. [CrossRef] [PubMed]
14. Seehaus, F.; Emmerich, J.; Kaptein, B.L.; Windhagen, H.; Hurschler, C. Experimental analysis of Model-Based Roentgen Stereophotogrammetric Analysis (MBRSA) on four typical prosthesis components. *J. Biomech. Eng.* **2009**, *131*, 041004. [CrossRef] [PubMed]
15. Hurschler, C.; Seehaus, F.; Emmerich, J.; Kaptein, B.L.; Windhagen, H. Comparison of the model-based and marker-based roentgen stereophotogrammetry methods in a typical clinical setting. *J. Arthroplast.* **2009**, *24*, 594–606. [CrossRef] [PubMed]
16. Li, Y.; Rohrl, S.M.; Boe, B.; Nordsletten, L. Comparison of two different Radiostereometric analysis (RSA) systems with markerless elementary geometrical shape modeling for the measurement of stem migration. *Clin. Biomech.* **2014**, *29*, 950–955. [CrossRef]
17. Xu, J.; Sonntag, R.; Kretzer, J.P.; Taylor, D.; Forst, R.; Seehaus, F. Model-Based Roentgen Stereophotogrammetric Analysis to Monitor the Head-Taper Junction in Total Hip Arthroplasty in Vivo-And They Do Move. *Materials* **2020**, *13*, 1543. [CrossRef]
18. Seehaus, F.; Schwarze, M.; Flörkemeier, T.; von Lewinski, G.; Kaptein, B.L.; Jakubowitz, E.; Hurschler, C. Use of single-representative reverse-engineered surface-models for RSA does not affect measurement accuracy and precision. *J. Orthop. Res.* **2016**, *34*, 903–910. [CrossRef]
19. Hurschler, C.; Seehaus, F.; Emmerich, J.; Kaptein, B.L.; Windhagen, H. Accuracy of model-based RSA contour reduction in a typical clinical application. *Clin. Orthop. Relat. Res.* **2008**, *466*, 1978–1986. [CrossRef]

20. Kaptein, B.; Valstar, E.; Stoel, B.; Rozing, P.; Reiber, J. A new model-based RSA method validated using CAD models and models from reversed engineering. *J. Biomech.* **2003**, *36*, 873–882. [CrossRef]
21. Hu, C.Y.; Yoon, T.R. Recent updates for biomaterials used in total hip arthroplasty. *Biomater. Res.* **2018**, *22*, 33. [CrossRef]
22. Vrooman, H.A.; Valstar, E.R.; Brand, G.J.; Admiraal, D.R.; Rozing, P.M.; Reiber, J.H. Fast and accurate automated measurements in digitized stereophotogrammetric radiographs. *J. Biomech.* **1998**, *31*, 491–498. [CrossRef]
23. Sesselmann, S.; Hong, Y.; Schlemmer, F.; Wiendieck, K.; Söder, S.; Hussnaetter, I.; Müller, L.A.; Forst, R.; Wierer, T. Migration measurement of the cemented Lubinus SP II hip stem–a 10-year follow-up using radiostereometric analysis. *Biomed. Tech.* **2017**, *62*, 271–278. [CrossRef] [PubMed]
24. RSAcore. *Model-Based RSA 4.1: User Manual*; Leiden University Medical Center: Leiden, The Netherlands, 2015.
25. Barnhart, H.X.; Kosinski, A.S.; Haber, M.J. Assessing individual agreement. *J. Biopharm. Stat.* **2007**, *17*, 697–719. [CrossRef] [PubMed]
26. U.S. Food and Drug Administration. *Guidance for Industry: Statistical Ppproaches to Establishing Bioequivalence, Food and Drug Administration*; Center for Drug Evaluation and Research: Silver Spring, MD, USA, 2001.
27. Cicchetti, D.V. Guidelines, criteria, and rules of thumb for evaluating normed and standardized assessment instruments in psychology. *Psychol. Assoc.* **1994**, *6*, 284–290. [CrossRef]
28. Norman, G.R.; Streiner, D.L. Analysis of Variance. In *Biostatistics: The Bare Essentials*, 3rd ed.; B.C. Decker: Hamilton, ON, Canada, 2008; pp. 77–80.
29. Karrholm, J.; Borssen, B.; Lowenhielm, G.; Snorrason, F. Does early micromotion of femoral stem prostheses matter? 4–7-year stereoradiographic follow-up of 84 cemented prostheses. *J. Bone Jt. Surg. Br.* **1994**, *76*, 912–917. [CrossRef]
30. Ryd, L.; Albrektsson, B.; Carlsson, L.; Dansgard, F.; Herberts, P.; Lindstrand, A.; Regner, L.; Toksvig-Larsen, S. Roentgen stereophotogrammetric analysis as a predictor of mechanical loosening of knee prostheses. *J. Bone Joint Surg. Br.* **1995**, *77*, 377–383. [CrossRef] [PubMed]
31. Van der Voort, P.; Pijls, B.G.; Nieuwenhuijse, M.J.; Jasper, J.; Fiocco, M.; Plevier, J.W.; Middeldorp, S.; Valstar, E.R.; Nelissen, R.G. Early subsidence of shape-closed hip arthroplasty stems is associated with late revision. A systematic review and meta-analysis of 24 RSA studies and 56 survival studies. *Acta Orthop.* **2015**, *86*, 575–585. [CrossRef]
32. R Core Team. *R: A Language and Environment for Statistical Computing*; R Foundation for Statistical Computing: Vienna, Austria, 2018.
33. Olofsson, K.; Digas, G.; Karrholm, J. Influence of design variations on early migration of a cemented stem in THA. *Clin. Orthop. Relat. Res.* **2006**, *448*, 67–72. [CrossRef]
34. Kjærgaard, K.; Ding, M.; Jensen, C.; Bragdon, C.; Malchau, H.; Andreasen, C.M.; Ovesen, O.; Hofbauer, C.; Overgaard, S. Vitamin E-doped total hip arthroplasty liners show similar head penetration to highly cross-linked polyethylene at five years: A multi-arm randomized controlled trial. *Bone Jt. J.* **2020**, *102*, 1303–1310. [CrossRef]
35. Nieuwenhuijse, M.J.; Vehmeijer, S.B.W.; Mathijsen, N.M.C.; Keizer, S.B. Fixation of the short global tissue-sparing hip stem. *Bone Jt. J.* **2020**, *102*, 699–708. [CrossRef]
36. Tabori-Jensen, S.; Mosegaard, S.B.; Hansen, T.B.; Stilling, M. Inferior stabilization of cementless compared with cemented dual-mobility cups in elderly osteoarthrosis patients: A randomized controlled radiostereometry study on 60 patients with 2 years' follow-up. *Acta Orthop.* **2020**, *91*, 246–253. [CrossRef]
37. Hasan, S.; van Hamersveld, K.T.; Marang-van de Mheen, P.J.; Kaptein, B.L.; Nelissen, R.; Toksvig-Larsen, S. Migration of a novel 3D-printed cementless versus a cemented total knee arthroplasty: Two-year results of a randomized controlled trial using radiostereometric analysis. *Bone Jt. J.* **2020**, *102*, 1016–1024. [CrossRef] [PubMed]
38. Hasan, S.; Marang-Van De Mheen, P.J.; Kaptein, B.L.; Nelissen, R.G.H.H.; Toksvig-Larsen, S. All-polyethylene versus metal-backed posterior stabilized total knee arthroplasty: Similar 2-year results of a randomized radiostereometric analysis study. *Acta Orthop.* **2019**, *90*, 590–595. [CrossRef] [PubMed]
39. Marrelli, M.; Maletta, C.; Inchingolo, F.; Alfano, M.; Tatullo, M. Three-point bending tests of zirconia core/veneer ceramics for dental restorations. *Int. J. Dent.* **2013**, *2013*, 831976. [CrossRef] [PubMed]

40. Seehaus, F.; Sonntag, R.; Schwarze, M.; Jakubowitz, E.; Sesselmann, S.; Kretzer, J.P.; Hurschler, C. Früherkennung des Risikos der späteren Implantatlockerung mittels der Röntgen Stereophotogrammetrischen Analyse (RSA). *Der Orthopäde* **2020**, *49*, 1042–1048. [CrossRef] [PubMed]
41. Nelissen, R.G.; Pijls, B.G.; Karrholm, J.; Malchau, H.; Nieuwenhuijse, M.J.; Valstar, E.R. RSA and registries: The quest for phased introduction of new implants. *J. Bone Jt. Surg. Am.* **2011**, *93* (Suppl. 3), 62–65. [CrossRef]
42. European Union. *Regulation (EU) 2017/745 of the European Parliament and of the Council of 5 April 2017 on Medical Devices, Amending Directive 2001/83/EC, Regulation (EC) No 178/2002 and Regulation (EC) No 1223/2009 and Repealing Council Directives 90/385/EEC and 93/42/EEC*; European Union: Brussels, Belgium, 2017.
43. Pijls, B.G.; Plevier, J.W.M.; Nelissen, R. RSA migration of total knee replacements. *Acta Orthop.* **2018**, *89*, 320–328. [CrossRef]
44. Laende, E.K.; Richardson, C.G.; Dunbar, M.J. Predictive value of short-term migration in determining long-term stable fixation in cemented and cementless total knee arthroplasties. *Bone Jt. J.* **2019**, *101*, 55–60. [CrossRef]
45. Galea, V.P.; Connelly, J.W.; Shareghi, B.; Karrholm, J.; Skoldenberg, O.; Salemyr, M.; Laursen, M.B.; Muratoglu, O.; Bragdon, C.; Malchau, H. Evaluation of in vivo wear of vitamin E-diffused highly crosslinked polyethylene at five years: A multicentre radiostereometric analysis study. *Bone Jt. J.* **2018**, *100*, 1592–1599. [CrossRef]
46. Johanson, P.-E.; Shareghi, B.; Eriksson, M.; Kärrholm, J. Wear measurements with use of radiostereometric analysis in total hip arthroplasty with obscured femoral head. *J. Orthop. Res.* **2020**. [CrossRef]
47. Gascoyne, T.; Parashin, S.; Teeter, M.; Bohm, E.; Laende, E.; Dunbar, M.; Turgeon, T. In vivo wear measurement in a modern total knee arthroplasty with model-based radiostereometric analysis. *Bone Jt. J.* **2019**, *101*, 1348–1355. [CrossRef]
48. Hansen, L.; De Raedt, S.; Jørgensen, P.B.; Mygind-Klavsen, B.; Kaptein, B.; Stilling, M. Marker free model-based radiostereometric analysis for evaluation of hip joint kinematics. *Bone Jt. Res.* **2018**, *7*, 379–387. [CrossRef] [PubMed]
49. Hansen, L.; de Raedt, S.; Jørgensen, P.B.; Mygind-Klavsen, B.; Kaptein, B.; Stilling, M. Dynamic radiostereometric analysis for evaluation of hip joint pathomechanics. *J. Exp. Orthop.* **2017**, *4*, 20. [CrossRef] [PubMed]
50. Humadi, A.; Dawood, S.; Halldin, K.; Freeman, B. RSA in Spine: A Review. *Glob. Spine J.* **2017**, *7*, 811–820. [CrossRef] [PubMed]
51. Fraser, A.N.; Tsukanaka, M.; Fjalestad, T.; Madsen, J.E.; Röhrl, S.M. Model-based RSA is suitable for clinical trials on the glenoid component of reverse total shoulder arthroplasty. *J. Orthop. Res.* **2018**, *36*, 3299–3307. [CrossRef]

Publisher's Note: MDPI stays neutral with regard to jurisdictional claims in published maps and institutional affiliations.

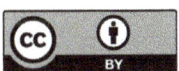

© 2020 by the authors. Licensee MDPI, Basel, Switzerland. This article is an open access article distributed under the terms and conditions of the Creative Commons Attribution (CC BY) license (http://creativecommons.org/licenses/by/4.0/).

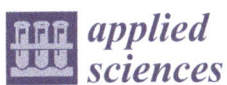

Article

Determination of Leg Alignment in Hip Osteoarthritis Patients with the EOS® System and the Effect on External Joint Moments during Gait

Stefan van Drongelen [1,*], Hanna Kaldowski [2], Benjamin Fey [2], Timur Tarhan [2], Ayman Assi [3], Felix Stief [2,4,*,†] and Andrea Meurer [2,†]

1 Dr. Rolf M. Schwiete Research Unit for Osteoarthritis, Orthopaedic University Hospital Friedrichsheim gGmbH, 60528 Frankfurt/Main, Germany
2 Orthopaedic University Hospital Friedrichsheim gGmbH, 60528 Frankfurt/Main, Germany; hannakaldowski@msn.com (H.K.); b.fey@friedrichsheim.de (B.F.); t.tarhan@friedrichsheim.de (T.T.); a.meurer@friedrichsheim.de (A.M.)
3 Laboratory of Biomechanics and Medical Imaging, Faculty of Medicine, University of Saint-Joseph, Beirut, Lebanon; ayman.assi@gmail.com
4 Faculty of Psychology and Sports Sciences, Goethe University Frankfurt, 60323 Frankfurt/Main, Germany
* Correspondence: s.vandrongelen@friedrichsheim.de (S.v.D.); f.stief@friedrichsheim.de (F.S.); Tel.: +49-69-6705-1903 (S.v.D.); +49-69-6705-862 (F.S.)
† These authors contributed equally to this work.

Received: 2 October 2020; Accepted: 29 October 2020; Published: 3 November 2020

Featured Application: Surgeons performing total hip replacements should know that they have a direct influence on leg alignment and knee adduction moments by implanting a new joint.

Abstract: The present study considered the entire leg alignment and links static parameters to the external joint moments during gait in patients with hip osteoarthritis. Eighteen patients with unilateral hip osteoarthritis were measured using the EOS® system. Clinical leg alignment and femoral parameters were extracted from the 3D reconstruction of the EOS images. A 3D gait analysis was performed and external knee and hip adduction moments were computed and compared to 18 healthy controls in the same age group. The knee adduction moments of the involved leg were strongly correlated to the femoral offset and the varus/valgus alignment. These parameters alone explained over 50% of the variance in the knee adduction moments. Adding the pelvic drop of the contralateral side increased the model of femoral offset and varus/valgus alignment and explained 78% of the knee adduction moment during the first half of the stance phase. The hip adduction moments were best associated with the hip kinematics and not the leg alignment.

Keywords: leg alignment; unilateral hip osteoarthritis; gait analysis; joint loading; external joint moments

1. Introduction

Hip osteoarthritis (OA) is a frequent musculoskeletal degenerative disease [1], initially causing pain during movement, which then progresses on to also include pain at rest. While the mechanism of the development of hip OA is not fully understood, some studies claim that anatomical deviations, especially of the acetabulum and the geometric relation between the head and the shaft, may play a role in the initiation and the course of hip OA [2,3]. In hip OA patients, Bendaya et al. [4] reported changes in leg alignment with a significantly higher sacral slope and a higher femoral mechanical angle. More studies have already reported on the causal relationship between leg alignment and knee OA. A varus alignment of the knee seems to worsen OA in the medial compartment, whereas a valgus alignment contributes to the development of lateral knee OA [5,6]. Furthermore, a smaller femoral offset (FO) and a larger neck–shaft angle (NSA) have been correlated to the incidence of OA in the lateral knee compartment [7].

Measurements of clinical leg parameters from radiographic images can be affected by how the leg is positioned, i.e., horizontal dimensional parameters, such as the femoral offset, are highly influenced by the rotation of the femur [8]. These measurement errors can be minimized by using 3D EOS® technology [9]. An important benefit of EOS is that images are captured with patients in an upright standing position, unlike in conventional hip X-rays, where patients are supine. This upright standing position allows for a more accurate recording of the patient's functional weight-bearing leg alignment [10]. Furthermore, EOS images provide information on the whole leg, not just a pelvic overview, and the patient is exposed to a lower radiation dose than with a conventional X-ray [11,12]. Hence, it is possible to extract clinical leg parameters that have not been previously studied in relation to gait.

Hip OA patients usually adjust their gait pattern in order to reduce pain, which leads to altered joint kinematics and kinetics [13–15]. It has been shown that hip OA patients show a significantly lower knee adduction moment (KAM) on the involved side compared to healthy subjects [14] and compared to their non-involved side [14,15]. It is suggested that a reduced KAM shifts the knee joint load from the medial to the lateral compartment [14,16], which supports the finding that lateral knee OA is often associated with hip OA [17]. Beyond the lower frontal knee moments, lower hip adduction moments (HAMs) on the involved side were also shown in unilateral hip OA patients [14,18].

Joint kinematics have a direct influence on the joint load. This has not only been shown in various simulation studies [19,20] but also in multiple studies in hip OA patients [14,21]. Patients walking with less hip adduction showed a reduced HAM [21]. Regarding the KAM, it was found that patients walking with a reduced knee flexion–extension and a greater foot progression angle (FPA) had a smaller KAM [14]. Schmidt et al. [14] found that the knee range of motion (RoM) in the sagittal plane and the FPA explained 39% of the KAM alterations of the involved limb during the second half of the stance phase.

Another aspect that can directly influence the external joint moments during gait is leg morphology. Leg alignment has previously been presented as a key factor in the load distribution of the knee. Hurwitz et al. [22] pointed out that the mechanical axis (varus/valgus configuration, calculated via the hip, knee, and ankle joints) is the best single predictor for alterations in the KAM. The abovementioned results point toward an influence of leg alignment on the joint load distribution of the knee and likely also of the hip. The question of whether leg alignment and femoral parameters explain the pathological joint adduction moments in unilateral hip OA patients has not been answered yet.

How clinical leg parameters (leg alignment and femoral parameters) impact the external knee and hip adduction moments in patients with unilateral hip OA was the subject of this research. The goal of this study was (1) to test whether there were differences in clinical leg parameters measured with the EOS system between the involved and non-involved side of unilateral hip OA patients and a healthy control group, (2) to confirm that patients with unilateral hip OA showed a deviating gait pattern to healthy controls walking at a similar walking speed, (3) to test whether the clinical leg parameters measured using the EOS system correlated with external joint moment alterations during gait in unilateral hip OA patients, and finally, (4) to test whether the external joint moment alterations were best associated to a combination of clinical leg parameters and gait kinematics.

2. Materials and Methods

This study was registered under the number DRKS00015053 with the German Clinical Trials Register (DRKS).

2.1. Patients

Eighteen patients (9 male, 9 female) with unilateral hip OA and planned for total hip replacement (THR) entered the study (Table 1). The standard exclusion criteria for measuring preoperative hip OA patients, published previously [14,23], were applied.

Table 1. Anthropometric data and walking speed.

Parameter	Patients (n = 17)	Healthy Controls Gait (n = 18)	p-Values Patients vs. Healthy Controls Gait	Healthy Controls Leg Alignment (n = 53)	p-Values Patients vs. Healthy Controls Leg Alignment
Age (years)	60.5 (9.9)	60.4 (8.0)	0.963	41.8 (8.2)	<0.001
Height (m)	1.72 (0.09)	1.73 (0.09)	0.684	1.69 (0.10)	0.302
Weight (kg)	83.3 (15.9)	72.0 (13.9)	**0.032**	74.3 (13.7)	**0.028**
BMI (kg/m^2)	28.1 (4.9)	23.9 (3.2)	**0.004**	25.9 (3.5)	**0.047**
Speed (m/s)	1.06 (0.17)	0.97 (0.07)	0.054	-	-
Gender (M/F)	9/8	11/7	0.625	26/27	0.780

Values are represented as mean value (standard deviation). Significant differences are highlighted in bold. Abbreviations: BMI—body mass index.

Reference gait data were collected from 18 healthy subjects (11 male, 7 female) with a comparable age distribution to the patients (Table 1) [14]. All participants gave written informed consent prior to participation. The protocol was approved by the medical ethics committee of the Department of Medicine of the Goethe University Frankfurt (reference number 497/15).

Since radiographic measurements of healthy controls are not permitted in our clinic, the clinical leg parameters were compared to data of 53 asymptomatic healthy adults, collected as part of a large study in Lebanon [24].

2.2. Radiographic Measurements

Preoperatively, biplane radiographic images were captured in a standing position with the EOS® system (EOS imaging, SA, Paris, France) for all patients [11,12]. An accurate 3D model of the lower extremities was reconstructed for each patient from the lateral and anterior images, as described and validated in previous studies [25]. The 3D model was made using sterEOS® (EOS imaging, SA, Paris, France) and was then used for planning the prosthesis (hipEOS®, EOS imaging, SA, Paris, France). From the 3D reconstruction, five clinical leg parameters, which were described in detail elsewhere [25,26], were considered to assess the leg alignment (Figure 1).

- Hip–knee–shaft angle (HKS): This was measured on the frontal plane, considering the femoral mechanical axis (which connects the centers of the femoral head and the trochlea) and the femoral anatomical axis (axis from the center of the trochlea to the center of the distal diaphysis of the femur).
- Femoral offset (FO): The distance defined by the center of the femoral head and the orthogonal projection of this point on the femoral anatomical axis.
- Neck–shaft angle (NSA): The angle measured between the axis going from the center of the femoral head through the femoral neck and the line drawn down the center of the femur's diaphysis.
- Hip–knee angle (HKA): The angle in the frontal femoral plane between the mechanical axes of the femur and the tibia (the line from the center of the tibial plateau to the center of the distal articular surface of the tibia). Valgus > 180°, varus < 180°.
- Femoral mechanical angle (FMA): The angle that is defined in the frontal plane between the femoral mechanical axis and the line through the medial and lateral condyles (the two most distal points).

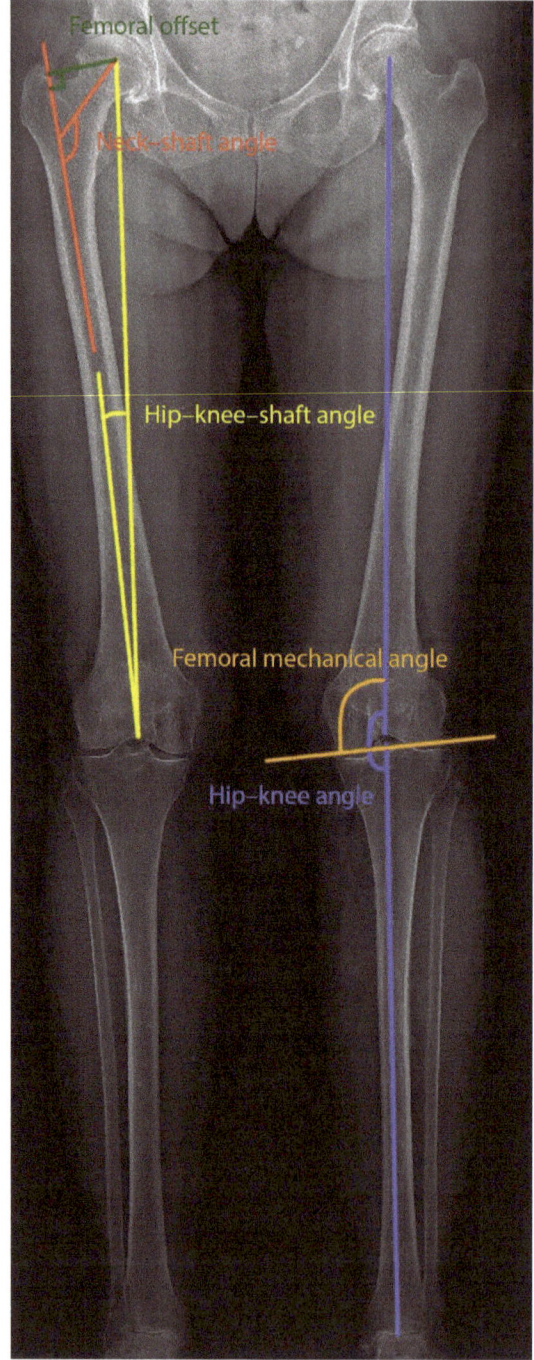

Figure 1. Clinical leg parameters overlaid on the frontal EOS image.

2.3. Gait Analysis

Patients walked barefoot at a self-selected speed in the gait laboratory. Kinematic data (8 MX T10 cameras, VICON Motion Systems, Oxford, UK) were collected synchronously to kinetic data (two OR-6-7-2000 force plates, Advanced Mechanical Technology, Inc., Watertown, MA, USA). Markers were placed on anatomical landmarks according to a modified version of the Plug-in-Gait model to improve the reliability and accuracy of the gait data in the frontal plane [27]. Of all the obtained trials, those in which one foot was completely on the force plate and no markers were missing were classified as good. Five good trials for each subject were selected for further processing. Control subjects walked at their own speed and at a slow walking speed ($\approx$1.0 m/s) which was similar to patients' walking speed shortly before surgery [14]. Since no significant differences were detected between the left and right sides in the control subjects, the left side was chosen for further analysis and for comparison with the involved and non-involved sides of the patient group.

Kinematic and kinetic gait variables were calculated using the inverse dynamics equations [28] in Vicon Nexus (version 2.5, VICON Motion Systems, Oxford, UK). In these equations, the hip joint center was obtained according to a geometrical prediction method [28] and the external joint moments are calculated from the force plate data and the mathematically derived joint centers. Kinematic and kinetic data were exported to Matlab (version R2018b, The Mathworks Inc., Natick, MA, USA) to normalize the data over the gait cycle. The peak external knee and hip adduction moment during the first (KAM1 and HAM1) and second (KAM2 and HAM2) half of the stance phase were computed for each trial (normalized to body weight and expressed in newton meters per kilogram) and averaged over the trials. As has been published previously [26], kinematic parameters during the stance phase of gait were also extracted (a) for the hip: the maximum adduction angle in the frontal plane, the maximum flexion and extension angle, and the hip RoM in the sagittal plane; (b) for the knee: the maximum flexion and extension angle, as well as the RoM in the sagittal plane (the difference between the maximum flexion in the first half and the maximum extension during the second half of the stance phase); (c) for the trunk: maximum sideward displacement (LTD—lateral displacement of the trunk relative to the supporting limb); (d) for the foot: mean progression angle in the transverse plane (FPA—the angle of the long axis of the foot segment relative to the direction of walking). Furthermore, the pelvic drop of the contralateral leg during the swing phase was determined. The gait speed was defined as the average value over the included trials.

2.4. Statistical Analysis

Statistical analyses were performed using SPSS Statistics (IBM SPSS Statistics for Windows, version 26, IBM Corp., Armonk, NY, USA). Anthropometrics were normally distributed, as confirmed by Shapiro–Wilk tests; therefore, differences in anthropometrics between patients and healthy controls were investigated with independent sample Students' t-tests. The comparison of the gender distribution over the two groups was studied using a chi-squared test.

The clinical leg alignment parameters of the patients were normally distributed; however, the FO, FMA, and HKS of the healthy controls were not normally distributed, and as such, Wilcoxon signed ranks test (involved vs. non-involved leg) and Mann–Whitney tests (involved/non-involved leg vs. healthy controls) were used to test for differences.

All kinetic and kinematic gait parameters, except the FPA of the involved side, were normally distributed; therefore, paired sample Students' t-tests were used to test for differences between the involved and non-involved sides for all parameters, except for the FPA, which was analyzed using Wilcoxon signed-rank tests. The involved/non-involved legs were tested against the healthy controls using Mann–Whitney tests for the FPA and using independent sample Students' t-tests for all other parameters.

For the involved and non-involved legs, Pearson's correlation coefficients were calculated between the external knee and hip moments in the frontal plane (adduction moments) and the calculated leg parameters/gait kinematics, as well as among the clinical leg parameters themselves. Multiple regression analysis was performed afterward with the parameters, which correlated significantly with the external joint adduction moments. Leg alignment parameters that showed too strong of a correlation ($R > 0.7$) between each other were excluded from the stepwise regression.

The effect size Cohen's d [29] was calculated (G*Power, version 3.1.9.2, Faul et al., University Kiel, Germany) [30] and p-values ≤ 0.05 were considered significant for all analyses.

3. Results

The data of 17 patients were included in the analysis as one patient had trouble walking without walking aids and walked at half the speed of the other patients. The subject characteristics and gait speed of all participants are displayed in Table 1. The patients had a significantly higher body mass and body mass index (BMI) in comparison to the healthy controls. The individuals of the healthy control group regarding the leg alignment were significantly younger and had a lower body mass and BMI than the patients. All patients had hip osteoarthritis of at least 2 on the Kellgren–Lawrence scale [31] and all patients expressed pain.

As shown in Table 2, no differences could be found between the involved and non-involved sides for all clinical leg alignment parameters. Only the FMA was significantly larger in the healthy control group compared to the patients' involved side ($p = 0.046$).

Table 2. Clinical leg parameters for the involved and non-involved sides, as well as for healthy controls.

Parameter	Involved Side	Non-Involved Side	Healthy Controls Leg Alignment	p-Values Involved vs. Non-Involved	p-Values Involved vs. Healthy Controls	p-Values Non-Involved vs. Healthy Controls
HKS (°)	4.67 (3.99–5.95)	4.75 (4.03–5.69)	4.63 (4.01–5.17)	0.943	0.326	0.505
FO (mm)	41.24 (34.70–46.94)	41.26 (37.37–48.18)	39.97 (35.42–43.01)	0.407	0.272	0.095
NSA (°)	127.12 (119.98–132.49)	125.66 (122.24–130.40)	127.83 (124.97–130.54)	0.906	0.660	0.162
HKA (°)	178.30 (177.18–181.55)	178.60 (175.99–181.59)	178.92 (177.22–181.12)	0.435	0.815	0.613
FMA (°)	91.49 (91.13–92.80)	92.18 (90.17–93.58)	92.66 (91.54–94.12)	0.356	**0.046**	0.218

Values are represented as median values with the 25th and 75th percentiles. The significant difference is highlighted in bold. Abbreviations: HKS—hip-knee-shaft angle; FO—femoral offset; NSA—neck-shaft angle; HKA—hip-knee angle; FMA—femoral mechanical angle.

For KAM1, no significant differences between the involved side/non-involved side and healthy control data could be observed. KAM2 of the involved side was significantly smaller compared to the non-involved side (0.30 vs. 0.40 Nm/kg, $p = 0.011$, $d = 0.68$) and compared to the healthy controls (0.30 vs. 0.45 Nm/kg, $p = 0.004$, $d = 1.07$), as can be seen in Table 3. For the hip, only differences between the non-involved side and healthy controls were found: HAM1 (0.99 vs. 0.80 Nm/kg, $p = 0.014$, $d = 0.90$) and HAM2 (0.94 vs. 0.75 Nm/kg, $p = 0.017$, $d = 0.95$) of the non-involved leg were significantly higher.

For the kinematics, significant differences were found between the involved and non-involved legs for the maximum knee flexion, maximum knee extension, knee RoM, LTD, maximum hip flexion, maximum hip extension, and hip RoM (Table 3). Differences in the maximum knee extension, knee RoM, LTD, hip extension, hip RoM, and the pelvic drop in the swing phase were found between the involved leg and the healthy control group (Table 3). The comparison between the non-involved leg and the healthy controls only showed significant differences in the knee RoM, hip flexion, and hip RoM.

For the involved side, significant correlations between leg alignment parameters were found (Table 4). A very strong (inverse) correlation was detected between the FO and the NSA ($R = -0.895$, $p < 0.001$), where a larger FO resulted in a narrower NSA. The HKA showed a positive correlation with both the NSA and the FMA, meaning that when the HKA appeared to be larger (more valgus alignment), the NSA and the FMA were larger as well, and vice versa. Furthermore, the HKA showed an inverse correlation to the FO, which means that with a smaller HKA (more varus alignment), the FO was larger, and vice versa. For the non-involved side, similar correlations were found for the involved side (Table 5).

Table 3. Kinetics and kinematics during the stance phase of gait for both the involved and non-involved sides and for healthy controls.

Parameter	Involved Side	Non-Involved Side	Healthy Controls Gait	p-Values Involved vs. Non-Involved	p-Values Involved vs. Healthy Controls	p-Values Non-Involved vs. Healthy Controls
Kinetics						
KAM1 (Nm/kg)	0.41 (0.17)	0.45 (0.14)	0.46 (0.15)	0.313	0.361	0.908
KAM2 (Nm/kg)	0.30 (0.14)	0.40 (0.12)	0.45 (0.14)	**0.011**	**0.004**	0.329
HAM1 (Nm/kg)	0.93 (0.22)	0.99 (0.26)	0.80 (0.16)	0.286	0.051	**0.014**
HAM2 (Nm/kg)	0.85 (0.22)	0.94 (0.26)	0.75 (0.14)	0.079	0.137	**0.017**
Kinematics						
FPA (°)	−7.7 (−11.2 to −4.2)	−7.7 (−10.8 to −4.4)	−7.2 (−9.9 to −3.4)	0.586	0.757	0.807
Knee_Flex (°)	16.1 (5.6)	20.8 (6.6)	16.2 (3.4)	**0.005**	0.909	**0.017**
Knee_Ext (°)	9.0 (6.6)	3.8 (5.2)	3.9 (3.4)	**<0.001**	**0.008**	0.954
Knee_RoM (°)	7.0 (4.5)	17.0 (5.3)	12.4 (4.3)	**<0.001**	**<0.001**	**0.007**
LTD (°)	−3.7 (2.4)	−1.3 (2.8)	−1.1 (2.1)	**0.050**	**0.002**	0.806
Hip_Add1 (°)	7.7 (4.5)	6.0 (5.8)	5.7 (4.9)	0.297	0.224	0.873
Hip_Add2 (°)	6.2 (4.3)	5.2 (4.6)	3.8 (4.5)	0.469	0.106	0.346
Hip_Flex (°)	28.6 (8.7)	36.5 (10.6)	30.1 (5.2)	**<0.001**	0.533	**0.036**
Hip_Ext (°)	2.0 (13.2)	−11.2 (9.5)	−9.2 (7.0)	**<0.001**	**0.005**	0.485
Hip_RoM (°)	26.6 (8.1)	47.7 (6.8)	39.3 (3.7)	**<0.001**	**<0.001**	**<0.001**
Pelvic_Drop (°)	−1.1 (2.7)	−2.6 (2.3)	−3.8 (1.7)	0.212	**0.002**	0.074

Values are represented as mean value (standard deviation), except for FPA, where the median and the 25th and 75th percentiles are displayed. Significant differences are highlighted in bold. Abbreviations: maximum external adduction moment for the knee and hip in the first half of the stance phase (KAM1, HAM1) and the second half of the stance phase (KAM2, HAM2); FPA—mean foot progression angle (external rotation as negative); Knee_Flex—maximum knee flexion (flexion as positive); Knee_Ext—maximum knee extension (extension as negative); Knee_RoM—knee range of motion in the sagittal plane; LTD—maximum lateral trunk displacement in the frontal plane (toward the stance limb as negative); maximum hip adduction during first (Hip_Add1) and second (Hip_Add2) halves of the stance phase (adduction as positive); Hip_Flex—maximum hip flexion (flexion as positive); Hip_Ext—maximum hip extension (extension as negative); Hip_RoM—hip range of motion in the sagittal plane; Pelvic_Drop—minimal pelvic obliquity in the frontal plane (swing phase of the contralateral leg and increased pelvic drop as negative).

Table 4. Correlations between the joint adduction moments, joint kinematics, and the clinical leg parameters for the involved leg.

	KAM1	KAM2	HAM1	HAM2	FO	HKA	HKS	NSA	FMA
FO	**0.686 ****	**0.706 ****	0.270	0.253	1.000	**−0.512 ***	0.457	**−0.895 *****	−0.345
HKA	**−0.676 ****	−0.480	−0.376	−0.070	**−0.512 ***	1.000	−0.384	**0.532 ***	**0.594 ***
HKS	0.407	0.345	0.201	0.157	0.457	−0.384	1.000	−0.386	**−0.780 *****
NSA	**−0.626 ****	**−0.535 ***	−0.205	−0.198	**−0.895 *****	**0.532 ***	−0.386	1.000	0.285
FMA	−0.477	−0.353	−0.445	−0.227	−0.345	**0.594 ***	**−0.780 *****	0.285	1.000
FPA	−0.273	−0.085	−0.205	−0.090	−0.077	0.424	0.347	0.191	−0.029
Knee_Flex	−0.019	0.047	−0.354	−0.407	0.001	−0.265	0.250	0.016	−0.182
Knee_Ext	−0.081	−0.043	−0.396	**−0.558 ***	0.073	−0.301	0.164	−0.093	−0.164
Knee_RoM	0.095	0.121	0.137	0.307	−0.104	0.110	0.072	0.156	0.013
LTD	0.264	0.243	−0.007	−0.219	0.200	−0.335	0.131	0.049	−0.248
Hip_Add1	0.060	0.044	**0.761 *****	**0.687 ****	−0.095	−0.072	0.050	0.112	−0.087
Hip_Add2	0.163	0.180	**0.759 *****	**0.732 *****	0.051	−0.095	0.085	−0.056	−0.085
Hip_Flex	0.105	0.106	−0.355	−0.446	0.251	**−0.601 ***	0.178	−0.329	−0.266
Hip_Ext	0.175	0.139	−0.287	−0.408	0.424	**−0.492 ***	0.166	**−0.493 ***	−0.242
Hip_RoM	−0.172	−0.113	0.086	0.186	−0.421	0.156	−0.080	0.451	0.109
Pelvic_Drop	**−0.621 ****	−0.461	**−0.552 ***	−0.425	−0.164	0.406	−0.095	0.181	0.062

Significant correlations are highlighted in bold. * $p \leq 0.05$, ** $p \leq 0.01$, *** $p \leq 0.001$. Abbreviations: maximum external adduction moment for knee and hip in the first half of the stance phase (KAM1, HAM1) and the second half of the stance phase (KAM2, HAM2); FO—femoral offset; HKA—hip-knee angle; HKS—hip-knee-shaft angle; NSA—neck-shaft angle; FPA—mean foot progression angle (external rotation as negative); Knee_Flex—maximum knee flexion (flexion as positive); Knee_Ext—maximum knee extension (extension as negative); Knee_RoM—knee range of motion in the sagittal plane; LTD—maximum lateral trunk displacement in the frontal plane (toward the stance limb as negative); maximum hip adduction during first (Hip_Add1) and second (Hip_Add2) halves of the stance phase (adduction as positive); Hip_Flex—maximum hip flexion (flexion as positive); Hip_Ext—maximum hip extension (extension as negative); Hip_RoM—hip range of motion in the sagittal plane; Pelvic_Drop—minimal pelvic obliquity in the frontal plane (swing phase of the contralateral leg and increased pelvic drop as negative).

Table 5. Correlations between the joint adduction moments, joint kinematics, and the clinical leg parameters for the non-involved leg.

	KAM1	KAM2	HAM1	HAM2	FO	HKA	HKS	NSA	FMA
FO	0.180	0.214	0.015	0.178	1.000	−0.733 ***	0.397	−0.874 ***	−0.340
HKA	−0.313	−0.323	0.303	0.276	−0.733 ***	1.000	−0.315	0.833 ***	0.435
HKS	0.542 *	0.433	0.182	0.064	0.397	−0.315	1.000	−0.388	−0.758 ***
NSA	−0.280	−0.282	0.120	0.004	−0.874 ***	0.833 ***	−0.388	1.000	0.394
FMA	−0.775 ***	−0.518 *	−0.109	0.059	−0.340	0.435	−0.758 ***	0.394	1.000
FPA	0.278	−0.027	0.375	0.238	−0.228	0.453	0.282	0.304	−0.222
Knee_Flex	0.177	0.051	−0.061	−0.149	0.253	−0.167	0.322	−0.384	−0.134
Knee_Ext	0.083	−0.290	−0.305	−0.207	0.332	−0.269	0.182	−0.378	−0.270
Knee_RoM	0.139	0.348	0.222	0.018	−0.011	0.056	0.222	−0.107	0.098
LTD	0.262	0.133	0.056	−0.117	−0.298	0.084	0.070	0.212	−0.392
Hip_Add1	−0.139	−0.165	0.779 ***	0.686 **	−0.321	0.677 **	0.070	0.556 *	0.091
Hip_Add2	−0.083	−0.128	0.790 ***	0.784 ***	−0.199	0.641 **	0.144	0.448	−0.010
Hip_Flex	0.299	0.149	−0.385	−0.392	0.676 **	−0.880 ***	0.371	−0.826 ***	−0.481 *
Hip_Ext	0.190	0.022	−0.360	−0.367	0.432	−0.687 **	0.173	−0.458	−0.415
Hip_RoM	0.203	0.203	−0.100	−0.101	0.457	−0.419	0.341	−0.655 **	−0.174
Pelvic_Drop	−0.181	−0.093	−0.175	0.031	0.452	−0.432	−0.136	−0.632 **	0.111

Significant correlations are highlighted in bold: * $p \leq 0.05$, ** $p \leq 0.01$, *** $p \leq 0.001$. Abbreviations: maximum external adduction moment for knee and hip in the first half of the stance phase (KAM1, HAM1) and the second half of the stance phase (KAM2, HAM2); FO—femoral offset; HKA—hip–knee angle; HKS—hip–knee–shaft angle; NSA—neck–shaft angle; FPA—mean foot progression angle (external rotation as negative); Knee_Flex—maximum knee flexion (flexion as positive); Knee_Ext—maximum knee extension (extension as negative); Knee_RoM—knee range of motion in the sagittal plane; LTD—maximum lateral trunk displacement in the frontal plane (toward the stance limb as negative); maximum hip adduction during first (Hip_Add1) and second (Hip_Add2) halves of the stance phase (adduction as positive); Hip_Flex—maximum hip flexion (flexion as positive); Hip_Ext—maximum hip extension (extension as negative); Hip_RoM—hip range of motion in the sagittal plane; Pelvic_Drop—minimal pelvic obliquity in the frontal plane (swing phase of the contralateral leg and increased pelvic drop as negative).

The correlations between the clinical leg parameters, the kinematics, and the external joint adduction moments for the involved and non-involved legs are also shown in Tables 4 and 5. For the involved side, the parameters FO, HKA, and NSA showed a significant correlation with KAM1, whereas only the FO and the NSA showed a correlation with KAM2. The FMA and the HKA showed a trend toward a significant correlation with KAM1 and KAM2, respectively ($p < 0.053$). For the non-involved leg, the HKS and the FMA showed significant correlations with KAM1. The FMA also showed a significant correlation with KAM2 of the non-involved leg. The HKS and the FO showed a positive correlation to the KAM, which means that with a larger FO and a larger HKS angle, the knee adduction moment was higher. The NSA, the HKA, and the FMA showed a negative correlation such that with a smaller NSA, HKA (more varus), and FMA, the knee adduction moment increased, and vice versa. No correlations between the clinical leg parameters and the HAM were found for the involved or for the non-involved side.

Furthermore, moderate-to-strong correlations between the hip adduction moments and the maximum hip adduction angles were found for both the involved and non-involved legs (R values between 0.686 and 0.790). For the involved leg, moderate correlations were found between KAM1 and HAM1 and the pelvic drop of the contralateral leg, as well as between the knee extension and HAM2. For the non-involved leg, no other correlations were found between the kinematics and the kinetics; however, more significant correlations were found between the kinematic gait parameters and the leg alignment parameters (Table 5).

For the involved leg, a multiple regression analysis revealed that the FO explained 47% of KAM1 ($R^2 = 0.471$; $F = 13.370$; $p = 0.002$; Table 6). Including the HKA significantly improved the model to 61% ($\Delta R^2 = 0.143$, $\Delta F = 5.194$, $p = 0.039$), whereas the NSA was excluded due to a strong correlation with the FO. Adding the pelvic drop of the contralateral side improved the model of the FO and the HKA even more and explained 78% of KAM1 ($\Delta R^2 = 0.162$, $\Delta F = 9.368$, $p = 0.009$; Table 6).

Table 6. Coefficients of determination (R^2 values (%)) for the external joint moments of the involved side as a function of the single correlating leg alignment or kinematic gait analysis parameters and coefficients of determination (Rm^2 values (%)) fitted as a function of all the significantly contributing parameters.

Parameter	First Coefficient of Determination	Second Coefficient of Determination	Third Coefficient of Determination	Multiple Regression
KAM1	FO * $R^2 = 47.1$	HKA * $R^2 = 45.7$	Pelvic_Drop * $R^2 = 38.6$	$Rm^2 = 77.6$
KAM2	FO * $R^2 = 49.91$			
HAM1	Hip_Add1 * $R^2 = 57.9$	Pelvic_Drop $R^2 = 30.5$		
HAM2	Hip_Add2 * $R^2 = 53.6$	Knee_Ext $R^2 = 31.1$		

* Statistically significant ($p \leq 0.05$) contribution that caused Rm^2 to change due to the inclusion of the new predictor. Abbreviations: maximum external adduction moment for the knee and hip in the first half of the stance phase (KAM1, HAM1) and the second half of the stance phase (KAM2, HAM2); femoral offset (FO); hip–knee angle (HKA); minimal pelvic obliquity in the frontal plane during the swing phase of the contralateral leg (Pelvic_Drop); maximum hip adduction during the first (Hip_Add1) and second (Hip_Add2) halves of the stance phase; maximum knee extension (Knee_Ext).

The FO explained 50% of KAM2 ($R^2 = 0.499$, $F = 14.927$, $p = 0.002$). No other parameters were included as the NSA was again excluded due to a too strong correlation with the FO.

The hip joint moments HAM1 and HAM2 were explained by the maximum hip adduction in the corresponding phases of the stance phase (HAM1: 58%, $R^2 = 0.579$, $F = 20.592$, $p < 0.001$; HAM2: 54%, $R^2 = 0.536$, $F = 17.359$, $p = 0.001$; Table 6). The pelvic drop on the contralateral side did not increase the model for HAM1 any further ($p = 0.498$), whereas the knee extension did not increase the model for HAM2 ($p = 0.069$).

For the non-involved leg, multiple regression analyses could not be performed because for KAM1, the HKS (the second parameter with a significant correlation) showed too strong of a correlation with the FMA (the parameter with the strongest significant correlation).

4. Discussion

In the present study, the aim was to determine whether clinical leg parameters (leg alignment and femoral parameters) were different in patients with unilateral hip OA and could be correlated to the altered hip and knee adduction moments. These results could help to better understand the initiation and progression of hip OA and the initiation of knee OA in hip OA patients.

In the last decade, the EOS system has been proven to be a reliable system for the determination of lower limb length and angle measurements [25], with lower radiation exposure in a weight-bearing position. In the present study, except for FMA, no differences were found in leg parameters between the involved and non-involved legs of hip OA patients and healthy controls. As in the present study, Bendaya et al. [4] found significant differences in the FMA and other pelvic parameters in OA patients; however, they could not conclude whether these differences were degenerative over time or were inherent differences between the individuals, or whether they contributed to the progression of OA. The orientation of the axis of the femur (FMA) might become important when planning a knee replacement. Although the risk for contralateral knee OA is higher in patients with a unilateral hip replacement for end-stage OA, the ipsilateral knee is not spared [32,33]. Than et al. [34] found a reduced NSA in their hip OA patients compared to the healthy controls and suggested that it might be due to the younger age of the healthy controls, as the NSA decreased over time. However, our patients showed a similar NSA to the healthy controls and to the controls of the study of Than, despite the significant age differences. Another study found similar values for the femoral offset and the HKA, but a significantly higher NSA in hip OA patients [35]. However, these patients were measured with standard radiography, whereas the present study used EOS images.

The present study confirmed that patients with unilateral hip OA showed a deviating gait pattern compared to healthy controls walking at a similar walking speed. Regarding joint loading, only KAM2 of the involved side was found to be significantly smaller compared to healthy controls (approximately 33%) and the non-involved side (25%), as was found by Shakoor et al [36]. A significantly lower KAM2 indicates a medial-to-lateral shift in the knee load [14,16] and might lead to increased degenerative cartilage wear. The load in the non-involved hip joint was slightly higher compared to the involved hip joint, as was found in preoperative hip OA patients [13,14]. Although these differences were not significant, they might be due to a learned gait pattern to reduce the load on the OA side. The significant differences compared to the healthy control group confirmed the extra load on the non-involved side.

The question of whether leg alignment and femoral parameters explain the pathological joint adduction moments in unilateral hip OA patients has not been answered before. The clinical leg parameters FO, HKA, NSA, and FMA showed a significant correlation (or a trend toward significance) with the knee adduction moments. The positive correlation between the KAM and the FO means that a larger FO implicated a larger KAM, and vice versa. The negative correlation of the KAM with the NSA, the HKA, and the FMA means that a varus leg (a smaller HKA) led to higher knee adduction moments. A larger NSA, and therefore a more valgus leg, was associated with a decreased KAM. Indeed, varus malalignment has been known to be a predictor for the peak knee adduction moments in patients with knee OA [22], and leg malalignment is thought to be one of the main risk factors contributing to the progression of knee OA [5]. Weidow et al. [17] showed that the hip and pelvic anatomy had an influence on the occurrence of medial and lateral knee OA. A decreased NSA, which leads to a more varus leg, was associated with medial knee OA. These results were supported by the present results, as a smaller NSA increased the knee adduction moments during gait. The clinical leg parameters explained 61% of the variance in KAM1 and 50% of the variance of KAM2. For the hip adduction moments, no correlations were found with the clinical leg parameters. In the previous literature, the effect of the FO on gait was discussed. A lower FO led to an asymmetrical gait pattern with a reduction in the knee RoM [37]. Rüdiger et al. [38] showed that with a smaller FO, the abductor muscle force must increase to preserve a normal gait pattern. These results agree with Mahmood et al. [37], who reported that a reduction in the offset was related to a reduction in the abductor muscle strength (moment-generating capacity) of the operated hip. As was found in clinical studies [39,40], the gait pattern is more influenced by a decrease than by an increase in the FO. The effect of the NSA on the hip moments has recently been shown in patients after a THR [41].

In this research, we also studied whether the clinical leg parameters in combination with the gait kinematics were better associated with the pathological hip and knee adduction moments. Till now, only the gait kinematics have been related to the pathological adduction moments in unilateral hip OA patients: Schmidt et al. [14] found a significantly more outward rotation of the foot in their patients, where the FPA, together with the knee RoM, explained 39% of the KAM2 alterations. In the present study, no correlation between KAM2 and the FPA was found. The severity of OA might explain the lack of correlation between KAM2 and the FPA. Rutherford et al. [42] found that only for asymptomatic and mild-to-moderate knee OA patients, the FPA was associated with alterations in the knee adduction moments. In the present study, all patients were symptomatic and severely affected. In the present study, a significant reduced knee RoM during gait was found in the involved limb compared to the non-involved limb and healthy controls. It might be that hip OA patients stiffen the knee on the involved side and flex the knee more on the non-involved side to compensate for leg length differences [14,43]; however, an accurate determination of leg length difference was not part of this study and thus this hypothesis cannot be confirmed.

The gait kinematics showed only a few correlations to the joint adduction moments: the peak hip adduction corresponded strongly to the HAM in the corresponding part of the stance phase and explained 58% and 54% of HAM1 and HAM2, respectively. These correlations were shown previously by Wesseling et al. [20], who showed in a simulation study that increased hip adduction increases the hip adduction moments, as well as the hip contact forces. An increased contralateral pelvic drop had a negative impact (it leads to increased adduction moments) on both KAM1 [44] and HAM1 [45].

The contralateral pelvic drop increased the model for KAM1, and in combination with the FO and the HKA, it explained 78% of the KAM1 alteration. Although a significant correlation was found between the contralateral drop and the external knee joint moments, no differences were found between the patients and healthy controls. Our patients showed a gait pattern with an increased ipsilateral trunk lean that was associated with a reduced pelvic drop. A gait compensation pattern of a stable or elevated pelvis, in combination with an increased trunk lean toward the involved side, was shown by Thurston [46] in individuals with hip OA and by Westhoff et al. [47] in children with Legg Calvé Perthes disease as a compensating strategy to reduce the hip load. However, an increased contralateral trunk lean associated with an increased pelvic drop was also shown in individuals with hip OA [46,48]; hence, the presence of these different combined movements may have confounded the correlation between the single movements and the external hip joint moments. Furthermore, Linley et al. [49] found that only a thorough biomechanical analysis using a principal component analysis could reveal differences in the trunk and pelvic leans.

This study represents the first step in a detailed analysis of the influence of leg alignment on joint adduction moments in unilateral hip OA patients. Nevertheless, our results should be read in light of some limitations. The small sample size used might have restricted the ability to detect significant differences between our groups. Due to the low number of cases, we were not able to take gender into account in our study, as was done by Than et al. [34], who found differences between the sexes in terms of leg alignment. Furthermore, Foucher et al. [50] and Allison et al. [48] were able to report higher hip adduction moments in women compared to men with hip OA. The hip and knee adduction moments are still the gold standards for assessing the load in the frontal plane; however, the joint contact force, calculated using musculoskeletal modeling, is likely a better indicator of joint load compared to joint moments. In the present study, only the effects morphology and kinematics have on joint adduction moments in hip OA patients are discussed. A joint load expressed by joint moments can also be influenced by the abductor muscle force [50] and leg length differences [51] (due to the destructive effect of OA on the hip joint); however, including leg length and abductor function were beyond the scope of the present study. The descriptive models are only valid for the included cohort of patients. In recognizing our limitations to conclusively discuss causality, we recommend that future longitudinal studies be designed to test the development of the leg alignment in patients with hip OA and its effects on hip and knee adduction moments.

5. Conclusions

No differences in the clinical leg parameters between the involved and non-involved legs of hip OA patients could be detected using the EOS system. This could suggest that in our study collective, the leg alignment per se was not the crucial factor for the development of hip OA or that the progression of hip OA did not depend on leg alignment. The last was supported by the present results, as no correlations between the hip adduction moments and leg alignment were found. The present study confirmed that patients with unilateral hip OA walked with a deviating gait pattern and showed lower adduction moments at the involved knee and higher adduction moments at the non-involved hip joint. The current results also confirmed that the varus alignment of the knee (HKA), as well as the femoral parameters (especially the FO), had an influence on the knee adduction moments in unilateral hip OA patients. These two clinical leg parameters explained 61% of the variance in KAM1, and the FO alone explained 50% of the variance of KAM2. A combination of static alignment and gait kinematics explained the knee adduction moments during gait even better in unilateral hip OA patients: adding the pelvic drop of the contralateral side increased the model with the FO and the HKA and explained 78% of KAM1. The hip adduction moments were best explained by the hip kinematics and not by the leg alignment.

Author Contributions: Conceptualization, S.v.D., F.S., and A.M.; methodology, S.v.D. and F.S.; validation, S.v.D. and F.S.; formal analysis, S.v.D., H.K., B.F., T.T., and A.A.; investigation, S.v.D., H.K., A.A., and F.S.; resources, B.F. and T.T.; data curation, S.v.D. and H.K.; writing—original draft preparation, S.v.D. and H.K.;

writing—review and editing, S.v.D., H.K., B.F., T.T., A.A., F.S., and A.M.; visualization, S.v.D.; supervision, A.M.; project administration, S.v.D. and H.K. All authors have read and agreed to the published version of the manuscript.

Funding: This research received no external funding.

Conflicts of Interest: The authors declare no conflict of interest. EOS Imaging (Paris, France) provided support for this study. EOS Imaging had no role in the design, execution, interpretation, or writing of the study.

References

1. Fuchs, J.; Rabenberg, M.; Scheidt-Nave, C. Prevalence of selected musculoskeletal conditions in Germany—Results of the German Health Interview and Examination Survey for Adults (DEGS1). *Bundesgesundheitsblatt* **2013**, *56*, 723–732. [CrossRef]
2. Sharma, L.; Song, J.; Felson, D.T.; Cahue, S.; Shamiyeh, E.; Dunlop, D.D. The role of knee alignment in disease progression and functional decline in knee osteoarthritis. *JAMA* **2001**, *286*, 188–195. [CrossRef]
3. Zeng, W.N.; Wang, F.Y.; Chen, C.; Zhang, Y.; Gong, X.Y.; Zhou, K.; Chen, Z.; Wang, D.; Zhou, Z.K.; Yang, L. Investigation of association between hip morphology and prevalence of osteoarthritis. *Sci. Rep.* **2016**, *6*, 23477. [CrossRef]
4. Bendaya, S.; Lazennec, J.Y.; Anglin, C.; Allena, R.; Sellam, N.; Thoumie, P.; Skalli, W. Healthy vs. osteoarthritic hips: A comparison of hip, pelvis and femoral parameters and relationships using the EOS®system. *Clin. Biomech. (Bristol, Avon)* **2015**, *30*, 195–204. [CrossRef]
5. Felson, D.T.; Niu, J.; Gross, K.D.; Englund, M.; Sharma, L.; Cooke, T.D.V.; Guermazi, A.; Roemer, F.W.; Segal, N.; Goggins, J.M.; et al. Valgus malalignment is a risk factor for lateral knee osteoarthritis incidence and progression: Findings from MOST and the Osteoarthritis Initiative. *Arthritis Rheum.* **2013**, *65*, 355–362. [CrossRef] [PubMed]
6. Sharma, L.; Song, J.; Dunlop, D.; Felson, D.; Lewis, C.E.; Segal, N.; Torner, J.; Cooke, T.D.V.; Hietpas, J.; Lynch, J.; et al. Varus and valgus alignment and incident and progressive knee osteoarthritis. *Ann. Rheum. Dis.* **2010**, *69*, 1940–1945. [CrossRef]
7. Boissonneault, A.; Lynch, J.A.; Wise, B.L.; Segal, N.A.; Gross, K.D.; Murray, D.W.; Nevitt, M.C.; Pandit, H.G. Association of hip and pelvic geometry with tibiofemoral osteoarthritis: Multicenter osteoarthritis study (MOST). *Osteoarthr. Cartil.* **2014**, *22*, 1129–1135. [CrossRef]
8. Lecerf, G.; Fessy, M.H.; Philippot, R.; Massin, P.; Giraud, F.; Flecher, X.; Girard, J.; Mertl, P.; Marchetti, E.; Stindel, E. Femoral offset: Anatomical concept, definition, assessment, implications for preoperative templating and hip arthroplasty. *Orthop. Traumatol. Surg. Res.* **2009**, *95*, 210–219. [CrossRef]
9. Wybier, M.; Bossard, P. Musculoskeletal imaging in progress: The EOS imaging system. *Jt. Bone Spine* **2013**, *80*, 238–243. [CrossRef] [PubMed]
10. McKenna, C.; Wade, R.; Faria, R.; Yang, H.; Stirk, L.; Gummerson, N.; Sculpher, M.; Woolacott, N. EOS 2D/3D X-ray imaging system: A systematic review and economic evaluation. *Health Technol. Assess.* **2012**, *16*. [CrossRef]
11. Charpak, G. Electronic imaging of ionizing radiation with limited avalanches in gases. *Rev. Mod. Phys.* **1993**, *65*, 591–598. [CrossRef]
12. Escott, B.G.; Ravi, B.; Weathermon, A.C.; Acharya, J.; Gordon, C.L.; Babyn, P.S.; Kelley, S.P.; Narayanan, U.G. EOS low-dose radiography: A reliable and accurate upright assessment of lower-limb lengths. *J. Bone Joint Surg. Am.* **2013**, *95*, e1831–e1837. [CrossRef] [PubMed]
13. Foucher, K.C.; Wimmer, M.A. Contralateral hip and knee gait biomechanics are unchanged by total hip replacement for unilateral hip osteoarthritis. *Gait. Posture* **2012**, *35*, 61–65. [CrossRef]
14. Schmidt, A.; Meurer, A.; Lenarz, K.; Vogt, L.; Froemel, D.; Lutz, F.; Barker, J.; Stief, F. Unilateral hip osteoarthritis: The effect of compensation strategies and anatomic measurements on frontal plane joint loading. *J. Orthop. Res.* **2017**, *35*, 1764–1773. [CrossRef]
15. Shakoor, N.; Dua, A.; Thorp, L.E.; Mikolaitis, R.A.; Wimmer, M.A.; Foucher, K.C.; Fogg, L.F.; Block, J.A. Asymmetric loading and bone mineral density at the asymptomatic knees of patients with unilateral hip osteoarthritis. *Arthritis Rheum.* **2011**, *63*, 3853–3858. [CrossRef]
16. Andriacchi, T.P. Valgus alignment and lateral compartment knee osteoarthritis: A biomechanical paradox or new insight into knee osteoarthritis? *Arthritis Rheum.* **2013**, *65*, 310–313. [CrossRef]

17. Weidow, J.; Mars, I.; Karrholm, J. Medial and lateral osteoarthritis of the knee is related to variations of hip and pelvic anatomy. *Osteoarthr. Cartil.* **2005**, *13*, 471–477. [CrossRef] [PubMed]
18. Hurwitz, D.E.; Hulet, C.H.; Andriacchi, T.P.; Rosenberg, A.G.; Galante, J.O. Gait compensations in patients with osteoarthritis of the hip and their relationship to pain and passive hip motion. *J. Orthop. Res.* **1997**, *15*, 629–635. [CrossRef]
19. Ardestani, M.M.; Moazen, M.; Jin, Z. Sensitivity analysis of human lower extremity joint moments due to changes in joint kinematics. *Med. Eng. Phys.* **2015**, *37*, 165–174. [CrossRef]
20. Wesseling, M.; de Groote, F.; Meyer, C.; Corten, K.; Simon, J.P.; Desloovere, K.; Jonkers, I. Gait alterations to effectively reduce hip contact forces. *J. Orthop. Res.* **2015**, *33*, 1094–1102. [CrossRef]
21. Meyer, C.A.G.; Wesseling, M.; Corten, K.; Nieuwenhuys, A.; Monari, D.; Simon, J.P.; Jonkers, I.; Desloovere, K. Hip movement pathomechanics of patients with hip osteoarthritis aim at reducing hip joint loading on the osteoarthritic side. *Gait. Posture* **2018**, *59*, 11–17. [CrossRef]
22. Hurwitz, D.E.; Ryals, A.B.; Case, J.P.; Block, J.A.; Andriacchi, T.P. The knee adduction moment during gait in subjects with knee osteoarthritis is more closely correlated with static alignment than radiographic disease severity, toe out angle and pain. *J. Orthop. Res.* **2002**, *20*, 101–107. [CrossRef]
23. Van Drongelen, S.; Wesseling, M.; Holder, J.; Meurer, A.; Stief, F. Knee load distribution in hip osteoarthritis patients after total hip replacement. *Front. Bioeng. Biotechnol.* **2020**, *8*. [CrossRef]
24. Bakouny, Z.; Assi, A.; Yared, F.; Bizdikian, A.J.; Otayek, J.; Nacouzi, R.; Lafage, V.; Lafage, R.; Ghanem, I.; Kreichati, G. Normative spino-pelvic sagittal alignment of Lebanese asymptomatic adults: Comparisons with different ethnicities. *Orthop. Traumatol. Surg. Res.* **2018**, *104*, 557–564. [CrossRef]
25. Guenoun, B.; Zadegan, F.; Aim, F.; Hannouche, D.; Nizard, R. Reliability of a new method for lower-extremity measurements based on stereoradiographic three-dimensional reconstruction. *Orthop. Traumatol. Surg. Res.* **2012**, *98*, 506–513. [CrossRef]
26. Van Drongelen, S.; Kaldowski, H.; Tarhan, T.; Assi, A.; Meurer, A.; Stief, F. Are changes in radiological leg alignment and femoral parameters after total hip replacement responsible for joint loading during gait? *BMC Musculoskelet. Disord.* **2019**, *20*, 526. [CrossRef]
27. Stief, F.; Böhm, H.; Michel, K.; Schwirtz, A.; Döderlein, L. Reliability and accuracy in three-dimensional gait analysis: A comparison of two lower body protocols. *J. Appl. Biomech.* **2013**, *29*, 105–111. [CrossRef]
28. Davis, R.B.; Õunpuu, S.; Tyburski, D.; Gage, J.R. A gait analysis data collection and reduction technique. *Hum. Mov. Sci.* **1991**, *10*, 575–587. [CrossRef]
29. Cohen, J. *Statistical Power Analysis for the Behavioral Sciences*, 2nd ed.; Routledge: New York, NY, USA, 2013; p. 567.
30. Faul, F.; Erdfelder, E.; Lang, A.G.; Buchner, A. G*power 3: A flexible statistical power analysis program for the social, behavioral, and biomedical sciences. *Behav. Res. Methods* **2007**, *39*, 175–191. [CrossRef]
31. Kellgren, J.H.; Lawrence, J.S. Radiological assessment of osteo-arthrosis. *Ann. Rheum. Dis.* **1957**, *16*, 494–502. [CrossRef] [PubMed]
32. Shakoor, N.; Block, J.A.; Shott, S.; Case, J.P. Nonrandom evolution of end-stage osteoarthritis of the lower limbs. *Arthritis Rheum.* **2002**, *46*, 3185–3189. [CrossRef] [PubMed]
33. Gillam, M.H.; Lie, S.A.; Salter, A.; Furnes, O.; Graves, S.E.; Havelin, L.I.; Ryan, P. The progression of end-stage osteoarthritis: Analysis of data from the Australian and Norwegian joint replacement registries using a multi-state model. *Osteoarthr. Cartil.* **2013**, *21*, 405–412. [CrossRef]
34. Than, P.; Szuper, K.; Somoskeoy, S.; Warta, V.; Illes, T. Geometrical values of the normal and arthritic hip and knee detected with the EOS imaging system. *Int. Orthop.* **2012**, *36*, 1291–1297. [CrossRef]
35. Ollivier, M.; Parratte, S.; Lecoz, L.; Flecher, X.; Argenson, J.N. Relation between lower extremity alignment and proximal femur anatomy. Parameters during total hip arthroplasty. *Orthop. Traumatol. Surg. Res.* **2013**, *99*, 493–500. [CrossRef] [PubMed]
36. Shakoor, N.; Hurwitz, D.E.; Block, J.A.; Shott, S.; Case, J.P. Asymmetric knee loading in advanced unilateral hip osteoarthritis. *Arthritis Rheum.* **2003**, *48*, 1556–1561. [CrossRef]
37. Sariali, E.; Klouche, S.; Mouttet, A.; Pascal-Moussellard, H. The effect of femoral offset modification on gait after total hip arthroplasty. *Acta Orthop.* **2014**, *85*, 123–127. [CrossRef]
38. Rüdiger, H.A.; Guillemin, M.; Latypova, A.; Terrier, A. Effect of changes of femoral offset on abductor and joint reaction forces in total hip arthroplasty. *Arch. Orthop. Trauma Surg.* **2017**, *137*, 1579–1585. [CrossRef]

39. Cassidy, K.A.; Noticewala, M.S.; Macaulay, W.; Lee, J.H.; Geller, J.A. Effect of femoral offset on pain and function after total hip arthroplasty. *J. Arthroplasty* **2012**, *27*, 1863–1869. [CrossRef] [PubMed]
40. Mahmood, S.S.; Mukka, S.S.; Crnalic, S.; Wretenberg, P.; Sayed-Noor, A.S. Association between changes in global femoral offset after total hip arthroplasty and function, quality of life, and abductor muscle strength. A prospective cohort study of 222 patients. *Acta Orthop.* **2016**, *87*, 36–41. [CrossRef] [PubMed]
41. Stief, F.; van Drongelen, S.; Brenneis, M.; Tarhan, T.; Fey, B.; Meurer, A. Influence of hip geometry reconstruction on frontal plane hip and knee joint moments during walking following primary total hip replacement. *J. Arthroplasty* **2019**, *34*, 3106–3113. [CrossRef]
42. Rutherford, D.J.; Hubley-Kozey, C.L.; Deluzio, K.J.; Stanish, W.D.; Dunbar, M. Foot progression angle and the knee adduction moment: A cross-sectional investigation in knee osteoarthritis. *Osteoarthr. Cartil.* **2008**, *16*, 883–889. [CrossRef] [PubMed]
43. Walsh, M.; Connolly, P.; Jenkinson, A.; O'Brien, T. Leg length discrepancy—An experimental study of compensatory changes in three dimensions using gait analysis. *Gait Posture* **2000**, *12*, 156–161. [CrossRef]
44. Dunphy, C.; Casey, S.; Lomond, A.; Rutherford, D. Contralateral pelvic drop during gait increases knee adduction moments of asymptomatic individuals. *Hum. Mov. Sci.* **2016**, *49*, 27–35. [CrossRef]
45. Tateuchi, H.; Akiyama, H.; Goto, K.; So, K.; Kuroda, Y.; Ichihashi, N. Gait kinematics of the hip, pelvis, and trunk associated with external hip adduction moment in patients with secondary hip osteoarthritis: Toward determination of the key point in gait modification. *BMC Musculoskelet. Disord.* **2020**, *21*, 8. [CrossRef] [PubMed]
46. Thurston, A.J. Spinal and pelvic kinematics in osteoarthrosis of the hip joint. *Spine* **1985**, *10*, 467–471. [CrossRef]
47. Westhoff, B.; Petermann, A.; Hirsch, M.A.; Willers, R.; Krauspe, R. Computerized gait analysis in Legg Calvé Perthes disease—Analysis of the frontal plane. *Gait Posture* **2006**, *24*, 196–202. [CrossRef]
48. Allison, K.; Hall, M.; Wrigley, T.V.; Pua, Y.H.; Metcalf, B.; Bennell, K.L. Sex-specific walking kinematics and kinetics in individuals with unilateral, symptomatic hip osteoarthritis: A cross sectional study. *Gait Posture* **2018**, *65*, 234–239. [CrossRef]
49. Linley, H.S.; Sled, E.A.; Culham, E.G.; Deluzio, K.J. A biomechanical analysis of trunk and pelvis motion during gait in subjects with knee osteoarthritis compared to control subjects. *Clin. Biomech. (Bristol, Avon)* **2010**, *25*, 1003–1010. [CrossRef] [PubMed]
50. Foucher, K.C. Sex-specific hip osteoarthritis-associated gait abnormalities: Alterations in dynamic hip abductor function differ in men and women. *Clin. Biomech. (Bristol, Avon)* **2017**, *48*, 24–29. [CrossRef]
51. Khamis, S.; Carmeli, E. The effect of simulated leg length discrepancy on lower limb biomechanics during gait. *Gait Posture* **2018**, *61*, 73–80. [CrossRef]

Publisher's Note: MDPI stays neutral with regard to jurisdictional claims in published maps and institutional affiliations.

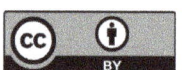

© 2020 by the authors. Licensee MDPI, Basel, Switzerland. This article is an open access article distributed under the terms and conditions of the Creative Commons Attribution (CC BY) license (http://creativecommons.org/licenses/by/4.0/).

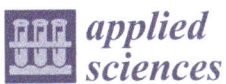

Article

Biomechanical Comparison of Posterior Fixation Combinations with an Allograft Spacer between the Lateral Mass and Pedicle Screws

Soo-Bin Lee [1,2], Hwan-Mo Lee [2], Tae-Hyun Park [3], Sung Jae Lee [3], Young-Woo Kwon [3], Seong-Hwan Moon [2] and Byung Ho Lee [2,*]

1. Department of Orthopedic Surgery, Bundang Jesaeng General Hospital, Daejin Medical Center, Seongnam 13590, Korea; sumanzzz@naver.com
2. Department of Orthopedic Surgery, Yonsei University College of Medicine, Seoul 03722, Korea; hwanlee@yuhs.ac (H.-M.L.); shmoon@yuhs.ac (S.-H.M.)
3. Department of Biomedical Engineering, College of Biomedical Science & Engineering, Inje University, Gyeongnam 621749, Korea; thyun06@gmail.com (T.-H.P.); sjl@bme.inje.ac.kr (S.J.L.); voicians0908@gmail.com (Y.-W.K.)
* Correspondence: bhlee96@yuhs.ac; Tel.: +82-2-2228-2180

Received: 23 September 2020; Accepted: 14 October 2020; Published: 19 October 2020

Abstract: Background: There are a few biomechanical studies that describe posterior fixation methods with pedicle screws (PS) and lateral mass screws (LMS); the combination of both screw types and their effect on an allograft spacer in a surgically treated cervical segment is unknown. Methods: Finite element model (FEM) analyses were used to investigate the effects of a hybrid technique using posterior PS and LMS. Stress distribution and subsidence risk from a combination of screws under hybrid motion control conditions, including flexion, extension, axial rotation, and lateral bending, were investigated to evaluate the biomechanical characteristics of different six-screw combinations. Findings: The load sharing on the allograft spacer in flexion mode was highest in the LMS model (74.6%) and lowest in the PS model (35.1%). The likelihood of subsidence of allograft spacer on C6 was highest in the screws from the distal LMS (type 5) model during flexion and extension (4.902 MPa, 30.1% and 2.189 MPa, 13.4%). In lateral bending, the left unilateral LMS (type 4) model screws on C5 (3.726 MPa, 22.9%) and C6 (2.994 MPa, 18.4%) yielded the greatest subsidence risks, because the lateral bending forces were supported by the LMS. In counterclockwise axial rotation, the left unilateral LMS (type 4) model screws on C5 (3.092 MPa, 19.0%) and C6 (3.076 MPa, 18.9%) demonstrated the highest subsidence risks. Conclusion: The asymmetrical ipsilateral use of LMS and posterior PS in lateral bending and axial rotation demonstrated the lowest stability and greatest subsidence risk. We recommend bilateral symmetrical insertion of LMS or posterior PS and posterior PS on distal vertebrae for increased stability and reduced risk of allograft spacer subsidence.

Keywords: cervical spine surgery; allograft spacer; lateral mass; pedicle screws; finite element model

---

1. Introduction

Advanced surgical techniques for combined anterior and posterior surgery to treat complex cervical conditions that are associated with deformity and neurologic deficiencies are increasing [1,2]. To improve biomechanical outcomes, an intraoperative radiologic device such as O-arm could be used in a hybrid technique with posterior pedicle screws (PS) and lateral mass screws (LMS) [3]. In a clinical setting, asymmetrical cervical pedicle screw placement is not uncommon and depends on both the vertebral artery anomaly and the pedicle anatomy [4,5]. Although there are a few biomechanical studies that describe posterior fixation methods with LMS and posterior PS [6–9], the combination of both screw types and their effect on an allograft spacer in a surgically treated cervical segment is unknown.

Here, we used finite element model (FEM) analyses to investigate the load sharing ratio between allograft spacers and different posterior fixation method combinations that are known to be closely associated with the fusion rate. We compared stability by analyzing the Peak von Mises stress of the allograft spacers and the yielding risk of peri-screw bone under hybrid motion control conditions, including flexion, extension, axial rotation, and lateral bending.

2. Materials and Methods

2.1. FEM of an Intact Cervical Spine

A previously validated three-dimensional intact cervical spinal segment model of C3–6 in a 54-year-old male subject was used [9,10]. The geometrical data of the multi-segmental cervical model were reconstructed from computed tomography (CT) images. The scanner operated at the following settings: ultra-high resolution with a transverse slice thickness of 0.5, and width of the pixel was 0.429 mm.

The cervical Finite Element (FE) model included cortical bone, cancellous bone, posterior elements, annulus fibrosus, nucleus pulposus, and facet. In addition, anterior longitudinal ligaments, posterior longitudinal ligaments, intraspinous ligaments, ligament flava, and capsular ligaments were included. Ligament insertion points were matched from CT image. The spinal ligaments adopted the nonlinear load-displacement material property for the physiological nonlinear behavior of the ligaments (Table 1) [10,11]. The cortical bone of the vertebrae was separately modeled from the inner cancellous bone because of its high stiffness. Although the thickness of the cortical bone varies depending on each vertebral body and on the location, an average value of 0.5 mm was used for the shell thickness in this study [12]. The vertebrae and discs were meshed using "eight-node brick" elements, and the posterior element was meshed using for-node brick elements. The material properties were assumed to be homogeneous and isotropic (Table 2) [13–15]. The mesh convergence was performed to confirm adequate mesh density among variable element sizes from 0.1 to 2.0 mm. Finally, a 0.5-mm element size was applied in our surgical model for the prediction of FE analysis results (implant and periphery, element size—0.5 mm; the others, 2 mm). No unusual stress patterns were presented in this study for this setting.

Table 1. The nonlinear material properties of the ligaments used in the Finite Element model [10].

ALL		PLL		LF		ISL		CL	
Load (N)	Disp. (mm)	Load (N)	Disp. (mm)	Load (N)	Disp. (mm)	Load (N)	Disp. (mm)	Load (N)	Disp. (mm)
0	0	0	0	0	0	0	0	0	0
32	1.2	28	1.2	30	1.8	8.5	1.3	1.5	1.7
60	2.5	50	2.2	55	3.5	10	2.8	29	3.6
81	3.7	66	3.2	71	5.1	23	4.1	52	5
100	4.8	79	3.4	95	6.9	28	5.5	86	7.5
115	6	88	5	105	8	32	7	104	9.5

ALL = anterior longitudinal ligament, PLL = posterior longitudinal ligament, LF = ligament flavum, ISL = interspinous ligament, CL = capsule ligament, and Disp. = displacement.

The intervertebral disc was consisted of an annulus fibrosus and a nucleus pulposus bounded by the endplates. The fiber contents in the annulus fibrosus were modeled using tension-only truss elements, which carry only tensile forces. The annulus fiber was arranged in an alternating crisscross manner with an about 25° orientation [16,17]. The facet cartilage joints were modeled 45° from the horizontal plane and soft frictionless, with an initial gap of 0.5 mm based upon CT imaging [16]. The segment angles used to create the cervical spine curvature for the model were as follows: C3–4: 4.5°, C4–5: 1.87°, and C5–6: 3.94° [18]. For this study, the general-purpose Finite element analysis (FEA) package ABAQUS (Abaqus 2017, Dassault Systèmes Simulia Corp., Providence, RI, USA.) nonlinear geometry parameter (NLGEON = ON) in the ABAQUS step module was used.

Table 2. Material properties.

Component Name	Young's Modulus (MPa)	Poisson's Ratio (ν)	Ref.
Cortical bone	12,000	0.3	[16]
Cancellous bone	100	0.29	[13]
End plate	500	0.4	[17]
Pedicle	5000	0.3	[19]
Posterior element	3500	0.29	[11]
Annulus matrix	4.2	0.45	[17]
Annulus Fibers	500	Cross-sectional Area 0.1(mm^2)	[14]
Nucleus pulposus	1.0	0.499(Incompressible)	[17]
Allospacer(Femoral cortical bone)	18,200	0.38	[20]
Allospacer(Femoral cancellous bone)	389	0.3	[20]
Posterior screw(Ti6Al4V ELI)	110,000	0.35	[21]

2.2. LMS and PS Combination Model with Allograft Spacer

The allograft spacer was constructed based on measuring the Cornerstone™ ASR (Medtronic Sofamor Danek, Memphis, TN, USA) using SolidWorks CAD drawings (Solidworks 2013, Dassault Systemes Solidworks Corporation, Waltham, MA, USA) and imported into ABAQUS to generate elements of 3D geometry. The mesh size of the allograft spacer was 0.5 mm. The boundary condition of the allograft spacer between the cortical bone and cancellous bone was accomplished through a "tie". Then, the meshed allograft spacer model was inserted into the C5–6 disc space of the previously constructed intact cervical FEM. The spacer had a length of 14 mm, a height of 7 mm, and a lordotic angle of 7°, which were the best dimensions to fit the vertebral anatomy at the C5–6 level for the cervical model being used.

The allograft spacers were inserted via an anterior surgical approach, which was previously described [22–24]. By simulating the surgical procedure, the anterior longitudinal ligament, the posterior longitudinal ligament, the superior and inferior endplates, and the anterior and posterior portions of the annulus fibrosus were excised. Then, the allograft spacer was positioned at the anterior margin of the vertebral body. Since our model was aimed at simulating the biomechanical behaviors after bony fusion, specific constraint conditions were imposed, especially at the bone-implant interface. In this study, the interface behavior was accomplished via a "tie" contact condition, which enabled the allograft spacer and vertebrae to be permanently bonded together and fully constrained.

By incorporating the Poseidon cervical pedicle screw system (Medyssey, Jecheon, Korea) for posterior fixation, each lateral mass screw, pedicle screw, and their combination models were set. The PS was 28 mm in length and 3.5 mm in diameter, and the LMS was 14 mm in length and 3.5 mm in diameter. The rod had a thickness of 3.7 mm. Each screw was inserted as described below. The LMS position was defined as 1-mm medial and 1-mm cephalad in relation to the midpoint of the lateral mass. The insertion angle was set to 28° in the lateral direction and 15° in the superior direction. The PS position was set to 1-mm lateral to the center of the articular mass and near the end of the superior articular process. The C5–C6 segment was 40° medial and sagittally parallel to the inferior endplate [25,26].

Six types of postoperative posterior fixation models (Type 1: all LMS, Type 2: all pedicle screws (PS), Type 3: left (Lt) PS and right (Rt) LMS combination, Type 4: Lt LMS and Rt PS, Type 5: upper PS and lower LMS, and Type 6: upper LMS and lower PS) were constructed by modifying the intact model to simulate device implantation at C5–C6 (Figure 1).

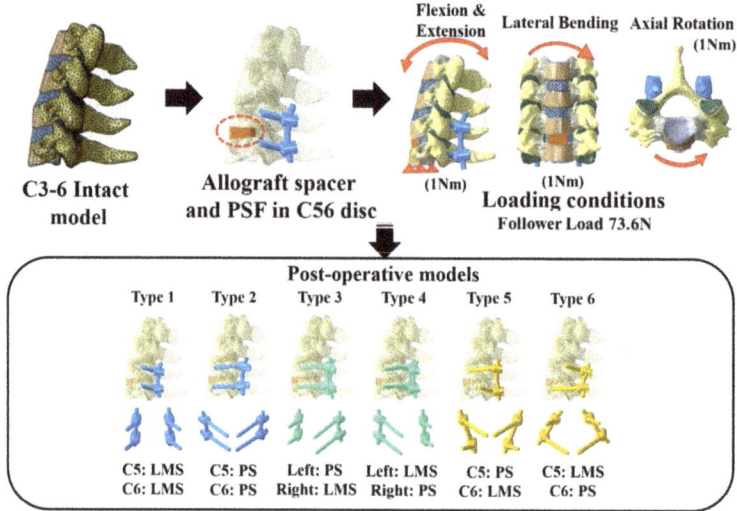

Figure 1. Finite element model and the six models with lateral mass screws (LMS) and pedicle screws (PS). Type 1: all LMS, Type 2: all PS, Type 3: left (Lt) PS and right (Rt) LMS, Type 4: Lt LMS and Rt PS, Type 5: upper PS and lower LMS, and Type 6: upper LMS and lower PS.

2.3. Loading and Boundary Conditions

The inferior endplate of the most caudal vertebra (C7) was fixed in all degrees of freedom, while loads were applied to the superior endplate of the most cephalic vertebra (C3). A compressive load of 73.6 N was used to approximate the weight of the head and local muscle stabilization during daily activity [27,28]. Six constrained degrees of freedom (translation and moment) at C6 were investigated after first applying a compressive load of 73.6 N and then a pure moment of 1.0 Nm. We divided the anterior (allograft spacer, annulus matrix, and fibers) and posterior sections (facet joint and posterior fixation constructs (PFCs)) and calculated the ratio after measuring the normal force in the x, y, and z directions of each surface node. In addition, the stability of the allograft spacer and bone was confirmed by measuring the Peak von Mises Stress (PVMS) of the allograft spacer and the maximum principle strain of the peri-screw bone. To confirm the subsidence potential of the treatment devices, the PVMS of the bone surface in contact with the treatment device was analyzed assuming a bone yield stress ratio of 16.3 MPa [9,29].

3. Results

3.1. Load Sharing Between Posterior Fixation Constructs and the Allograft Spacer

In flexion mode, the load sharing on the allograft spacer was highest in the Type 1 model (74.6%; Figure 2). When combined with any number of PS, the load sharing on the allograft spacer decreased. In extension mode, the load sharing on the allograft spacer was lowest in the Type 5 (14.4%) model and highest in the Type 1 LMS-only model (25.3%). In the lateral bending mode, the load sharing on the allograft spacer was highest in the Type 6 model (60.9%) and lowest in the Type 3 model (23.5%), where the compressed side during lateral bending was supported by the PS. In the counterclockwise axial rotation mode, all models except Type 2 demonstrated increased physiologic loading on the allograft spacers. The load sharing on the allograft spacer was highest in the Type 1 model (42.2%) and lowest in the Type 2 model (19.9%).

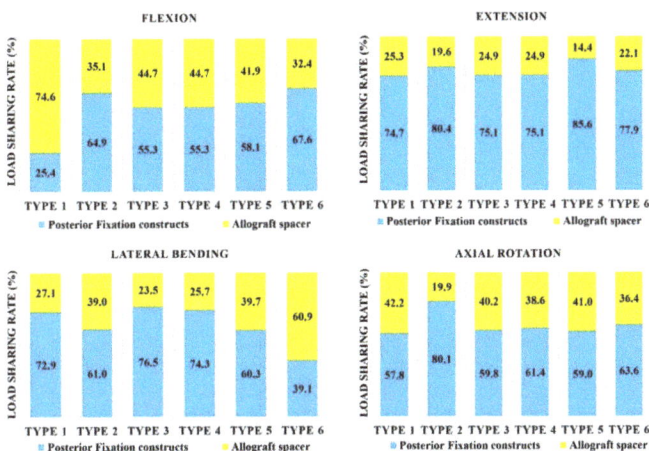

Figure 2. Load sharing on allograft spacers and posterior fixation constructs. Type 1: all LMS, Type 2: all PS, Type 3: left (Lt) PS and right (Rt) LMS, Type 4: Lt LMS and Rt PS, Type 5: upper PS and lower LMS, and Type 6: upper LMS and lower PS.

3.2. Effect of LMS and PS Combinations on the Allograft Spacer and Posterior Fixation Stress Distributions

In flexion mode, the PVMSs of the allograft spacer and PFCs were lowest in the Type 2 model (Figure 3). In extension mode, the PVMS was highest in the allograft spacers in the Type 3 and 4 models and the PFCs in the Type 5 and 6 models. During lateral bending, the PVMSs of the allograft spacers and PFCs were lowest in the Type 2 and 3 models. In the axial rotation mode, the PVMSs of the allograft spacers and PFCs were lowest in the Type 2 model. The PVMSs were highest in type 3 of the PFCs and in Type 4 of the allospacer.

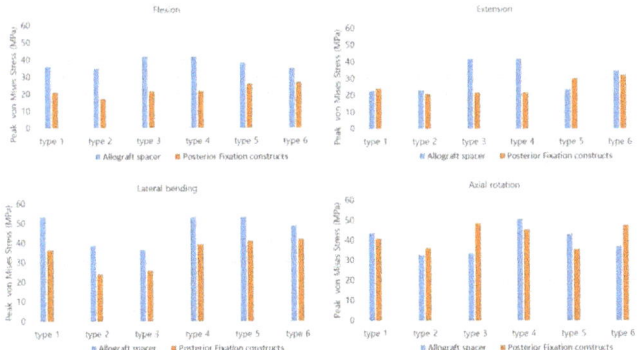

Figure 3. The Peak von Mises stress on the allograft spacers and posterior fixation constructs were dependent on the plate-screw combination. Type 1: all LMS, Type 2: all PS, Type 3: left (Lt) PS and right (Rt) LMS, Type 4: Lt LMS and Rt PS, Type 5: upper PS and lower LMS, and Type 6: upper LMS and lower PS.

3.3. Effect of Posterior Fixation Constructs on Allograft Spacer Subsidence Risk

In general, the vertebra with LMS exhibited a higher risk of subsidence independent of the vertebra level. The likelihood of subsidence of the allograft spacer was calculated on the basis of the yield strength of the C5 and C6 vertebral body cancellous bone of 16.3 MPa (Figure 4).

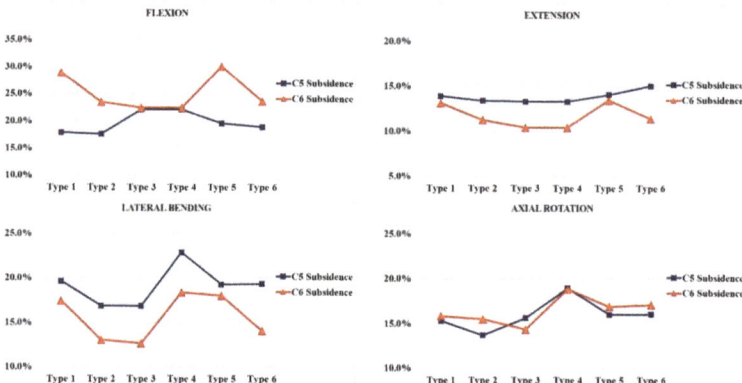

Figure 4. The subsidence risk analysis of the allograft spacers on C5 and C6. Type 1: all LMS, Type 2: all PS, Type 3: left (Lt) PS and right (Rt) LMS, Type 4: Lt LMS and Rt PS, Type 5: upper PS and lower LMS, and Type 6: upper LMS and lower PS.

In flexion modes, the allograft spacer subsidence risk on C6 was highest in the Type 5 (4.902 MPa, 30.1%) model, where the LMS were bilaterally inserted in the lower vertebra. On the C5 vertebra, Type 3 and 4 (ipsilateral hybrid models) (3.598 MPa, 22.1%) had the highest subsidence risks due to asymmetric physical loading and the weaker support from LMS compared to PS.

In the extension mode, the Type 6 model (2.45 MPa, 15.0%) yielded the highest subsidence risk on C5, and the Type 5 model (2.189 MPa, 13.4%) yielded the highest subsidence risk on the C6. During lateral bending, the Type 3 model (2.746 MPa, 16.8%) had the lowest projected subsidence risk on C5 and (2.061 MPa, 12.6%), also, on C6. This can be explained by a PS counterforce opposing the lateral bending force. Contrarily, in the Type 4 model, the lateral bending force was supported by the lateral mass screw. Accordingly, the highest subsidence risks (3.726 MPa, 22.9%) on C5 and (2.994 MPa, 18.4%) C6 were associated with the Type 4 model, because asymmetry on the LMS side caused excessive LMS-side compression forces. In the counterclockwise axial rotation, the Type 4 model (3.092 MPa, 19.0%) had the highest risk of subsidence on C5 and (3.076 MPa, 18.9%) C6. This model had the PS and LMS parallel to the counterclockwise rotation force, which would enable pulling forces that could displace the screws. The Type 2 model, which was all PS, had the lowest subsidence risk during counterclockwise rotation.

3.4. Distribution of Screw-Bone Interface Stresses

In all models, no complete yield of cancellous bone occurred, which was related to screw loosening. The yield strain of cervical cancellous bone was 0.0081. The screw-bone interface stresses increased at the LMS insertion site near the cortex hole. In general, the whole-body stress distribution was on the LMS-inserted side within the same vertebra and the LMS-inserted vertebral body. The highest stress parts, which were dependent on the fixation and motion, are indicated with red arrows in Figure 5.

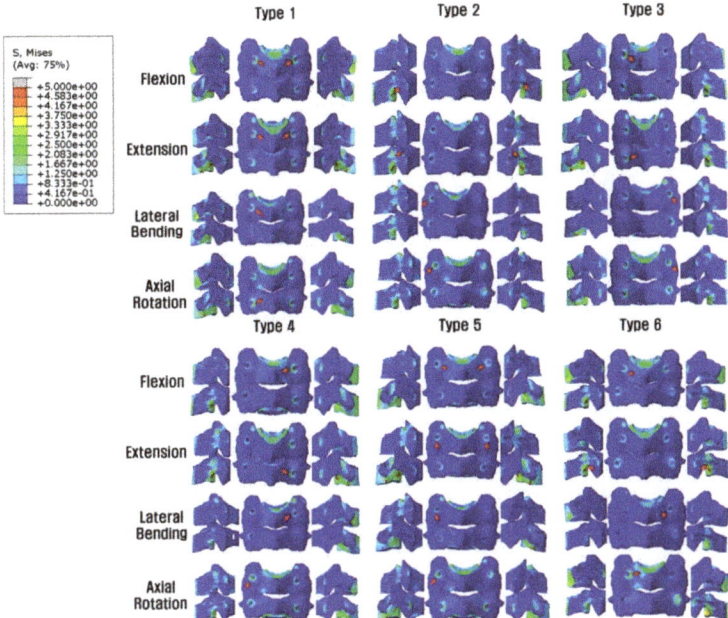

Figure 5. Posterior and lateral views of the Peak von Mises stress distributions on the screw-bone interface. On the LMS side, the stress load of the vertebral body is demonstrated, but on the PS side, the stress shielding of the vertebral body by PS is seen. *Red arrows indicate the highest stress distribution. Type 1: all LMS, Type 2: all PS, Type 3: left (Lt) PS and right (Rt) LMS, Type 4: Lt LMS and Rt PS, Type 5: upper PS and lower LMS, and Type 6: upper LMS and lower PS.

3.5. Distribution of the Peak von Mises Stress on Posterior Fixation Constructs

In general, the Peak von Mises stress of a screw was higher in the LMS than the PS (Figure 6). The Type 2 model had the lowest calculated PVMS in all motion modes. In flexion and extension modes, when both LMS and PS were included, the Type 3 and 4 models demonstrated the highest PVMS, which occurred around the C5 LMS neck area. In the lateral bending mode, the Type 6 model demonstrated the highest PVMS near the C6 PS rod. Additionally, in the lateral bending mode, the Type 2 model demonstrated the lowest PVMS, which occurred near the inlet of the vertebral body pedicle. During the axial rotation mode, the Type 3 model had the highest predicted PVMS around the LMS neck on the C6 area. In the Type 6 model, the PVMS was highest near the LMS neck on C5. In this area, the counterforce was applied counterclockwise against the rotation force. All of the models demonstrated very low values with respect to the yield of the strength of titanium (880 MPa).

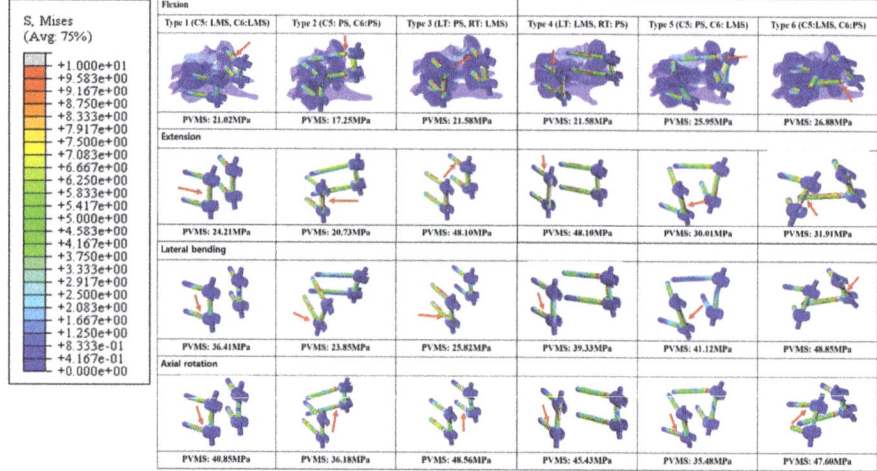

Figure 6. Posterior and lateral views of the Peak von Mises stress distributions on the screw-bone interface. *Red arrows indicate the highest stress distributions. Type 1: all LMS, Type 2: all PS, Type 3: left (Lt) PS and right (Rt) LMS, Type 4: Lt LMS and Rt PS, Type 5: upper PS and lower LMS, and Type 6: upper LMS and lower PS.

4. Discussion

The treatment for severe spondylotic cervical radiculomyelopathy patients is a combination of lateral mass and pedicle screws that are essential to ensure the biomechanical stability of a surgically treated bone-allograft spacer segment. The screw combination is based on patient-specific anatomical considerations and surgeon preferences [1,30]. Despite the variety of screw combinations that can be used, no study has analyzed how different combinations of lateral mass and posterior pedicle screws affects biomechanical stresses. We compared the different biomechanical stresses on allograft spacers, endplates, the bone-screw interface, and rod screws for different screw combinations.

The combination of a lateral mass and pedicle screw is expected to have different stabilization outcomes during flexion, extension, axial rotation, and lateral bending. Furthermore, deeper insertion of the pedicle screw results in better stabilization.

4.1. Load Distribution and PVMS on Posterior Fixation Constructs and Allograft Spacers

In the current study, the PFCs functioned better in extension than tension during the flexion mode regardless of the LMS and PS. The Type 2 model (PS-only) had lower overall loading on the allograft spacer when compared to other models, except during lateral bending. During flexion, the Type 1 model demonstrated the highest allograft spacer loading, which indicated that the LMS alone could be insufficient to support the vertebral body-allograft spacer constructs under specific circumstances, such as loading in osteoporosis patients. Interestingly, in lateral bending mode, the Type 3 and 4 models, which had support from the PS on the compressed side or the opposite side, demonstrated the lowest loading on the allograft spacers. These data suggest that, on both the compressive and distractive sides, the PS hold the C5–6-allograft spacer construct tightly and resist the lateral bending forces.

In axial rotation, the type 3 model had the highest PVMS on the PFCs, which occurred around the LMS neck due to the direction of the counterclockwise rotation force and relatively weaker support from the LMS on the opposite side. Therefore, the stress on the PS side increased to compensate the weaker support from the LMS. The stress on the PS side also increased but was widely distributed over the entire body of the PS. However, on the LMS side, in the near cortex, which was in contact with the LMS, there was increased bone-interface stress. In this area, screw toggling and loosening are expected (Figures 2, 3, 5 and 6). In contrast, for the Type 4 model, the PVMS on the allograft spacer was the highest. The PVMS on the PFC also increased near the LMS neck area due to the screw direction, which allowed for the counterclockwise rotation of the vertebra that could displace the screws.

It is anticipated that, in flexion mode, the allograft spacer PVMSs are higher than in the PFCs. However, in extension mode, after ipsilateral hybrid insertion of the LMS and the PS (Type 3 and 4 models), the allograft spacer PVMSs increased due to asymmetric physiologic loading when compared to the LMS and PS-only models. In the proximal and distal combinations (Type 5 and 6 models), however, both the PVMS on the allograft spacers and on the PFCs increased. For example, in the Type 6 model, the C6 PS had a stronger column fixation when compared to the C5 LMS. The C6 PS was a source of stiffness against LMS fixation, and the PVMS was highest on the rod near the PS head. In the Type 5 model, the PVMS on the PFCs was the highest on the rods near the distal screws (Figure 6). During lateral bending, the Type 2 and 3 models were supported by the PS on the compressed side and demonstrated the lowest PVMSs on both the allograft spacers and PFCs. When combined with the LMS or when the LMS was used alone on the compressed side, the PVMSs on the allograft spacers and PFCs increased (Figures 2 and 3).

The distribution patterns of the PVMSs on the PFCs are clinically meaningful (Figure 6). Most of LMS exhibited higher PVMSs around the LMS neck area (Type 1, 3, and 4 models), which is the most common area for bone-screw interface loosening. In the PS, the highest PVMSs regions were at the screw neck insertion point and at the pedicle screw–shaft interface. In contrast to the LMS, in the PS, the range of bone-screw contacts are wider and have a decreased risk of bone-screw failure caused by toggling motions.

4.2. Effect of Posterior Fixation Constructs on the Subsidence Risk of Allograft Spacers

The asymmetrical hybrid insertion of LMS and PS, especially in the Type 4 model, had worsening subsidence risks that were dependent on the applied forces, except for extension.

In flexion mode, the Type 1 and 5 models had the highest C6 subsidence risks These results indicate that LMS inserted at C6 are weaker than PS and less able to support the flexion force of the constructs, which would accompany the collapse of the C6 endplate. In contrast, the Type 3 and 4 ipsilateral hybrid models had an increased subsidence risk of C5 due to asymmetric physical loading and the weaker support from LMS compared to PS.

In the extension mode, the LMS demonstrated increase subsidence risk at the insertion level in Type 1, 5, and 6 models. When the LMS were inserted at lower levels, the weakest support resulted in increased C5 and C6 subsidence risks. The LMS on C6 in the Type 5 model are biomechanically insufficient to hold the PS inserted in the C5 vertebral body.

In lateral bending, the PS on the compression side provided the strongest support in the Type 2 and 3 models. However, in the Type 4 model, the asymmetry on the LMS side caused excessive LMS-side compression forces, which yielded the highest C5 and C6 subsidence risks. When the LMS was at a lower level (Type 1 and 5 models), it also led to increased concomitant C5 and C6 subsidence risks. In the axial rotation, the screw direction with respect to the rotational force and the bilateral positioning of the LMS affected the allograft spacer subsidence.

In the current study, as anticipated, the PS constructs were biomechanically stronger than the LMS constructs. As the number of PS added to a construct with LMS increased, the biomechanical stability increased. More specifically, the load distribution, especially in flexion, increased. The only exception was the Type 4 model during lateral bending. However, the results indicated that an asymmetric combination of PS and LMS caused an increased subsidence risk in the Type 4 model in the lateral bending and axial rotation. Therefore, when using a hybrid model with LMS and PS, a spine surgeon should understand that specific screw combinations could negatively affect the postoperative subsidence risk of allograft spacers.

This study had a few limitations that are related to the middle-aged 54-year-old male patient that was the basis for the FEM modeling, which have already been mentioned by other studies. The results do not reflect the condition of the discs and endplates in older female patients who undergo spinal surgery with cervical radiculomyelopathy. In addition, our FEM model only included an allograft spacer-vertebral body fusion model; it did take into account the immediate postoperative status of the allograft spacer-vertebral body interface before bony fusion occurs. Additionally, a 3D intact cervical FE model validated by range of motion (ROM) was utilized in the present study [9,10]. This approach confirmed that the kinematics of the developed FEM reflected real soft tissue functions. However, we evaluated the stress and strain of the peri-screw bone, which could be a different context for the use of this FEM. Therefore, this study could lack sufficient evidence to support the validation of this FEM. Nevertheless, in many biomechanical studies, ROM was utilized to validate and verify models, as well as to predict stress and forces reflective of real-world settings [31–37].

5. Conclusions

In conclusion, the asymmetrical ipsilateral hybrid use of LMS and PS in lateral bending and axial rotation yielded the worst mechanical stability and a higher allograft spacer subsidence risk. In addition, distal LMS insertion increased the subsidence risk of allograft spacers on C6 in both flexion and extension. Therefore, we recommend the bilateral symmetrical insertion of LMS or PS and PS insertion on distal vertebra for the improved stability and decreased risk of allograft spacer subsidence.

Author Contributions: Conceptualization, S.-B.L., B.H.L., S.-H.M., S.J.L.,T.-H.P., H.-M.L., and Y.-W.K.; methodology, S.-H.M., S.-B.L., Y.-W.K., B.H.L., S.J.L., T.-H.P., and H.-M.L.; software, H.-M.L., S.-B.L., T.-H.P., B.H.L., S.J.L., S.-H.M., and Y.-W.K.; validation, S.-B.L., T.-H.P., B.H.L., S.J.L., H.-M.L., Y.-W.K., and S.-H.M.; formal Analysis, T.-H.P., B.H.L., and S.J.L.; investigation, T.-H.P., S.J.L., and B.H.L.; resources, T.-H.P., B.H.L., and S.J.L.; data curation, S.J.L., T.-H.P., and B.H.L.; writing—original draft preparation, B.H.L.; writing—review and editing, B.H.L.; visualization, S.J.L., T.H.P, and B.H.L.; supervision, H.-M.L., S.J.L., S.-B.L., Y.-W.K., T.-H.P., S.-H.M., and B.H.L.; project administration, T.-H.P, B.H.L., and S.J.L.; and funding acquisition, B.H.L. All authors have read and agreed to the published version of the manuscript.

Funding: This research was funded by NRF-2017R1C1B5017402.

Conflicts of Interest: The authors declare no conflict of interest.

References

1. Bram, R.; Fiore, S.; Labiak, J.J.; Davis, R.P. Combined Anterior-Posterior Decompression and Fusion for Cervical Spondylotic Myelopathy. *Am. J. Orthop.* **2017**, *46*, E97–E104. [PubMed]
2. Sethy, S.S.; Ahuja, K.; Ifthekar, S.; Sarkar, B.; Kandwal, P. Is Anterior-Only Fixation Adequate for Three-Column Injuries of the Cervical Spine? *Asian Spine J.* **2020**. [CrossRef] [PubMed]
3. Ishikawa, Y.; Kanemura, T.; Yoshida, G.; Matsumoto, A.; Ito, Z.; Tauchi, R.; Muramoto, A.; Ohno, S.; Nishimura, Y. Intraoperative, full-rotation, three-dimensional image (O-arm)–based navigation system for cervical pedicle screw insertion. *J. Neurosurg. Spine.* **2011**, *15*, 472–478. [CrossRef] [PubMed]
4. Koller, H.; Hitzl, W.; Acosta, F.; Tauber, M.; Zenner, J.; Resch, H.; Yukawa, Y.; Meier, O.; Schmidt, R.; Mayer, M. In vitro study of accuracy of cervical pedicle screw insertion using an electronic conductivity device (ATPS part III). *Eur. Spine J.* **2009**, *18*, 1300–1313. [CrossRef] [PubMed]
5. Suda, K.; Taneichi, H.; Kajino, T.; Otomo, H.; Moridaira, H.; Toyoda, H.; Kaneda, K. P66. How to Avoid Fatal Vascular Complications Caused by Cervical Pedicle Screws: A New Surgical Strategy and Techniques for Safe Screw Placement. *Spine J.* **2006**, *6*. [CrossRef]
6. Duan, Y.; Wang, H.H.; Jin, A.M.; Zhang, L.; Min, S.X.; Liu, C.L.; Qiu, S.J.; Shu, Q.X. Finite element analysis of posterior cervical fixation. *Orthop. Traumatol. Surg. Res.* **2015**, *101*, 23–29. [CrossRef]
7. Duan, Y.; Zhang, H.; Min, S.X.; Zhang, L.; Jin, A.M. Posterior cervical fixation following laminectomy: A stress analysis of three techniques. *Eur. Spine J.* **2011**, *20*, 1552–1559. [CrossRef]
8. Hong, J.T.; Qasim, M.; Espinoza Orias, A.A.; Natarajan, R.N.; An, H.S. A biomechanical comparison of three different posterior fixation constructs used for C6–C7 cervical spine immobilization: A finite element study. *Neurol. Med. Chir.* **2013**, *54*, 727–735. [CrossRef]

9. Kwon, J.-W.; Bang, S.H.; Park, T.H.; Lee, S.-J.; Lee, H.-M.; Lee, S.-B.; Lee, B.H.; Moon, S.-H. Biomechanical comparison of cervical discectomy/fusion model using allograft spacers between anterior and posterior fixation methods (lateral mass and pedicle screw). *Clin. Biomech.* **2020**, *73*, 226–233. [CrossRef]
10. Jung, T.-G.; Woo, S.-H.; Park, K.-M.; Jang, J.-W.; Han, D.-W.; Lee, S.J. Biomechanical behavior of two different cervical total disc replacement designs in relation of concavity of articular surfaces: ProDisc-C® vs. Prestige-LP®. *Int. J. Precis. Eng. Manuf.* **2013**, *14*, 819–824. [CrossRef]
11. Galbusera, F.; Bellini, C.M.; Raimondi, M.T.; Fornari, M.; Assietti, R. Cervical spine biomechanics following implantation of a disc prosthesis. *Med. Eng. Phys.* **2008**, *30*, 1127–1133. [CrossRef] [PubMed]
12. Ritzel, H.; Amling, M.; Pösl, M.; Hahn, M.; Delling, G. The thickness of human vertebral cortical bone and its changes in aging and osteoporosis: A histomorphometric analysis of the complete spinal column from thirty-seven autopsy specimens. *J. Bone Miner. Res.* **1997**, *12*, 89–95. [CrossRef]
13. Zhang, Q.H.; Teo, E.C.; Ng, H.W.; Lee, V.S. Finite element analysis of moment-rotation relationships for human cervical spine. *J. Biomech.* **2006**, *39*, 189–193. [CrossRef]
14. Kim, J.-D.; Kim, N.-S.; Hong, C.-S.; Oh, C.-Y. Design optimization of a xenogeneic bone plate and screws using the Taguchi and finite element methods. *Int. J. Precis. Eng. Manuf.* **2011**, *12*, 1119–1124. [CrossRef]
15. Whyne, C.M.; Hu, S.S.; Klisch, S.; Lotz, J.C. Effect of the pedicle and posterior arch on vertebral body strength predictions in finite element modeling. *Spine* **1998**, *23*, 899–907. [CrossRef]
16. Faizan, A.; Goel, V.K.; Garfin, S.R.; Bono, C.M.; Serhan, H.; Biyani, A.; Elgafy, H.; Krishna, M.; Friesem, T. Do design variations in the artificial disc influence cervical spine biomechanics? A finite element investigation. *Eur. Spine J.* **2012**, *21*, 653–662. [CrossRef]
17. Ha, S.K. Finite element modeling of multi-level cervical spinal segments (C3–C6) and biomechanical analysis of an elastomer-type prosthetic disc. *Med. Eng. Phys.* **2006**, *28*, 534–541. [CrossRef] [PubMed]
18. Harrison, D.E.; Harrison, D.D.; Cailliet, R.; Troyanovich, S.J.; Janik, T.J.; Holland, B. Cobb method or Harrison posterior tangent method: Which to choose for lateral cervical radiographic analysis. *Spine* **2000**, *25*, 2072–2078. [CrossRef]
19. Wong, C.; Rasmussen, J.; Simonsen, E.; Hansen, L.; de Zee, M.; Dendorfer, S. The influence of muscle forces on the stress distribution in the lumbar spine. *Open Spine J.* **2011**, *3*, 21–26. [CrossRef]
20. Shi, D.; Wang, F.; Wang, D.; Li, X.; Wang, Q. 3-D finite element analysis of the influence of synovial condition in sacroiliac joint on the load transmission in human pelvic system. *Med. Eng. Phys.* **2014**, *36*, 745–753. [CrossRef]
21. Li, J.; Shang, J.; Zhou, Y.; Li, C.; Liu, H. Finite element analysis of a new pedicle screw-plate system for minimally invasive transforaminal lumbar interbody fusion. *PloS ONE* **2015**. [CrossRef]
22. Baker, A.D. The treatment of certain cervical-spine disorders by anterior removal of the intervertebral disc and interbody fusion. In *Classic Papers in Orthopaedics*; Banaszkiewicz, P., Kader, D., Eds.; Springer: London, UK, 2014.
23. Kwon, J.-W.; Lee, H.-M.; Park, T.-H.; Lee, S.J.; Kwon, J.-W.; Moon, S.-H.; Lee, B.H. Biomechanical Analysis of Allograft Spacer Failure as a Function of Cortical-Cancellous Ratio in Anterior Cervical Discectomy/Fusion: Allograft Spacer Alone Model. *Appl. Sci.* **2020**, *10*, 6413. [CrossRef]
24. Lee, J.C.; Jang, H.-D.; Ahn, J.; Choi, S.-W.; Kang, D.; Shin, B.-J. Comparison of cortical ring allograft and plate fixation with autologous iliac bone graft for anterior cervical discectomy and fusion. *Asian Spine J.* **2019**, *13*, 258–264. [CrossRef] [PubMed]
25. Abumi, K.; Itoh, H.; Taneichi, H.; Kaneda, K. Transpedicular screw fixation for traumatic lesions of the middle and lower cervical spine: Description of the techniques and preliminary report. *J. Spinal Disord.* **1994**, *7*, 19–28. [CrossRef] [PubMed]
26. Coe, J.D.; Vaccaro, A.R.; Dailey, A.T.; Skolasky, R.L., Jr.; Sasso, R.C.; Ludwig, S.C.; Brodt, E.D.; Dettori, J.R. Lateral mass screw fixation in the cervical spine. *J Bone Joint Surg. Am.* **2013**, *95*, 2136–2143. [CrossRef]
27. Goel, V.K.; Panjabi, M.M.; Patwardhan, A.G.; Dooris, A.P.; Serhan, H. Test protocols for evaluation of spinal implants. *J. Bone Joint Surg. Am.* **2006**, *88*, 103–109.
28. Panjabi, M.M. Hybrid multidirectional test method to evaluate spinal adjacent-level effects. *Clin. Biomech.* **2007**, *22*, 257–265. [CrossRef]
29. Kwon, J.-W.; Bang, S.-H.; Kwon, Y.-W.; Cho, J.-Y.; Park, T.-H.; Lee, S.-J.; Lee, H.-M.; Moon, S.-H.; Lee, B.H. Biomechanical comparison of the angle of inserted screws and the length of anterior cervical plate systems with allograft spacers. *Clin. Biomech.* **2020**, *76*, 105021. [CrossRef]

30. Wang, S.; Wang, C.; Leng, H.; Zhao, W.; Yan, M.; Zhou, H. Pedicle Screw Combined With Lateral Mass Screw Fixation in the Treatment of Basilar Invagination and Congenital C2–C3 Fusion. *Clin. Spine Surg.* **2016**, *29*, 448–453. [CrossRef]
31. Chiang, M.-F.; Teng, J.-M.; Huang, C.-H.; Cheng, C.-K.; Chen, C.-S.; Chang, T.-K.; Chao, S.-H. Finite element analysis of cage subsidence in cervical interbody fusion. *J. Med. Biol. Eng.* **2004**, *24*, 201–208.
32. Liu, N.; Lu, T.; Wang, Y.; Sun, Z.; Li, J.; He, X. Effects of new cage profiles on the improvement in biomechanical performance of multilevel anterior cervical Corpectomy and fusion: A finite element analysis. *World Neurosurg.* **2019**, *129*, e87–e96. [CrossRef] [PubMed]
33. Zhang, Y.; Zhou, J.; Guo, X.; Cai, Z.; Liu, H.; Xue, Y. Biomechanical effect of different graft heights on adjacent segment and graft segment following C4/C5 anterior cervical discectomy and fusion: A finite element analysis. *Med. Sci. Monit. Int. Med. J. Exp. Clin. Res.* **2019**, *25*, 4169–4175. [CrossRef] [PubMed]
34. Wang, J.; Qian, Z.; Ren, L. Biomechanical comparison of optimal shapes for the cervical intervertebral fusion cage for C5–C6 cervical fusion using the anterior cervical plate and cage (ACPC) fixation system: A finite element analysis. *Med. Sci. Monit. Int. Med. J. Exp. Clin. Res.* **2019**, *25*, 8379–8388. [CrossRef] [PubMed]
35. Lee, J.H.; Park, W.M.; Kim, Y.H.; Jahng, T.-A. A biomechanical analysis of an artificial disc with a shock-absorbing core property by using whole-cervical spine finite element analysis. *Spine* **2016**, *41*, E893–E901. [CrossRef]
36. Lee, S.-H.; Im, Y.-J.; Kim, K.-T.; Kim, Y.-H.; Park, W.-M.; Kim, K. Comparison of cervical spine biomechanics after fixed-and mobile-core artificial disc replacement: A finite element analysis. *Spine* **2011**, *36*, 700–708. [CrossRef]
37. Lin, C.-Y.; Chuang, S.-Y.; Chiang, C.-J.; Tsuang, Y.-H.; Chen, W.-P. Finite element analysis of cervical spine with different constrained types of total disc replacement. *J. Mech. Med. Biol.* **2014**, *14*, 1450038. [CrossRef]

Publisher's Note: MDPI stays neutral with regard to jurisdictional claims in published maps and institutional affiliations.

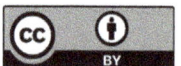

© 2020 by the authors. Licensee MDPI, Basel, Switzerland. This article is an open access article distributed under the terms and conditions of the Creative Commons Attribution (CC BY) license (http://creativecommons.org/licenses/by/4.0/).

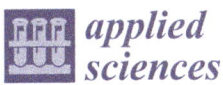

Article

Characterization of Gait and Postural Regulation in Late-Onset Pompe Disease

Ilka Schneider [1], Stephan Zierz [2], Stephan Schulze [3], Karl-Stefan Delank [3], Kevin G. Laudner [4], Richard Brill [5] and René Schwesig [3,*]

1. Clinic St. Georg, Delitzscher Str. 141, 04129 Leipzig, Germany; neurologie@sanktgeorg.de
2. Department of Neurology, Martin-Luther-University Halle-Wittenberg, Ernst-Grube-Str. 40, 06120 Halle (Saale), Germany; stephan.zierz@uk-halle.de
3. Department of Orthopaedic and Trauma Surgery, Martin-Luther-University Halle-Wittenberg, Ernst-Grube-Str. 40, 06120 Halle (Saale), Germany; stephan.schulze@uk-halle.de (S.S.); stefan.delank@uk-halle.de (K.-S.D.)
4. Department of Health Sciences, University of Colorado, Colorado Springs, CO 80918, USA; klaudner@uccs.edu
5. University Clinic and Policlinic of Radiology, Martin-Luther-University Halle-Wittenberg, Ernst-Grube-Str. 40, 06120 Halle (Saale), Germany; richard.brill@uk-halle.de
* Correspondence: rene.schwesig@uk-halle.de; Tel.: +49-345-557-1317; Fax: +49-345-557-4899

Received: 11 September 2020; Accepted: 7 October 2020; Published: 8 October 2020

Featured Application: Pompe disease is a neurological disease with significant impacts on gait and balance. Therefore, it is important to measure these characteristics in a functional, valid and reliable manner. This investigation used a cross-sectional study design utilizing gait analysis and posturography to quantify the difference between patients with late-onset Pompe disease (LOPD) and matched asymptomatic subjects. These results may be useful to develop more specific and efficient rehabilitation programs depending on the individual abilities of the patients.

Abstract: Pompe disease is a multisystemic disorder with the hallmark of progressive skeletal muscle weakness that often results in difficulties in walking and balance. However, detailed characterization of gait and postural regulation with this disease is lacking. The objective of this investigation was to determine if differences exist between the gait and postural regulation of LOPD patients and a matched control group. The gaits of 16 patients with LOPD were assessed using a gait analysis mobile system (RehaGait) and a dynamometric treadmill (FDM-T 1.8). The Interactive Balance System (IBS) was used to evaluate postural regulation and stability. All measures were compared to individual reference data. Demographic (age, gender), morphological (body height, body mass) and clinical data (muscle strength according to the Medical Research Council Scale (MRC Scale), as well as the 6-min walking test and a 10-m fast walk) were also recorded. Compared to individual reference data, LOPD patients presented with reduced gait velocity, cadence and time in single stand. A total of 87% of LOPD patients had abnormalities during posturographic analysis presenting with differences in postural subsystems. This study provides objective data demonstrating impaired gait and posture in LOPD patients. For follow-up analysis and as outcome measurements during medical or physiotherapeutic interventions, the findings of this investigation may be useful.

Keywords: glycogenosis type II; acid maltase deficiency; enzyme replacement therapy; posturography; balance

1. Introduction

Pompe disease (Online Mendelian Inheritance in Man (OMIM) 606800) is an autosomal recessive inherited orphan disease caused by mutations in the glucosidase alpha acid (GAA) gene. Resulting in deficient activity of the enzyme alpha-1,4-glucosidase that is located in cellular lysosoms involved in the degradation of glycogen. Consequently, glycogen accumulation occurs not only in skeletal muscle, but also in cardiac and smooth muscles [1].

The entrapment of lysosomal glycogen results in muscle damage by a number of pathogenic mechanisms, such as defective autophagy, calcium homeostasis, oxidative stress, and mitochondrial abnormalities [2]. Recently, metabolic abnormalities and energy deficits have also been shown to contribute to this pathogenic cascade [3]. The severity of clinical manifestations, tissue impairment and age of onset correlate with the residual enzymatic activity and can be classified into two forms: the Infantile Onset Pompe Disease (IOPD) or classical form has no or very low enzymatic activity levels, leading to severe general muscular weakness with floppy infant syndrome. Cardiomyopathy and respiratory failure usually lead to death within the first year of life. The late-onset Pompe disease (LOPD) or non-classical form has a higher residual enzyme activity. This disease progresses slowly and may start at any age after the first year of life. A common sign of LOPD is weakness of the proximal limbs, predominantly affecting the hip girdle. Axial muscles as well as respiratory muscles may also be impaired due to myopathy [4]. Patients often present clinically with back pain and exercise intolerance and dyspnea [5]. Recently, the systemic characteristics of this primary muscular disorder have been discovered: alteration of smooth muscles of the intestine and vessels, especially ectasia of vertebrobasial arteries, and the involvement of the nervous system (white matter lesions and small fiber neuropathy) widening the Pompe disease phenotype [6].

Since 2006, a causal treatment is available with enzyme replacement therapy (ERT) using recombinant human α-glucosidase. This treatment has been shown to improve patient survival and muscle strength to a variable extent [7]. It can also improve the quality of life of LOPD patients due to better mobility and participation in activities of daily life [8]. However, the actual ERT is not a cure for the disease and further therapeutic approaches are necessary. A detailed understanding of LOPD patients' gait patterns and balance may help improve physiotherapeutic strategies in the prevention of falls and preserving the patient's ambulatory status. Additionally, analysis of these features might be a tool for following up on future therapeutic strategies (i.e., next level ERT order gene therapy) [9]. There is a paucity in this research, with one study reporting reduced spatio-temporal parameters during gait in 22 LOPD patients on ERT [10] and another showing deficits in standing postural stability among five LOPD patients [11].

The aim of this study was to provide a systematic analysis of both gait parameters and postural abilities, as well as their interaction in patients with LOPD. These data were then compared to a group of matched healthy controls.

2. Materials and Methods

2.1. Subjects

All subjects provided written informed consent prior to data collection. This study protocol was approved by the local ethics committee (approval number: 2019-164). Sixteen ambulatory LOPD patients with a genetically confirmed diagnosis were included (9 women; mean age: 54.2 ± 15.3 years, range: 19–82 years, Table 1).

Table 1. Characteristics of late-onset Pompe disease (LOPD) patients. IVS1—first intervening sequence (of glucosidase alpha acid (GAA) gene).

Subject ID (No.)	Sex	GAA-Genotype		Age (y)	Disease Duration (y)	Duration ERT (mo)	NIV	Use of Ambulatory Aids
1	M	IVS1 (−13T > G)	p.C103G	58	14	135	Yes	None
2	F	IVS1 (−13T > G)	c.925G > A	62	2	9	No	None
3	M	IVS1 (−13T > G)	p.G309R	82	6	37	No	Rolling walker
4	F	IVS1 (−13T > G)	p.L552P	53	17	99	Yes	E-wheelchair
5	M	IVS1 (−13T > G)	IVS1 (−13T > G)	62	13	29	Yes	Rolling walker
6	M	IVS1 (−13T > G)	p.P493L	51	15	63	No	Walking sticks
7	F	IVS1 (−13T > G)	p.P493L	61	21	63	No	None
8	F	IVS1 (−13T > G)	IVS9 G > C)	26	15	67	No	None
9	F	IVS1 (−13T > G)	c307 T > G	50	23	119	Yes	Rolling walker
10	M	IVS1 (−13T > G)	c.832delC	46	6	17	Yes	None
11	F	IVS1 (−13T > G)	c.2481 + 102_2646 + 31del	54	19	48	No	None
12	F	IVS1 (−13T > G)	c.2481 + 102_2646 + 31del	57	18	44	No	Rolling walker
13	M	IVS1 (−13T > G)	c.525delT	19	19	132	No	None
14	F	IVS1 (−13T > G)	c.525delT	66	7	33	Yes	Rolling walker
15	M	IVS1 (−13T > G)	c.2136-7delGT	50	40	116	Yes	None
16	F	IVS1 (−13T > G)	c.1019T > C	70	20	0	No	Rolling walker

M—Male; F—Female; ERT—Enzyme replacement therapy; NIV—Non-invasive ventilation; y—years; mo—months.

Fifteen of sixteen patients (94%) were on ERT at the standard dose of 20 mg/kg biweekly (range: 9–135 months; mean: 67.4 months). The duration of the disease ranged from 2 years to 40 years (mean: 15.9 years). One female was tested before ERT was started. A total of 44% of the patients required temporarily non-invasive ventilation and 50% of the patients used walking aids. All LOPD patients were individually matched with healthy controls based on the relevant selection criteria sex, age, and body height to guarantee a valid comparison with asymptomatic subjects and to avoid the recruitment of an asymptomatic control group [12,13]. The reference data were obtained from 1860 subjects for mobile gait analysis [14], from 141 subjects for treadmill analysis [15] and from 1724 subjects for the posturographic parameters [16].

2.2. Clinical Analysis

Synopsis of the study protocol for each patient is depicted in Figure 1. All LOPD patients were examined clinically using MRC scale similar to previous trials with LOPD patients [11,17]. For lower limb assessment, the bilateral strength of the hip flexors and extensors, hip abductors and adductors, knee flexors and extensors, and ankle dorsiflexors and plantarflexors were assessed. For correlation analysis, the bilateral sum of the MRC scale was used for each individual strength variable, as well as the bilateral sum of all examined muscle groups were obtained. Furthermore, all LOPD patients completed a 6-min walking test and a 10-m fast walk [4]. Concomitant peripheral neuropathy was examined via a clinical screening for symptoms of polyneuropathy (e.g., reduction of distal sensibility and tendon reflexes, pain of distal legs) and confirmation by nerve conduction analyses.

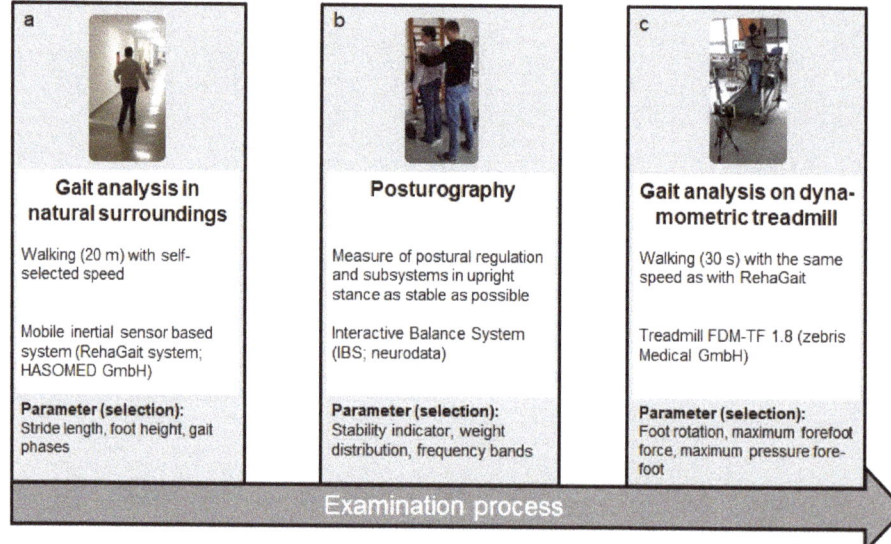

Figure 1. (a–c) Examination protocol.

2.3. Mobile Gait Analysis Using an Inertial Sensor Based System

Participants were initially equipped with a mobile inertial sensor-based system (RehaGait® HASOMED GmbH, Magdeburg, Germany) (Figure 1a). This system has been reported to have a high intraobserver reliability (intraclass correlation coefficients (ICCs) range: 0.691–0.959) [18]. Donath et al. [19] also reported good to excellent intraobserver reliability by testing 22 healthy subjects on two separate days (time interval: 7 days). Additionally, these authors confirmed the validity of this system by comparing it to the FDM-T system (zebris medical GmbH, Isny, Germany), which was also used in the present study. These authors captured spatio-temporal gait data simultaneously using both gait analysis systems and with the exception of speed and stride length at a slow speed (15% below habitual walking speed), both systems showed a high level of accordance. In line with the study of Donath et al. [19], each sensor (dimensions: 60 × 15 × 35 mm) contained a 3-axis accelerometer (±8 g), a 3-axis gyroscope (±1000 °/s) and a 3-axis compass (±1.3 Gs). The sensors were attached to the lateral aspect of the shoe using special straps to measure linear acceleration, angular velocity and the magnetic field of the foot (sampling rate: 500 Hz). Heel-strike was used to determine each gait cycle. All other gait events (full contact, heel-off, toe-off) were identified relative to heel-strike. These gait phases were then used to derive orientation and position and spatio-temporal gait parameters.

Since self-selected speed has been suggested to provide the most functionally relevant data [20], each subject was instructed to walk through a 20-m common hospital corridor (without any obstacles) at a self-preferred speed. LOPD patients wore their own personal walking shoes and the first walking trial was used for subjects to adjust to the test conditions. Data from the second trial were used for analysis. Each gait parameter for all recorded steps was analyzed.

2.4. Balance Measurement Using Posturography

Posturographic assessment was established with the IBS (neurodata GmbH, Vienna, Austria) (Figure 1b). The IBS consists of four independent force plates used to measure postural regulation at a sampling rate of 32 Hz. Sway intensities at different frequency ranges were determined using Fast Fourier Transformation (FFT). The raw signal (force-time signal) was subtracted from the mean value and then subjected to a FFT with a rectangular window. On the ordinate, the amplitude of the frequency components was exposed and, consequently, the ordinate was dimensionless in that the results of the FFT are proportional to the output signal [21]. Different functional frequency bands were used to delineate the postural subsystems (F1, F2–4, F5–6, F7–8) [22–24]:

1. F1: Frequency band 1 (0.01–0.03 Hz)—visual and nigrostriatal system;
2. F2–4: Frequency band 2–4 (0.03–0.5 Hz)—peripheral-vestibular system;
3. F5–6: Frequency band 5–6 (0.5–1.0 Hz)—somatosensory system;
4. F7–8: Frequency band 7–8 (>1.0 Hz)—cerebellar system.

Additionally, motor output was determined as:

1. Stability indicator (ST): The root mean square of successive differences in pressure signals. Greater instability is indicated by a greater ST.
2. Weight distribution index (WDI): Standard deviation of the weight distribution score.
3. Synchronization (Synch): Six values that describe the relationship of vibration patterns between plates calculated as a scalar product: 1000—complete coactivity; −1000—complete compensation; 0—no coactivity or compensation.
4. Forefoot–hindfoot ratio (Heel): Percentage of load distribution between the forefoot and hindfoot with an emphasis on heel loading.
5. Left–right ratio (Left): Percentage of load distribution between the left and right feet with an emphasis on left side loading.

Subjects were tested barefoot using a single trial (32 s) for each of the following test conditions:

1. Head straight, eyes open, without foam pads (NO);
2. Head straight, eyes closed, without foam pads (NC);
3. Head straight, eyes open, on foam pads (PO);
4. Head straight, eyes closed, on foam pads (PC);
5. Head rotated 45° to the right, eyes closed, without foam pads (HR);
6. Head rotated 45° to the left, eyes closed, without foam pads (HL);
7. Head up (dorsiflexed), eyes closed, without foam pads (HB);
8. Head up (plantarflexed), eyes closed, without foam pads (HF).

Initially, subjects were asked to stand upright, with their weight evenly distributed on the two force plates while focusing on a fixed target (placed at each subject's respective body height). In this starting position, subjects were then asked to stand freely and as still as possible. Positions, reliability, frequency bands, and parameters of motor output used in the IBS have been previously described in detail [12]. For example, the intraobserver reliability has been confirmed using both asymptomatic subjects [25] and patients [26,27]. ICCs for every parameter and all test positions have been reported from 0.71 to 0.95 [25–27]. In support of these previous reliability investigations, which showed that the reliability averaged over eight positions were clearly higher than from a single position, we also used the mean values captured in the eight test positions for all parameters.

2.5. Gait Analysis Using a Dynamometric Treadmill

Gait trials were performed on a dynamometric treadmill with a fall protector (h/p/cosmos/quasar, FDM-T, zebris medical GmbH, Isny, Germany, Figure 1c) [15]. This instrumented treadmill (length: 1.5 m; width: 0.5 m) contained an integrated pressure sensor mat comprising a matrix of high-quality capacitive force sensors (range, 1–120 N/cm^2; precision, 1–120 N/cm^2 ± 5 %; sensor area: 135.5 × 54.1 cm; resolution: 1.4 sensors per cm^2; total number of sensors: 10.240) and analysis software [19]. The assessment captures the dynamic pressure distribution under the feet while walking on the treadmill at a sampling rate of 300 Hz. Two mobile camera modules were positioned behind and beside the treadmill to confirm correct foot placement on the treadmill. Prior to data collection, the force plate was set to zero in order to calibrate the entire measurement system [28]. Spatio-temporal gait parameters were calculated automatically from the pressure data within the FDM-T software for the heel, midfoot, and forefoot. Based on the manufacturer's specifications, heel-strike was defined as initial contact (threshold: 1 N/cm^2), while toe-off was the final data frame before all foot pressures were sub-threshold. Furthermore, stride length was defined as the distance between two consecutive heel contact points (alternate sides), stride time was the time between two consecutive heel-strikes (same foot) and cadence is the number of steps taken per minute [19]. Each subject walked (30 s duration) at their self-selected gait speed, while wearing their own personal shoes.

2.6. Statistics

The balance and gait analysis results of the LOPD patients were defined as conspicuous when outside a reference range between the 10th percentile (P10) and the 90th percentile (P90) obtained from the matched control group.

Relationships between clinical predictors and the test parameters were calculated using Pearson bivariate two-sided product moment correlations, because the measures obtained were normally distributed. Correlation (r) was graded as: < 0.1, trivial; 0.1–0.3, small; 0.3–0.5, moderate; 0.5–0.7, large; 0.7–0.9, very large; and 0.9–1.0, nearly perfect [29].

Differences between groups (patients with and without polyneuropathy (PN)) were tested using a one-factor (group) univariate general linear model. Differences between means (group effect) were considered statistically significant if p-values were <0.05 or partial eta-squared (η_p^2) values were greater than 0.15. Due to the relatively small number of cases in each group (n < 10), decisions on significance were based on both statistical values.

All statistical analysis was performed using SPSS version 25.0 for Windows (IBM, Armonk, NY, USA).

3. Results

3.1. Gait Analysis with Mobile Device (Rehagait) and Dynamometric Treadmill Analysis

LOPD patients showed gait abnormalities in cadence (75%), velocity (69%) and percentage of time in double limb support (56%) compared to the matched references (Tables 2 and 3).

Table 2. Gait parameters of LOPD patients compared to reference data from matched controls. LOPD patients (ID: 1–16) with polyneuropathy (PN) are marked in bold.

Subject ID Number	Stride Length (m)		Walking Speed (m/s)		Cadence (steps/min)		Stance Phase (%)		Single Support (%)		Maximum Foot Height (m)	
	RR	Value	RR	Value	RR	Value	RR	Value	RR	Value	RR	Value
1	0.98–1.34	1.06	1.18–1.60	0.72 *	96–110	80 *	57–64	65 *	36–42	32 *	0.10–0.24	0.18
2	1.25–1.53	1.41	1.15–1.59	1.30	108–124	108	57–63	57	37–43	40	0.09–0.24	0.17
3	1.11–1.45	1.18	0.80–1.43	0.98	102–116	98 *	57–64	61	36–42	36	0.10–0.24	0.15
4	0.78–1.16	0.70 *	1.21–1.61	0.34 *	89–100	55 *	58–65	79 *	35–41	22 *	0.09–0.24	0.16
5	1.13–1.47	1.11 *	1.15–1.59	1.04 *	103–117	110	57–63	65 *	36–42	37	0.10–0.24	0.17
6	1.23–1.53	1.41	1.21–1.61	1.19 *	105–121	99 *	57–63	57	36–43	42	0.11–0.24	0.14
7	1.26–1.58	1.42	1.16–1.59	1.29	108–124	104 *	57–63	64 *	37–43	38	0.10–0.25	0.20
8	1.28–1.61	1.60	1.14–1.55	1.34	107–125	99 *	56–63	59	37–43	40	0.10–0.25	0.18
9	0.85–1.20	0.91	1.22–1.61	0.49 *	92–104	63 *	58–65	64	35–41	32 *	0.09–0.24	0.12
10	1.32–1.64	1.51	1.22–1.61	1.41	109–127	112	56–62	59	37–43	40	0.10–0.25	0.20
11	1.20–1.50	1.41	1.20–1.61	1.18 *	106–121	100 *	57–63	60	37–43	37	0.09–0.24	0.13
12	0.70–1.09	0.38 *	1.19–1.61	0.19 *	86–97	57 *	58–66	82 *	35–41	18 *	0.09–0.24	0.07 *
13	1.41–1.72	1.61	1.09–1.50	1.58 *	111–131	117	56–62	58	37–44	42	0.10–0.25	0.20
14	0.82–1.10	0.67 *	1.10–1.56	0.45 *	92–104	79 *	58–65	66 *	36–41	29 *	0.08–0.21	0.10
15	1.02–1.38	1.06	1.04–1.54	0.80 *	97–112	91 *	57–64	63	36–42	32 *	0.10–0.25	0.13
16	0.73–1.10	0.40 *	1.04–1.54	0.25 *	88–98	74 *	58–65	76 *	35–41	27 *	0.09–0.23	0.09
∑ * (n/%)	5/31%		11/69%		12/75%		7/44%		7/44%		1/6%	

RR—reference range; *—outside of reference data; percentage over 10% marked in bold.

Table 3. Gait analysis and clinical parameters of LOPD patients.

Subject ID	13	10	8	11	6	7	2	3	1	16	15	5	9	14	4	12
Mobile gait parameters using RehaGait																
Stride length (m)	-	-	-	-	-	-	-	-	-	X	-	-	-	X	X	X
Walking speed (m/s)	-	-	-	X	X	-	-	-	X	X	X	X	X	X	X	X
Cadence (steps/min)	-	-	X	X	X	X	X	X	X	X	X	-	X	X	X	X
Stance (%)	-	-	-	-	-	X	-	-	X	X	-	X	-	X	X	X
Single support (%)	-	-	-	-	-	-	-	-	X	X	X	-	X	X	X	X
Double support (%)	-	-	-	-	-	X	-	-	X	X	X	X	X	X	X	X
Maximum foot high (m)	-	-	-	-	-	-	-	-	-	-	-	-	-	-	-	X
Treadmill gait parameters using FDM-T system																
Foot rotation (°)	X	X	X	X	-	-	X	X	X	X	X	NA	-	-	NA	X
Step width (m)	-	X	X	-	-	X	X	-	-	-	X	NA	-	-	NA	-
Initial stance (%)	-	X	X	X	X	X	-	-	-	-	-	NA	X	-	NA	X
Mid stance (%)	X	X	X	-	X	X	X	-	X	-	-	NA	-	X	NA	X
Terminal stance (%)	X	X	X	-	X	X	X	-	X	-	-	NA	-	-	NA	X
Lateral displacement of Gait line (m)	X	-	-	-	X	X	X	X	X	X	X	NA	X	X	NA	-
Clinical data																
Muscle strength hip	-	X	X	X	X	X	X	X	X	-	X	X	X	X	X	X
Muscle strength knee	-	-	X	X	X	X	X	X	X	X	X	X	X	X	-	X
Muscle strength ankle	-	-	-	X	X	X	-	X	-	-	-	-	-	-	-	-
Polyneuropathy	-	-	-	X	-	X	-	X	X	-	-	X	-	X	-	-
6MWT (m)	800	590	470	445	420	370	323	318	315	265	254	200	125	114	105	NA
Time 10-m fast walk (s)	5	5.3	6.2	6.7	9.6	10.6	9.4	12	12.7	24	17	12.7	17.4	29	28	25

- indicates normal results (inside the reference range of matched controls). X indicates abnormal results (outside the reference range of matched controls). Gray highlight indicates results superior to those of references. Abnormal muscle force values were defined as any result <5 according to MRC grading for a single measurement. 6MWT—6-min walking test. NA—not available because patients were not able to perform the test.

Maximum foot height was reduced in 6% of LOPD patients, stride length in 25% and step widths in 36% (Table 3). Foot rotation and lateral displacement were conspicuous in 71% of the patients. In most patients (71%), pressure distribution across the heel, midfoot and forefoot regions were outside the inter-percentile range in one or more items (Tables 2 and 3).

There was a moderate relationship between overall hip muscle strength and the percentage of single limb support during the gait cycle ($r_{RehaGait} = 0.525$, $p = 0.037$). Step widths showed a moderate correlation with strength of hip muscles ($r_{treadmill} = -0.579$, $p = 0.030$) and total strength of the lower limbs ($r = -0.613$, $p = 0.020$). Performance on the 10-m fast walk was highly correlated with walking speed ($r_{RehaGait} = -0.919$, $p < 0.001$; $r_{treadmill} = -0.750$, $p = 0.002$) and stride length ($r_{RehaGait} = -0.779$, $p = 0.001$). There was also a moderate correlation between 10-m fast walk performance and the percentage of mid stance phase ($r_{RehaGait} = -0.589$, $p = 0.027$). Stride length correlated with the percentage of double support ($r_{RehaGait} = -0.749$, $p = 0.002$) and single support ($r_{RehaGait} = -0.907$, $p < 0.001$), as well as with forefoot pressure ($r_{treadmill} = 0.578$, $p = 0.031$), and heel pressure ($r_{treadmill} = 0.851$, $p < 0.001$).

Cadence was significantly correlated with hip flexion strength ($r_{RehaGait} = 0.575$, $p = 0.020$; $r_{treadmill} = 0.539$, $p = 0.047$) and hip adduction strength ($r_{RehaGait} = 0.623$, $p = 0.010$; $r_{treadmill} = 0.620$, $p = 0.018$). Furthermore, cadence was also highly correlated with performance during the 6-min walking test ($r_{RehaGait} = 0.742$, $p = 0.002$; $r_{treadmill} = 0.658$, $p = 0.014$).

3.2. Posturographic Analysis

Most LOPD patients (87%) showed abnormal results (Table 4) for balance and postural regulation. One patient (no. 15) was unable to perform the test. Frequency band analysis revealed abnormal results in 53% of the patients: regulations in F1 and F2–4 were most often affected in this cohort. Three patients presented with isolated abnormalities in F1 that detects for visual [22,24] and nigrostriatal [30] contribution to balance regulation. Postural stability (parameter: ST) and forefoot–heel coordination (parameter: Synch) were affected in 60% and 53%, respectively. Patient no. 5 had the lowest level of balance and postural regulation (Table 4) with abnormal results for all frequency bands combined with a disturbed gait pattern with the mobile gait analysis. This patient was not able to perform the gait treadmill test (Table 3). The muscle strength of the knee and forefoot–heel ratio correlated moderately. Results in F5–6 also correlated with performance in the 6-min walking test ($r = -0.517$, $p = 0.049$) and with ST ($r = 0.983$, $p < 0.001$).

Table 4. Posturographic analysis of LOPD patients compared to matched controls. Values are the means of eight test positions. LOPD patients (ID: 1–16) with PN are marked in bold.

Para-Meter ID	F1 RR	F1 Value	F2-4 RR	F2-4 Value	F5-6 RR	F5-6 Value	F7-8 RR	F7-8 Value	ST RR	ST Value	Synch RR	Synch Value	Heel (%) RR	Heel (%) Value	Left (%) RR	Left (%) Value
1	10.7–25.8	20.0	6.25–14.8	15.2 *	2.92–6.81	6.62	0.51–1.08	1.33 *	13.8–29.3	36.6 *	379–807	720	36.5–67.4	49.0	46.0–55.1	46.7
2	9.48–21.0	22.7 *	6.86–13.0	10.0	2.94–6.96	4.29	0.53–1.29	0.77	13.4–32.8	24.6	426–762	664	36.8–57.4	35.4 *	43.6–55.3	58.0 *
3	12.2–22.9	16.1	7.98–15.1	11.3	3.08–8.32	4.59	0.54–2.56	0.86	15.1–40.1	25.5	341–776	161 *	39.1–57.0	25.4 *	42.6–56.4	52.6
4	10.6–22.7	13.1	6.98–12.4	8.9	2.75–6.73	5.91	0.48–1.17	1.02	13.5–30.4	31.0 *	528–840	654	42.2–64.8	46.8	44.3–54.3	49.0
5	10.4–23.4	26.0 *	6.44–12.4	15.8 *	3.00–6.83	9.36 *	0.51–1.34	1.99 *	14.7–30.9	57.5 *	518–770	314 *	36.9–56.6	36.1 *	47.3–53.0	50.2
6	10.7–25.8	10.5 *	6.25–14.8	10.3	2.92–6.81	4.95	0.51–1.08	0.93	13.8–29.3	29.8 *	379–807	341 *	36.5–67.4	18.0 *	46.0–55.1	60.1 *
7	9.48–21.0	15.8	6.86–13.0	9.7	2.94–6.96	2.85 *	0.53–1.29	0.47 *	13.4–32.8	15.8	426–762	308 *	36.8–57.4	43.2	43.6–55.3	43.9
8	9.59–20.3	19.5	5.84–10.2	11.7 *	2.40–4.64	4.94 *	0.44–1.01	1.06 *	11.7–21.2	30.2 *	515–793	700	38.2–56.5	47.1	46.1–53.9	54.8 *
9	10.6–22.7	25.6 *	6.98–12.4	14.1 *	2.75–6.73	6.75 *	0.48–1.17	0.97	13.5–30.4	33.4 *	528–840	704	42.2–64.8	39.1 *	44.3–54.3	47.5
10	11.2–22.5	10.5 *	6.25–10.9	8.9	2.86–4.98	4.90	0.50–1.15	1.04	13.3–23.4	30.0 *	415–787	435	38.7–54.2	32.9 *	46.2–53.9	52.7
11	10.6–22.7	13.5	6.98–12.4	8.7	2.75–6.73	2.78	0.48–1.17	0.51	13.5–30.4	16.7	528–840	722	42.2–64.8	29.2 *	44.3–54.3	50.0
12	10.6–22.7	8.5 *	6.98–12.4	5.9 *	2.75–6.73	3.62	0.48–1.17	0.67	13.5–30.4	21.2	528–840	500 *	42.2–64.8	30.8 *	44.3–54.3	52.1
13	12.6–24.9	12.6	7.10–12.4	6.5 *	3.16–5.76	2.20 *	0.58–1.19	0.38 *	15.0–28.1	11.7 *	229–664	729 *	36.3–59.8	47.6	45.1–55.6	50.2
14	9.48–21.0	20.5	6.86–13.0	13.9 *	2.94–6.96	8.51 *	0.53–1.29	1.52 *	13.4–32.8	46.8 *	426–762	284 *	36.8–57.4	42.4	43.6–55.3	35.9 *
16	9.73–23.7	15.7	6.92–14.7	12.2	3.41–8.71	3.97	0.66–1.61	0.66	16.4–39.5	22.7	423–787	434	38.1–58.5	49.2	43.9–56.8	50.4
Σ * (n/%)	6/40%		7/47%		5/33%		6/40%		9/60%		7/44%		9/53%		4/27%	

RR—reference range. Gray highlighted—results superior to those of references. *—outside of reference data.

Figure 2 presents two examples for low and high gait and postural performances. Postural stability, measured by a stability indicator, and postural regulation, measured by frequency bands, are presented for posturographic analysis. Plantar pressure distribution and plantar forces regarding heel, midfoot and forefoot (left and right) and force–time curves depict different gait patterns.

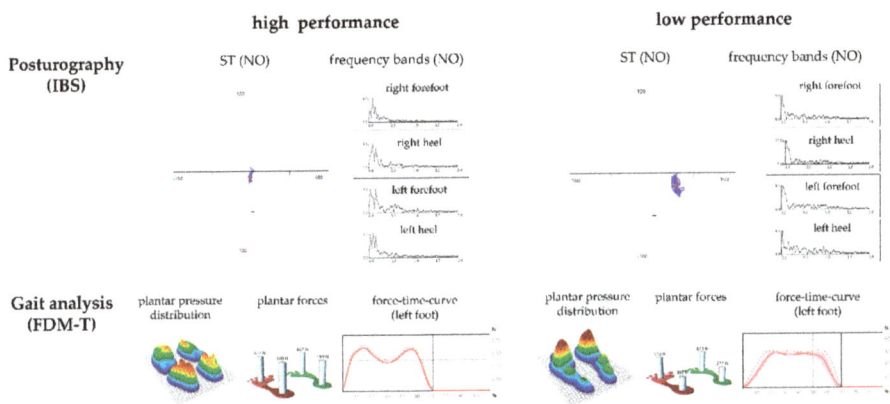

Figure 2. Examples for high and low performances concerning gait and posture stability and regulation.

3.3. Impact of Existence of Polyneuropathy on Posturographic Results

All posturographic parameters were sub-analyzed according to the presence of PN. Patients with PN had significantly more abnormalities in the synchronization ($p = 0.142$, $\eta_p^2 = 0.158$; Figure 3a) and in F2–4 ($p = 0.101$, $\eta_p^2 = 0.194$; Figure 3b) than those without PN.

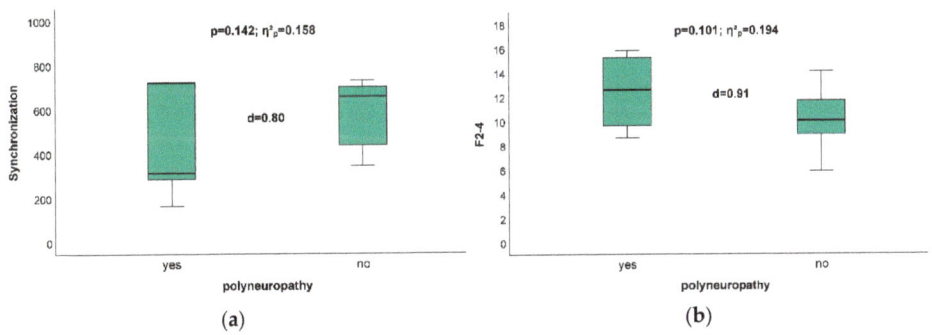

Figure 3. (a,b) Synchronization (a) and F2–4 (b) depending on polyneuropathy (yes: n = 6; no: n = 9).

No relevant correlations were detected between disease duration or ERT duration and any performance parameter (e.g., 6-min walking test, 10-m fast walk, walking speed, postural stability measured by a stability indicator). A total of 69% (n = 11) of the LOPD patients were classified with mild axial weakness (dimension: strength of the axial musculature).

4. Discussion

Gait abnormalities in LOPD patients included reduced gait velocity, reduced stride length and a shift from time in single stance phase towards double limb support, which support the previous findings of McIntosh et al. [10]. These abnormalities most likely result from proximal lower limb weakness common with this disease [31,32]. However, in the current study, the only strength characteristic that correlated with gait was for the association between hip strength with time in single leg support stance and step widths.

Postural stability and regulation were reduced in most patients in this study, similar to those of previous research [11]. This is believed to result from reduced muscle strength. However, in the present study, there was no significant correlation between muscle weakness and postural parameters except for knee-joint force and forefoot–heel coordination. There were no relevant correlations between gait performance and posturographic results. In contrast, two patients with marked gait impairment performed better than the reference cohort in isolated parameters of posturography. Therefore, other muscular determinants of gait and balance must exist.

It has previously been reported that postural regulation in LOPD patients is impaired when their eyes are closed and believed to result from sensory deficits [10]. Consistently in this study, LOPD patients with clinical PN had significantly more abnormalities in the postural synchronization than those without. However, no differences in sway between LOPD patients with or without PN were observed in F5–6 (averaged over all test positions), which has been shown to be affected in patients with diabetic polyneuropathy [23]. It is possible that, in LOPD patients, additional effects on the muscle spindles [33] or spinal cord [34] may contribute to alterations in sway rather than PN. A differentiated calculation (F5–6$_{NO + PO}$ = open eyes vs. F5–6$_{NC + PC + HR + HL + HB + HF}$ = closed eyes) based on an effect size (d) provided a significantly larger difference with open eyes (with PN: 4.26 ± 2.43 vs. without PN: 3.04 ± 0.88; d = 0.74) than with eyes closed (with PN: 6.29 ± 3.44 vs. without PN: 5.14 ± 1.55; d = 0.47). This finding may be explained by the neuroplasticity of biological systems and the model of selective compensatory optimization. The alteration of afferent sensory (proprioceptive) information, potentially caused by mechanoreceptor damage (PN, Anterior Cruciate Ligament (ACL) surgery, High Tibial Osteotomy (HTO) surgery), may contribute to disturbances of postural regulation [12,13]. In support of Brehme et al. [13] and in contrast to Bartels et al. [12], we showed hyperactivity of the somatosensory system in the presence of PN. This hyperactivity could also be observed in the cerebellar system (four patients had abnormal posturographic findings; Table 4). This may partially explain the close relationship between the somatosensory system and the spinocerebellum system as an important part of the cerebellum, which is responsible for processing afferent (somatosensory) information. Obviously, most of the PN patients developed hyperactivity of the somatosensory (2/3) and cerebellar (3/4) system, which should be interpreted as an ineffective and excessive function of these postural subsystems. Only one patient (ID 7; Table 4) developed suppression in both subsystems.

LOPD patients of this study also revealed balance deficiencies in visual and nigrostriatal regulation, cerebellar regulation, and in the vestibular subsystem with various interactions between the subsystems. This reflects the multi-systemic nature of Pompe disease since there are reports about cerebral [35,36] and vestibulocochlear affections [37] in LOPD patients. However, visual function has not yet been found when analyzed by evoked potentials [38]. Therefore, future research is necessary in this area.

When looking at the weak correlations between muscle strength, gait performance and balance in the LOPD patients of this study, the impact of factors other than those tested is possible. High-quality and frequent physiotherapy and individual training, as well as personal motivation, may result in better compensation of gait disturbances and balance. Furthermore, it has to be considered that each patient received physiotherapy in a non-standardized manner. Research has previously shown that the application of whole body vibration training with an oscillating platform was beneficial in LOPD patients for improving general muscle strength [39]. These authors speculated that this effect results from the stimulation of muscle spindles that might lead to reflex contraction of extrafusal muscle fibers [40]. However, influences of vibration on gait and posture have been shown to reduce the risk of falls by a more multimodal approach (e.g., ankle joint motion, sensation of foot plantar surface and fear) in older adults [41]. Finally, Corrado et al. [42] revealed that there is no research supporting the effectiveness of rehabilitation protocols among LOPD patients. Corrado et al. [42] performed a systematic review investigating current rehabilitation protocols for LOPD patients and concluded that studies with larger sample sizes and higher quality are necessary to reduce the lack of evidence surrounding rehabilitative treatments. The extremely large gait performance differences within LOPD patients (e.g., range of walking speed: 0.25–1.58 m/s; Table 2) and postural stability (e.g., range of ST: 11.7–57.5; Table 4) in our study may have also been a result of the small size of our cohort. At the same time, these large performance differences within LOPD patients are reasons for individualized physiotherapy. The gait and posturographic performances in some patients suggest that individualized physiotherapy has the potential to improve gait and balance performance in LOPD patients and may help prevent falls. As such, our study could be used as reference for future investigations using a lager patient cohort with a standardized physiotherapeutic program that would ideally be tested using a controlled randomized trial.

Another limitation of this study was that a lot of the LOPD patients did not have any experience walking on a treadmill. Consequently, this fact may be responsible for any deviating gait analyses. For this reason, we also conducted the mobile gait analysis in a more function environment in order to ensure a valid gait analysis. Based on our experience, the self-selected speed on the treadmill is typically slower than the speed used in a natural environment, because subjects feel more unstable when walking on a treadmill. Anxiety or depression could have caused a negative influence on the patient's performance. These data were not obtained in the present study and should be analyzed in further investigations.

5. Conclusions

This study found relevant impairment of gait and balance parameters in LOPD patients that showed a wide variability between patients. Therefore, these results can only be partially explained by reduced muscle strength as result of the underlying myopathy. Yet, there must be additional regulatory systems that might be affected in the context of the multisystemic character of Pompe disease and individual factors that were not analyzed in this study. The assessment of gait and posture should be used for designing individual rehabilitation programs to improve the patient's mobility. These findings also allow for detailed follow-up analysis and as outcome measurements for future medical and physiotherapeutic trials.

Author Contributions: Conceptualization, I.S., R.S., and S.Z.; methodology, I.S., R.S., and R.B.; formal analysis, K.S.D., R.S. and K.G.L.; investigation, S.S., I.S. and R.S.; resources, S.Z.; data curation, R.S.; writing—original draft preparation, I.S., R.S., R.B. and K.G.L.; writing—review and editing, I.S., R.S., K.G.L. and K.-S.D.; visualization, S.S.; supervision, S.Z. and I.S.; project administration, I.S., S.Z. and R.S. All authors have read and agreed to the published version of the manuscript.

Funding: This research received no external funding.

Acknowledgments: We are grateful to all the patients who participated after HTO surgery and made this study possible.

Conflicts of Interest: The authors declare no conflict of interest.

Ethical standards: All procedures performed in studies involving human participants or on human tissue were in accordance with the ethical standards of the institutional and/or national research committee and with the 1975 Helsinki declaration and its later amendments or comparable ethical standards. Informed consent was obtained from all individual participants included in the study.

References

1. Hobson-Webb, L.D.; Proia, A.D.; Thurberg, B.L.; Banugaria, S.; Prater, S.N.; Kishnani, P.S. Autopsy findings in late-onset Pompe disease: A case report and systematic review of the literature. *Mol. Genet. Metab.* **2012**, *106*, 462–469. [CrossRef]
2. Kohler, L.; Puertollano, R.; Raben, N. Pompe Disease: From Basic Science to Therapy. *Neurotherapeutics* **2018**, *15*, 928–942. [CrossRef]
3. Meena, N.K.; Ralston, E.; Raben, N.; Puertollano, R. Enzyme Replacement Therapy Can Reverse Pathogenic Cascade in Pompe Disease. *Mol. Ther. Methods Clin. Dev.* **2020**, *18*, 199–214. [CrossRef]

4. Cupler, E.J.; Berger, K.I.; Leshner, R.T.; Wolfe, G.I.; Han, J.J.; Barohn, R.J.; Kissel, J.T. AANEM Consensus Committee on Late-onset Pompe Disease. Consensus treatment recommendations for late-onset Pompe disease. *Muscle Nerve* **2012**, *45*, 319–333. [CrossRef] [PubMed]
5. Taverna, S.; Cammarata, G.; Colomba, P.; Sciarrino, S.; Zizzo, C.; Francofonte, D.; Zora, M.; Scalia, S.; Brando, C.; Lo Curto, A.; et al. Pompe disease: Pathogenesis, molecular genetics and diagnosis. *Aging (Albany N. Y.)* **2020**, *12*, 15856–15874. [CrossRef]
6. Toscano, A.; Rodolico, C.; Musumeci, O. Multisystem late onset Pompe disease (LOPD): An update on clinical aspects. *Ann. Transl. Med.* **2019**, *7*, 284. [CrossRef] [PubMed]
7. Schoser, B.; Stewart, A.; Kanters, S.; Hamed, A.; Jansen, J.; Chan, K.; Karamouzian, M.; Toscano, A. Survival and long-term outcomes in late-onset Pompe disease following alglucosidase alfa treatment: A systematic review and meta-analysis. *J. Neurol.* **2017**, *264*, 621–630. [CrossRef] [PubMed]
8. Gungor, D.; Kruijshaar, M.E.; Plug, I.; Rizopoulos, D.; Kanters, T.A.; Wens, S.C.; Reuser, A.J.J.; van Doorn, P.A.; van der Ploeg, A.T. Quality of life and participation in daily life of adults with Pompe disease receiving enzyme replacement therapy: 10 years of international follow-up. *J. Inherit. Metab. Dis.* **2016**, *39*, 253–260. [CrossRef] [PubMed]
9. Ronzitti, G.; Collaud, F.; Laforet, P.; Mingozzi, F. Progress and challenges of gene therapy for Pompe disease. *Ann. Transl. Med.* **2019**, *13*, 287. [CrossRef] [PubMed]
10. McIntosh, P.T.; Case, L.E.; Chan, J.M.; Austin, S.L.; Kishnani, P. Characterization of gait in late onset Pompe disease. *Mol. Genet. Metab.* **2015**, *116*, 152–156. [CrossRef] [PubMed]
11. Valle, M.S.; Casabona, A.; Fiumara, A.; Castiglione, D.; Sorge, G.; Cioni, M. Quantitative analysis of upright standing in adults with late-onset Pompe disease. *Sci. Rep.* **2016**, *6*, 37040. [CrossRef] [PubMed]
12. Bartels, T.; Brehme, K.; Pyschik, M.; Pollak, R.; Schaffrath, N.; Schulze, S.; Delank, K.S.; Laudner, K.G.; Schwesig, R. Postural stability and regulation before and after anterior cruciate ligament reconstruction—A two-years longitudinal study. *Phys. Ther. Sport* **2019**, *38*, 49–58. [CrossRef] [PubMed]
13. Brehme, K.; Bartels, T.; Pyschik, M.; Jenz, M.; Delank, K.S.; Laudner, K.G.; Schwesig, R. Postural stability and regulation before and after high tibial osteotomy and rehabilitation. *Appl. Sci.* **2020**, *10*, 6517. [CrossRef]
14. Schwesig, R.; Leuchte, S.; Fischer, D.; Ullmann, R.; Kluttig, A. Inertial sensor based reference gait data for healthy subjects. *Gait Posture* **2011**, *33*, 673–678. [CrossRef]
15. Lauenroth, A.; Laudner, K.G.; Schulze, S.; Delank, K.S.; Fieseler, G.; Schwesig, R. Treadmill-based gait reference data for healthy subjects. Dependence on functional and morphologic parameters. *Man. Med.* **2018**, *56*, 182–187. [CrossRef]
16. Schwesig, R.; Fischer, D.; Kluttig, A. Are there changes in postural regulation across the lifespan? *Somatosens. Mot. Res.* **2013**, *30*, 167–174. [CrossRef]
17. Regnery, C.; Kornblum, C.; Hanisch, F.; Vielhaber, S.; Strigl-Pill, N.; Grunert, B.; Müller-Felber, W.; Glocker, F.X.; Spranger, M.; Deschauer, M.; et al. 36 months observational clinical study of 38 adult Pompe disease patients under alglucosidase alfa enzyme replacement therapy. *J. Inherit. Metab. Dis.* **2012**, *35*, 837–845. [CrossRef]
18. Schwesig, R.; Kauert, R.; Wust, S.; Becker, S.; Leuchte, S. Reliability of the novel gait analysis system RehaWatch. *Biomed. Tech. (Berl)* **2010**, *55*, 109–115. [CrossRef]
19. Donath, L.; Faude, O.; Lichtenstein, E.; Nüesch, C.; Mündermann, A. Validity and reliability of a portable gait analysis system for measuring spatiotemporal gait characteristics: Comparison to an instrumented treadmill. *J. Neuroeng. Rehabil.* **2016**, *13*, 6. [CrossRef]
20. Auvinet, B.; Berrut, G.; Touzard, C.; Moutel, L.; Collet, N.; Chaleil, D.; Barrey, E. Reference data for normal subjects obtained with an accelerometric device. *Gait Posture* **2002**, *16*, 124–134. [CrossRef]
21. Reinhardt, L.; Heilmann, F.; Teicher, M.; Wollny, R.; Lauenroth, A.; Delank, K.S.; Schwesig, R.; Kurz, E. Comparison of posturographic outcomes between two different de-vices. *J. Biomech.* **2019**, *86*, 218–224. [CrossRef] [PubMed]
22. Friedrich, M.; Grein, H.J.; Wicher, C.; Schuetze, J.; Mueller, A.; Lauenroth, A.; Hottenrott, K.; Schwesig, R. Influence of pathologic and simulated visual dysfunctions on the postural system. *Exp. Brain Res.* **2008**, *186*, 305–314. [CrossRef] [PubMed]
23. Oppenheim, U.; Kohen-Raz, R.; Alex, D.; Kohen-Raz, A.; Azarya, M. Postural characteristics of diabetic neuropathy. *Diabetes Care* **1999**, *22*, 328–332. [CrossRef] [PubMed]
24. Schwesig, R.; Goldich, Y.; Hahn, A.; Muller, A.; Kohen-Raz, R.; Kluttig, A.; Morad, Y. Postural control in subjects with visual impairment. *Eur. J. Ophthalmol.* **2011**, *21*, 303–309. [CrossRef]

25. Schwesig, R.; Becker, S.; Fischer, D. Intraobserver reliability of posturography in healthy subjects. *Somatosens. Mot. Res.* **2014**, *31*, 16–22. [CrossRef]
26. Schwesig, R.; Fischer, D.; Becker, S.; Lauenroth, A. Intraobserver reliability of posturography in patients with vestibular neuritis. *Somatosens. Mot. Res.* **2014**, *31*, 28–34. [CrossRef]
27. Schwesig, R.; Hollstein, L.; Plontke, S.K.; Delank, K.S.; Fieseler, G.; Rahne, T. Comparison of intraobserver single-task reliabilities of the Interactive Balance System (IBS) and Vertiguard in asymptomatic subjects. *Somatosens. Mot. Res.* **2017**, *34*, 9–14. [CrossRef]
28. Schulze, S.; Schwesig, R.; Edel, M.; Fieseler, G.; Delank, K.S.; Hermassi, S.; Laudner, K.G. Treadmill based reference running data for healthy subjects is dependent on speed and morphological parameters. *Hum. Mov. Sci.* **2017**, *55*, 269–275. [CrossRef]
29. Hopkins, W.G. Measures of reliability in sports medicine and science. *Sports Med.* **2000**, *30*, 1–15. [CrossRef]
30. Schwesig, R.; Becker, S.; Lauenroth, A.; Kluttig, A.; Leuchte, S.; Esperer, H.D. A novel posturographic method to differentiate sway patterns of patients with Parkinson's disease from patients with cerebellar ataxia. *Biomed. Tech. (Berl.)* **2009**, *54*, 347–356. [CrossRef]
31. Chan, J.; Desai, A.K.; Kazi, Z.B.; Corey, K.; Austin, S.; Hobson-Webb, L.D.; Case, L.E.; Jones, H.N.; Kishnani, P.S. The emerging phenotype of late-onset Pompe disease: A systematic literature review. *Mol. Genet. Metab.* **2017**, *120*, 163–172. [CrossRef] [PubMed]
32. Schneider, I.; Zierz, S. Profile of alglucosidase alfa in the treatment of Pompe disease: Safety, efficacy, and patient acceptability. *Res. Rep. Endocr. Disord.* **2015**, *6*, 1–9. [CrossRef]
33. van der Walt, J.D.; Swash, M.; Leake, J.; Cox, E.L. The pattern of involvement of adult-onset acid maltase deficiency at autopsy. *Muscle Nerve* **1987**, *10*, 272–281. [CrossRef]
34. DeRuisseau, L.R.; Fuller, D.D.; Qiu, K.; DeRuisseau, K.C.; Donnelly, W.H., Jr.; Mah, C.; Reier, P.J.; Byrne, B.J. Neural deficits contribute to respiratory insufficiency in Pompe disease. *Proc. Natl. Acad. Sci. USA* **2009**, *106*, 9419–9424. [CrossRef] [PubMed]
35. Hensel, O.; Schneider, I.; Wieprecht, M.; Kraya, T.; Zierz, S. Decreased outlet angle of the superior cerebellar artery as indicator for dolichoectasia in late onset Pompe disease. *Orphanet J. Rare Dis.* **2018**, *13*, 57. [CrossRef] [PubMed]
36. Musumeci, O.; Marino, S.; Granata, F.; Morabito, R.; Bonanno, L.; Brizzi, T.; Lo Buono, V.; Corallo, F.; Longo, M.; Toscano, A. Central nervous system involvement in late-onset Pompe disease: Clues from neuroimaging and neuropsychological analysis. *Eur. J. Neurol.* **2019**, *26*, 442-e35. [CrossRef] [PubMed]
37. Hanisch, F.; Rahne, T.; Plontke, S.K. Prevalence of hearing loss in patients with late-onset Pompe disease: Audiological and otological consequences. *Int. J. Audiol.* **2013**, *52*, 816–823. [CrossRef]
38. Wirsching, A.; Muller-Felber, W.; Schoser, B. Are evoked potentials in patients with adult-onset pompe disease indicative of clinically relevant central nervous system involvement? *J. Clin. Neurophysiol.* **2014**, *31*, 362–366. [CrossRef]
39. Montagnese, F.; Thiele, S.; Wenninger, S.; Schoser, B. Long-term whole-body vibration training in two late-onset Pompe disease patients. *Neurol. Sci.* **2016**, *37*, 1357–1360. [CrossRef]
40. Vry, J.; Schubert, I.J.; Semler, O.; Haug, V.; Schonau, E.; Kirschner, J. Whole-body vibration training in children with Duchenne muscular dystrophy and spinal muscular atrophy. *Eur. J. Paediatr. Neurol.* **2014**, *18*, 140–149. [CrossRef]
41. Yang, F.; King, G.A.; Dillon, L.; Su, X. Controlled whole-body vibration training reduces risk of falls among community-dwelling older adults. *J. Biomech.* **2015**, *48*, 3206–3212. [CrossRef] [PubMed]
42. Corrado, B.; Ciardi, G.; Iammarrone, C.S. Rehabilitation management of Pompe disease, from childhood trough adulthood: A systematic review of the literature. *Neurol. Int.* **2019**, *11*, 7983. [CrossRef] [PubMed]

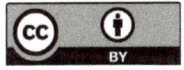

© 2020 by the authors. Licensee MDPI, Basel, Switzerland. This article is an open access article distributed under the terms and conditions of the Creative Commons Attribution (CC BY) license (http://creativecommons.org/licenses/by/4.0/).

 *applied sciences*

Article

Postural Stability and Regulation before and after High Tibial Osteotomy and Rehabilitation

Kay Brehme [1], Thomas Bartels [1], Martin Pyschik [1], Manuel Jenz [2], Karl-Stefan Delank [2], Kevin G. Laudner [3] and René Schwesig [2,*]

[1] Sports Clinic Halle, Center of Joint Surgery, 06108 Halle (Saale), Germany; kay.brehme@sportklinik-halle.de (K.B.); thomas.bartels@sportklinik-halle.de (T.B.); martin.pyschik@sportklinik-halle.de (M.P.)
[2] Department of Orthopaedic and Trauma Surgery, Martin-Luther-University Halle-Wittenberg, Ernst-Grube-Str. 40, 06120 Halle (Saale), Germany; manuel.jenz@freenet.de (M.J.); stefan.delank@uk-halle.de (K.-S.D.)
[3] Department of Health Sciences, University of Colorado, Colorado Springs, CO 80918, USA; klaudner@uccs.edu
* Correspondence: rene.schwesig@uk-halle.de; Tel.: +49-345-557-1317; Fax: +49-345-557-4899

Received: 31 August 2020; Accepted: 15 September 2020; Published: 18 September 2020

Featured Application: Knee osteoarthrosis (OA) is a common orthopedic problem often surgically treated using a high tibial osteotomy (HTO). Unfortunately, little is known regarding the effects of HTO on postural stability and regulation. The purpose of our study was to provide a better understanding of the underlying mechanisms of postural regulation, especially the potential change in postural subsystems following HTO.

Abstract: Knee osteoarthrosis (OA) is a widespread orthopedic problem and a high tibial osteotomy (HTO) is a common treatment to minimize degeneration of the affected compartment. The primary aim of this study was to evaluate the postural regulation and stability among patients who underwent HTO and rehabilitation. This prospective study included 32 patients (55.3 ± 5.57 years) diagnosed with medial tibiofemoral OA. Each subject completed postural regulation and stability testing (Interactive Balance System), as well as pain intensity (visual analogue scale) and quality of life questionnaires (SF-36) prior to HTO (exam 1), and at six weeks (exam 2), twelve weeks (exam 3) and six months (exam 4) post HTO. For postural comparison, all patients were matched (sex, age, height) with asymptomatic subjects. Significant time effects (exam 1 vs. exam 4) were found for weight distribution index (WDI; $\eta_p^2 = 0.152$), mediolateral weight distribution $\eta_p^2 = 0.163$) and anterior–posterior weight distribution $\eta_p^2 = 0.131$). The largest difference (exam 3: $\eta_p^2 = 0.251$) and the most significant differences to the matched sample were calculated for the stability indicator (exam 1: $\eta_p^2 = 0.237$; exam 2: $\eta_p^2 = 0.215$; exam 3: $\eta_p^2 = 0.251$; exam 4: $\eta_p^2 = 0.229$). Pain intensity showed a significant reduction ($\eta_p^2 = 0.438$) from exam 1 (50.7 ± 20.0 mm) to exam 4 (19.3 ± 16.0 mm). Physical pain was the quality of life parameter with the largest improvement between exams 1 and 4 ($\eta_p^2 = 0.560$). HTO allows patients to improve their mediolateral weight distribution, whereas postural stability is consistently lower than in asymptomatic subjects. This surgery leads to marked improvements in quality of life and pain.

Keywords: knee osteoarthrosis; surgery; posturography; postural subsystems; pain; quality of life

1. Introduction

For more than 25% of patients under the age of 70 years, knee osteoarthritis (OA) is a widespread orthopedic problem [1]. Kurtz et al. [2] reported a predicted increase in prevalence to 40% between 2005 and 2030 for Western Europe and North America.

High tibial osteotomy (HTO) is a well-established and often recommended surgical option for medial compartment knee OA in patients with varus malalignment [3,4]. This surgical intervention is indicated for varus deformities of 5° or greater in patients with cartilage defects and who are able to defer total knee arthroplasty (TKA) [5,6]. HTO has been shown to reduce pain, improve function and slow the progression of OA [7]. Previous research has investigated the effectiveness of using an opening-wedge HTO to evaluate cartilage quality [8–11] and compared HTO and knee joint distraction as an alternative surgical treatment for OA [6,12]. Bode et al. [5] compared the survival rates (defined as the absence for need of reintervention) of patients with less than 5° varus deformity when treated with autologous chondrocyte implantation and additional HTO compared to those treated with ACI alone. Bastard et al. [13] investigated the influence of HTO on return to sport at one year postoperative using the Tegner score (primary outcome) and quality of life questionnaire (SF-36).

Unfortunately, the effects of HTO on postural stability and regulation have received little attention. Hunt et al. [14] found that standing balance in patients with OA is not significantly different following HTO, but this was only assessed 12 months postoperative. Zhang et al. [15] evaluated the circadian rhythm of balance control in patients with OA using posturography and found reduced postural performance and pain in the morning compared to the early afternoon.

The current study is based on the longitudinal study design of Bartels et al. [16] with a postoperative follow-up of six months. Four hypotheses were proved:

(1) Medial tibiofemoral OA and HTO will induce unbalanced mediolateral weight distribution;
(2) Postural stability will be reduced before and after HTO;
(3) After medial tibiofemoral OA/HTO and compared to healthy matched individuals the cerebellar and somatosensory subsystem will display the largest changes;
(4) Pain perception and quality of life will significantly improve following HTO and rehabilitation.

2. Materials and Methods

2.1. Subjects

Thirty-two (84%) of an initial 38 included male patients completed all four examinations (exams). For the statistical analysis, only data from these 32 participants were included (Table 1).

Table 1. Demographic and anthropometric characteristics of patients (exam 1, n = 32).

Sex, Male:Female	32:0
Age (year)	55.3 ± 5.57 (42.0–62.0)
Height (m)	1.80 ± 0.07 (1.70–2.01)
Weight (kg)	99.4 ± 13.4 (77.8–129.1)
Body mass index (kg/m^2)	30.7 ± 3.65 (24.0–39.6)
Duration of pain (month)	28.3 ± 20.2 (4–96)
Affected side	n = 12 left; n = 20 right
Dominant and non-dominant leg	n = 13 left; n = 18 right (1 subject did not indicate dominance)

Results reported as mean ± standard deviation (range).

No relation (Chi-Quadrat: 2.306, $p = 0.129$) was calculated between the side of diagnosis and the side of the dominant or non-dominant leg. All included patients had moderate OA (Kellgren–Lawrence grade: 3). Prior to data collection, all participants provided written consent to participate after being informed of all study procedures and risks. The study was approved by the ethical committee of Martin-Luther-University Halle-Wittenberg (approval number: 2018-66).

2.2. Measurement Set-Up

Figure 1 shows the prospective and longitudinal design used for this study. All patients had been diagnosed with medial knee compartmental OA verified by MRI, arthroscopy of the knee and clinical check performed by an experienced (30–40 HTO surgeries yearly) orthopedist. Only one surgeon was included in this examination to ensure the highest level of observation equality.

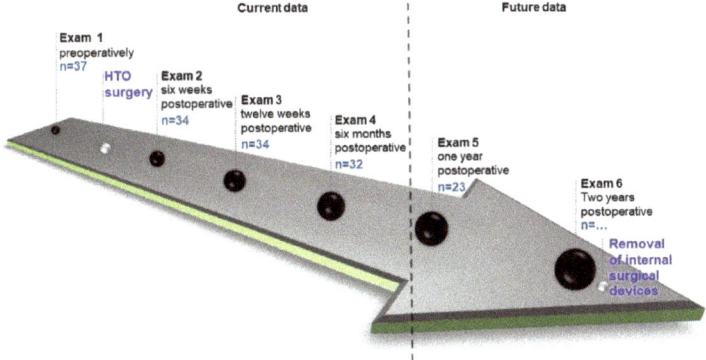

Figure 1. Flow chart of the longitudinal study design.

In total, 37 patients with symptomatic medial knee compartmental OA were initially (exam 1) recruited between May 2018 and August 2019 in this single-center (SportsClinic Halle) controlled trial. The following inclusion criteria were used:

- A body mass index (BMI) of less than 40 kg/m^2 based on an age range from 18 to 70 years;
- A tibiofemoral angle of less than 10° of varus;
- Intact knee ligaments;
- An asymptomatic range of motion (minimum of 120° flexion);
- Chronic knee pain during rest and motion.

Patients with instability of the knee ligaments and contralateral knee OA requiring treatment were excluded, as were those with primary patellofemoral OA, bi-compartmental OA, tibial or femoral osteonecrosis and those with a history of an inflammatory rheumatic disease. The patients did not participate in the study if they were unable to perform the balance tests (posturography) owing to pain or limited motion of the lower limb [17].

Patients were assessed initially (exam 1) and then again postoperatively at six weeks (exam 2), twelve weeks (exam 3) and six months (exam 4) (authors are currently investigating 2-year follow-up). Between exam 1 and exam 2, the HTO surgery was conducted. The time between exam 1 and HTO surgery was on average 6.38 ± 10.2 days (range: 0–40 days). Overall, 34% (11/32) of patients had surgery and exam 1 on the same day; 22% (7/32) of patients had a time interval of at least seven days. The primary reasons for these deviations were mostly organizational issues and the short-term illnesses of patients. The aim of this study was to determine the long-term impacts of HTO and the subsequent standardized rehabilitation and individual treatment (Figure 1, Table A1). All measurements were performed at the same time of day and in a quiet room to minimize any disruptions during testing.

2.3. Surgery and Medication

The surgical procedure used consisted of a bi-plane medial-based opening-wedge HTO, including a distal release of the superficial medial collateral ligament fibers. The aim was to shift the weight-bearing line laterally, with the post-operative mechanical axis running laterally through the tibial plateau at 62% of its entire width (measured from the medial side) [6]. Only one surgeon (KB) was used for all procedures to avoid any surgeon bias. The LOQTEQ Osteotomy Plate system (aap Implants Inc. Dover, DE, USA) was used for fixation.

Using standing whole leg radiographs, the amount of needed correction was determined using the Miniaci method [18]. The x-raying of the knee joint (bi-plane) was performed at two weeks and four weeks postoperatively in order to judge the process of bone healing. The axis control using standing whole leg radiographs was only conducted preoperatively, because it had no impact on the rehabilitation process.

Concerning medication, Mono-embolex (a low molecular heparin) was given for 20 days postoperative to reduce the risk of thrombosis. Diclofenbeta and Imbun (non-steroidal anti-inflammatory/antirheumatic drugs) were used for perioperative pain management (Diclofenbeta: three times for three days and afterwards once per day until removing sutures; Imbun: if necessary, one-two times per day). The pain management (Imbun) ended after a 20-day postoperative period.

2.4. Assessments

2.4.1. Posturography

Postural regulation and stability were measured using the Interactive Balance System (IBS, neurodata, Vienna, Austria). This system provides a comprehensive and sufficient reference database of asymptomatic subjects (n = 1724) stratified by age and gender [19]. The IBS is well established and commonly used in scientific research, and considered as valid [20–23] and reliable [24–26]. For example, the intraobserver reliability calculated by intraclass correlation coefficients moved from 0.71 to 0.95 for all parameter and tests.

For a valid comparison with asymptomatic subjects, we performed a matched-pairs technique [16] using the parameters age ($p = 0.412$), gender ($p = 1.000$) and body height ($p = 0.272$). For this reason, recruitment of an asymptomatic control group was not necessary.

All participants were tested by the same investigator (MJ) on the vertical force platform (IBS). All measurements were conducted at the same time of day and in a quiet room to minimize any disruptions during testing.

The IBS consists of four independent force plates (acquisition frequency: 32 Hz, recording time per trial: 32 s) in order to measure forefoot and heel forces separately. A detailed description regarding parameters (including interpretation and explanation of functional frequency bands), test positions/conditions and instructions for subjects has already been published [16,23,27,28].

2.4.2. Pain Assessment (Visual Analogue Scale)

To evaluate pain intensity of the affected limb, the Visual Analogue Scale (VAS) was used [29]. The VAS consists of a 100-mm line whose endpoints were declared as "no pain" (at 0 mm) and "insupportable pain" (at 100 mm). The patients were asked before the posturography to locate the level of pain on the line with a small vertical mark [15].

2.4.3. Quality of Life Assessment (SF-36)

Health-related quality of life (HRQL) was evaluated using the SF-36 questionnaire (German version) [30,31]. Mc Horney et al. [32] reported an Intraclass correlation coefficient (ICC) of 0.85. Psychometric validation of the German SF-36 revealed comparable results concerning reliability, and construct validity with other European samples [30,31,33]. Based on 36 questions, eight different subscales describing physical and mental health can be assessed. These subscales include Physical Functioning (PF), Role Physical (RP), Bodily Pain (BP), and General Health (GH), which represent the physical aspect, Vitality (VT), Social Functioning (SF), Role Emotional (RE), and Mental Health (MH) represent the mental aspect. Finally, and in order to allow for interpretation and discussion of the results of this study, a transformation of the subscales into a physical health component summary score (PCS) and a mental health component summary score (MCS) was performed [34].

2.4.4. Statistics

An a priori power analysis (nQuery 4.0, Statistical solutions Ltd., Cork, Ireland) was performed to determine the sample size using a two-sided hypothesis test at an alpha level of 0.05. In line with other authors [6,12] the sample size calculation was performed based on noninferiority using a power of 80%. Van der Woude et al. [6] recommended studies account for possible attrition and/or insufficient data quality. Therefore, the sample size was increased by 15%.

For all parameters, mean, standard deviation, 95% confidence intervals were reported. In the run-up to the inference statistical analyses, all variables were tested for normal distribution (Shapiro–Wilk Test). Mean differences between exams (1–4) and groups (HTO patients vs. matched subjects) were tested using a one-factorial (time or group) univariate general linear model. The variance analysis was divided into three parts according to and described in detail in Bartels et al. [16].

The critical level of significance was adjusted using the Bonferroni correction. After this correction, a significance level (p) of 0.05 was divided by the number of posturographic tests (9). Differences between means were considered as statistically significant if p values were <0.006 or partial eta squared (partial-η^2 (η_p^2)) values were greater than 0.10 [35].

All statistical analyses were performed using SPSS version 25.0 for Windows (SPSS Inc., Chicago, IL, USA).

3. Results

3.1. Normal Distribution and Variance Homogeneity

Only the variable BMI ($p = 0.063$) had a normal distribution. Regarding variance homogeneity, one parameter (stability indicator: $p = 0.005$) did not show variance homogeneity. Otherwise, all p-values were higher than 0.078 (synchronization) indicating that the variances from all other variables were not significantly different.

No significant differences between patients and asymptomatic references were calculated for age ($p = 0.412$, $\eta_p^2 = 0.011$) and height ($p = 0.272$, $\eta_p^2 = 0.019$). In contrast, significant mean differences were detected for weight ($p = 0.001$, $\eta_p^2 = 0.152$) and BMI ($p = 0.007$, $\eta_p^2 = 0.110$). The body weight for the patients was clearly higher (patients: 99.4 ± 13.4 kg vs. reference group: 88.4 ± 13.1 kg) than for the reference group and was stable over the six-month period ($p = 0.567$, $\eta_p^2 = 0.018$).

3.2. Longitudinal Analysis

Longitudinal analysis within the HTO patients can be viewed in Tables 2 and 3, and in Figures 2–4. For posturographic parameters, we only found a significant main effect for time (preoperative vs. six months post-operation) in weight distribution index (WDI) (Table 2; Figure 3B).

Table 2. Descriptive comparison of five examinations and analysis of variance, calculation of effect size (η_p^2) only for bilateral posturographic parameters (n = 32). Grey marked the descriptive values (mean ± standard deviation in column 1) and four cross-sectional comparisons with the reference matched sample (p/η_p^2).

Parameter	Examinations (Exam)				Variance Analysis		
	Exam 1 Preoperative	Exam 2 6 Weeks Postoperative	Exam 3 12 Weeks Postoperative	Exam 4 6 Months Postoperative	Comparison of Exam 1 vs. Exam 4		Comparison of Adjacent Exams
Matched Sample					p	η_p^2	η_p^2
Visual and Nigrostriatal 16.6 ± 6.44	18.4 ± 5.44 0.213/0.025	20.9 ± 22.1 0.289/0.018	21.6 ± 22.0 0.220/0.024	17.7 ± 5.07 0.431/0.010	0.635	0.014	reference matched sample
Peripheral-vestibular 9.67 ± 3.46	10.3 ± 3.13 0.416/0.011	9.78 ± 2.15 0.872/0.000	**9.65 ± 2.00** 0.983/0.000	9.93 ± 2.01 0.708/0.002	0.145	0.059	reference matched sample
Somatosensory 4.18 ± 1.39	4.81 ± 1.50 0.086/0.047	**4.48 ± 1.35** 0.382/0.012	4.62 ± 1.17 0.175/0.029	4.62 ± 1.36 0.198/0.027	0.114	0.062	1 vs. 2 (0.152) reference matched sample
Cerebellar 0.75 ± 0.22	**0.90 ± 0.27** 0.015/0.092	0.91 ± 0.30 0.017/0.088	0.91 ± 0.24 **0.005/0.118**	0.93 ± 0.32 **0.010/0.103**	0.810	0.008	reference matched sample
Stability indicator 19.2 ± 5.40	**<0.001/0.237** 27.1 ± 8.59	26.3 ± 8.03 **<0.001/0.215**	26.5 ± 7.31 **<0.001/0.251**	26.7 ± 8.20 **<0.001/0.229**	0.728	0.012	reference matched sample
Weight distribution index 6.11 ± 3.80	6.60 ± 1.78 0.513/0.007	7.13 ± 2.26 0.198/0.027	6.01 ± 2.05 0.896/0.000	6.01 ± 2.09 0.897/0.000	**0.003**	**0.152**	2 vs. 3 (0.297) reference matched sample
Synchronization 623 ± 157	622 ± 108 0.978/0.000	589 ± 142 0.368/0.013	610 ± 136 0.722/0.002	**628 ± 143** 0.901/0.000	0.390	0.031	reference matched sample
Anterior-posterior 0.58 ± 10.7	**5.30 ± 8.16** 0.051/0.060	7.54 ± 6.93 **0.003/0.134**	5.81 ± 6.91 0.023/0.080	7.44 ± 6.57 **0.003/0.134**	**0.031**	0.095	1 vs. 2 (0.170) 3 vs. 4 (0.124) reference matched sample
Mediolateral 0.31 ± 5.55	−0.35 ± 5.42 0.628/0.004	−0.19 ± 7.93 0.769/0.001	−0.26 ± 5.27 0.675/0.003	−0.58 ± 4.13 0.469/0.008	0.966	0.002	reference matched sample

Values are given as mean ± standard deviation. Significance level: $p < 0.006$ or $\eta_p^2 \geq 0.10$. Significant differences and performance maxima marked in bold.

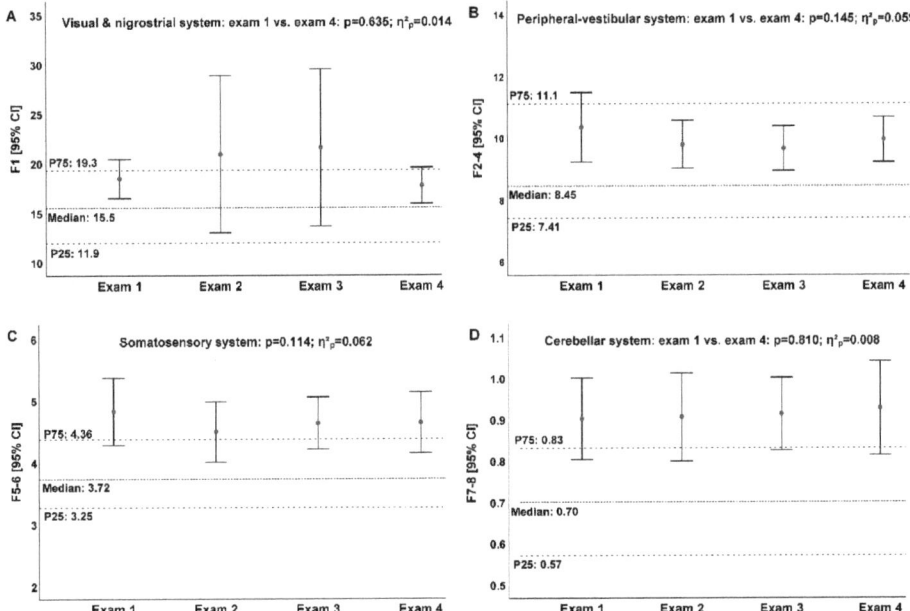

Figure 2. (**A**–**D**) Longitudinal changes of the postural subsystems compared with the matched reference sample based on percentile (P25, P50, P75) analysis. Total effects and relevant ($\eta_p^2 \geq 0.10$) partial effects are reported.

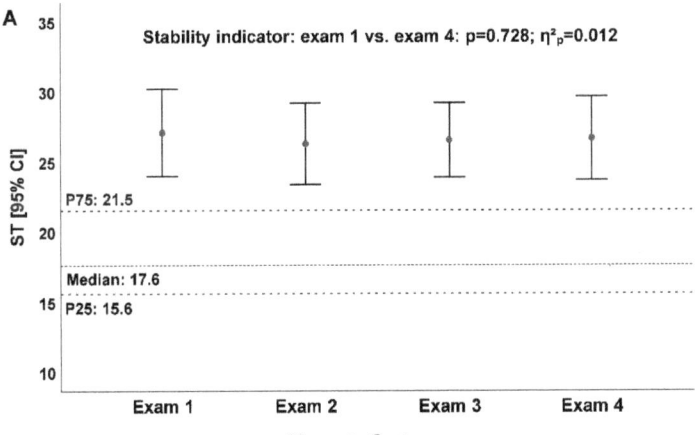

Figure 3. *Cont.*

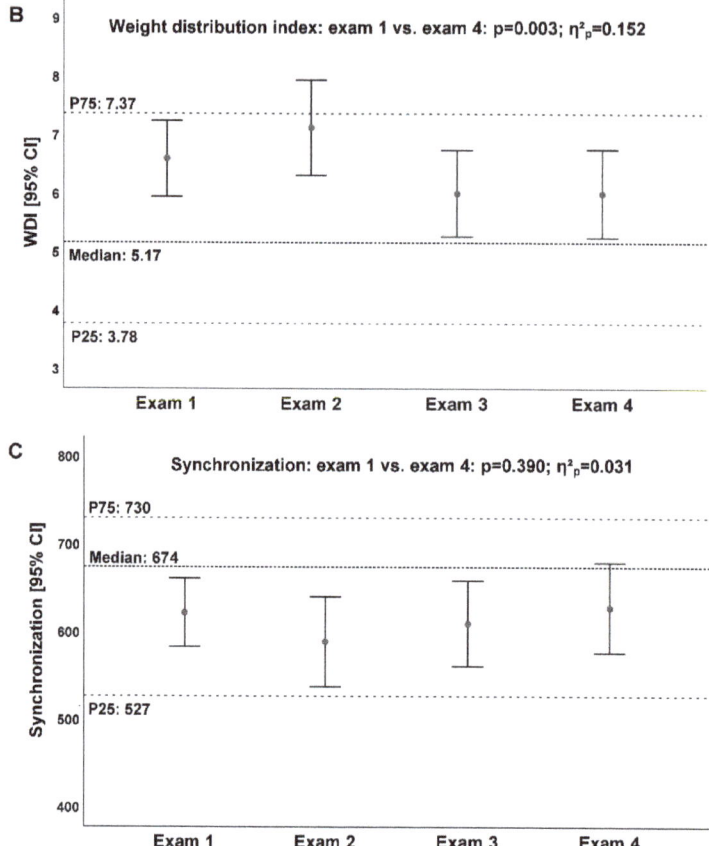

Figure 3. (A–C) Longitudinal changes of bilateral (stability indicator (ST) weight distribution index (WDI); synchronization (Synch)) posturographic parameters compared with the matched reference sample based on percentile (P25, P50, P75) analysis. Total effects and relevant ($\eta_p^2 \geq 0.10$) partial effects are reported.

The WDI was the parameter with the largest improvement ($\eta_p^2 = 0.152$) over the total time of the investigation. The HTO induced a short-term enhancement of the forefoot load (exam 1: 54.2 vs. exam 2: 57.2%, $\eta_p^2 = 0.272$; Table 3, Figure 4A) and the load of the unaffected side (left-sided load, injury on the right side: exam 1: 52.9 vs. exam 2: 54.5%; Table 3).

Table 3. Descriptive longitudinal comparison, analysis of variance and calculation of effect size (η_p^2) for unilateral Interactive Balance System (IBS) parameters depending on the side of injury/correction (left: n = 12; right: n = 20). Based on the comparison of adjacent examinations only significant differences are reported.

Parameter (%)	Examinations (Exam)				Variance Analysis		
	Exam 1	Exam 2	Exam 3	Exam 4	Comparison of Exam 1 vs. Exam 4		Comparison of Adjacent Exams
	Preoperative	6 Weeks Postoperative	12 Weeks Postoperative	6 Months Postoperative	p	η_p^2	η_p^2
Patients with left-sided injury (n = 12)							
Heel	42.9 ± 5.78	41.9 ± 6.11	42.8 ± 4.56	41.4 ± 4.87	0.594	0.051	3 vs. 4 (0.145)
Left	46.2 ± 4.25	43.1 ± 6.23	47.9 ± 3.68	50.2 ± 3.28	0.001	0.547	1 vs. 2 (0.219)
							2 vs. 3 (0.636)
							3 vs. 4 (0.486)
Patients with right-sided injury (n = 20)							
Heel	45.8 ± 9.28	42.8 ± 7.51	45.0 ± 7.99	43.3 ± 7.44	0.052	0.131	1 vs. 2 (0.272)
							2 vs. 3 (0.122)
							3 vs. 4 (0.118)
Left	52.9 ± 4.43	54.5 ± 5.42	51.7 ± 5.64	50.8 ± 4.64	0.031	0.163	2 vs. 3 (0.420)

Values are given as mean ± standard deviation. Heel: percentage of weight distribution forefoot vs. heel with description of heel loading; Left: percentage of weight distribution left vs. right with description of left side loading. Significance level: $p < 0.006$ or $\eta_p^2 \geq 0.10$. Significant differences and performance maxima marked in bold.

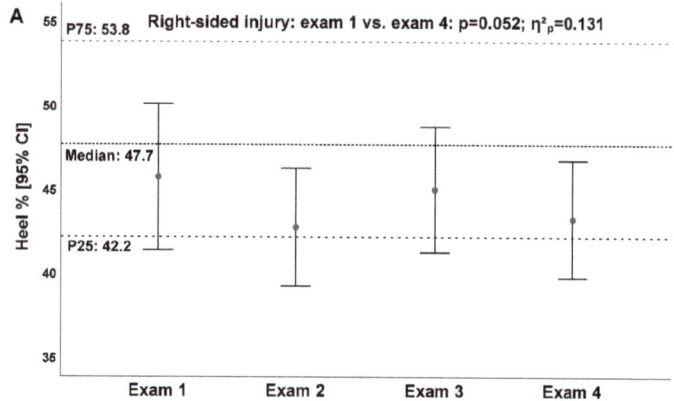
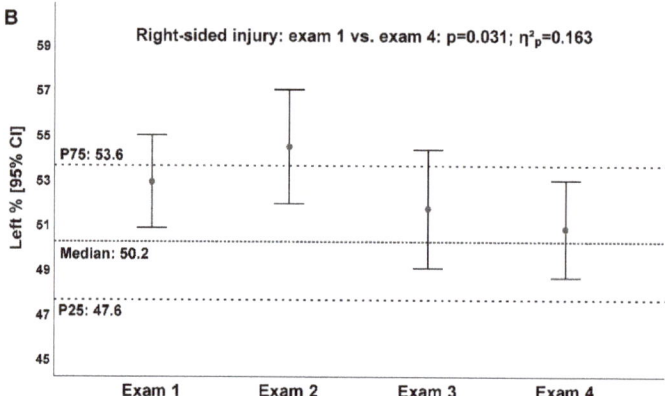

Figure 4. (**A**,**B**) Longitudinal changes of unilateral (heel, left) posturographic parameters compared with the matched reference sample based on percentile (P25, P50, P75) analysis for the patients with right-sided injury (n = 20). Total effects and relevant ($\eta_p^2 \geq 0.10$) partial effects are reported.

The highest time effects between adjacent examinations (patients with left-sided injury) were detected for the mediolateral weight distribution between exam 2 vs. exam 3 postoperatively ($\eta_p^2 = 0.636$) and exam 2 vs. exam 4 ($\eta_p^2 = 0.486$; Table 3). From exam 2 to exam 3, both subsamples showed the largest improvements (left-sided injury: 4.8%, $\eta_p^2 = 0.636$; right-sided injury: 2.8%, $\eta_p^2 = 0.420$) concerning the mediolateral weight distribution in the sense of a more powerful balance. Concerning postural regulation, no postural subsystems showed main effects for time (Table 2). There was only one partial time effect for the somatosensory subsystem between exam 1 (4.81 ± 1.50) and exam 2 (4.48 ± 1.35) detected ($\eta_p^2 = 0.152$).

3.3. Cross-Sectional Analysis—Comparison of HTO Patients with Matched Subjects

The comparison of HTO patients with matched individuals can be viewed in Tables 2 and 3, and in Figures 2–4. The largest difference (exam 3: $\eta_p^2 = 0.251$) to the matched sample was calculated for the stability indicator (ST, Figure 3A). The most (4) significant differences to the matched sample were also observed for ST (preoperative: $\eta_p^2 = 0.237$; exam 2: $\eta_p^2 = 0.215$; exam 3: $\eta_p^2 = 0.251$; exam 4: $\eta_p^2 = 0.229$; Table 2).

At six months post-HTO, the mediolateral load distribution moved on the "healthy" level (Figure 4B, Table 3). In contrast, the postural stability, measured by stability indicator was completely outside (above the percentile 75) the interquartile range of the healthy subjects (Figure 3A). The peripheral–vestibular system (Figure 2B) was the postural subsystem with the smallest difference to the median of the healthy subjects over the whole six-month period. Conversely, the activity of the cerebellar system (Figure 2D) was consistently above the 75th percentile of the healthy subjects for all examinations. Two significant differences (twelve weeks postoperative: $\eta_p^2 = 0.118$; six months postoperative: $\eta_p^2 = 0.103$) compared with the matched subjects were observed. The somatosensory system (Figure 2C) showed a similar pattern, but without significant differences at any examination.

3.4. Comparison of Patients Depending on the Side of Injury/HTO

A significant rise in mediolateral weight distribution was observed on the injured side after HTO (Table 3). This effect was much stronger in the patients with left-sided injury (exam 1 vs. 4: $\eta_p^2 = 0.547$ vs. $\eta_p^2 = 0.163$). Simultaneously, this was one of the largest observed main time effects. The left-side load in the HTO left-sided injury patients was the only parameter with significant changes in all three postoperative observation periods (Table 3). A peak was calculated between exam 2 and 3 ($\eta_p^2 = 0.636$). In contrast, the changes concerning anteroposterior weight distribution were much lower in both patient groups, especially for the left-sided HTO injury patients (exam 1 vs. 4: $\eta_p^2 = 0.051$ vs. 0.131). At six months post-operation, there was still an enhanced forefoot load (59 and 57%; Table 3) with the same difference (1.5%) between exam 1 and 4 for both patient groups.

3.5. Pain Assessment (VAS)

Pain perception over the entirety of the study (Figure 5) sharply decreased (main time effect: $p < 0.001$, $\eta_p^2 = 0.438$), especially from exam 1 to exam 2 (50.7 ± 20.0 vs. 33.9 ± 17.1; $\eta_p^2 = 0.339$).

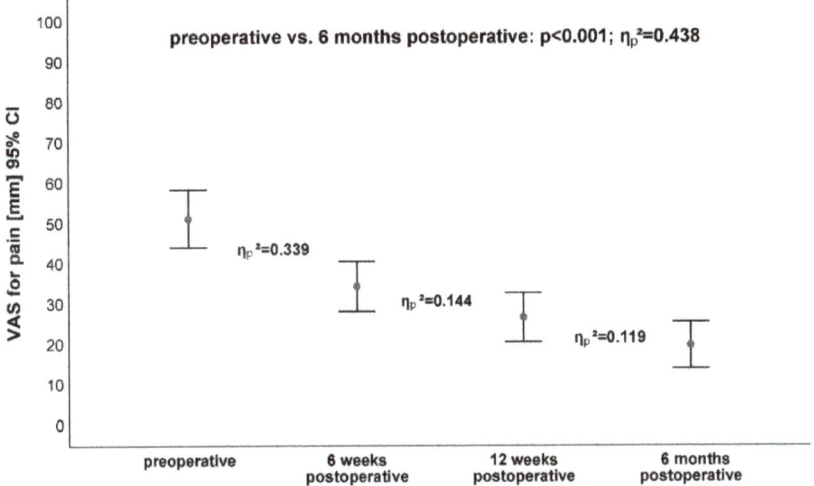

Figure 5. Descriptive, longitudinal changes for visual analogue scale (VAS), analysis of variance and calculation of effect size (η_p^2). Total effects and relevant ($\eta_p^2 \geq 0.10$) partial time effects are reported.

Significant changes were found for all investigated time intervals with the smallest significant difference displayed between exams 3 and 4 (26.2 ± 16.8 vs. 19.3 ± 16.0; $\eta_p^2 = 0.119$).

3.6. Quality of Life Assessment (SF-36)

With the exception of mental health ($\eta_p^2 = 0.016$), all other subscales showed significant improvements (Table 4).

Table 4. Descriptive longitudinal comparison, analysis of variance and calculation of effect size (η_p^2) for quality of life parameters. Based on the comparison of adjacent examinations only significant differences are reported.

Parameter	Examinations (Exam); n = 32					Variance Analysis		
	Exam 1 Preoperative	Exam 2 6 Weeks Postoperative	Exam 3 12 Weeks Postoperative	Exam 4 6 Months Postoperative		Comparison of Exam 1 vs. Exam 4		Comparison of Adjacent Exams η_p^2
						p	η_p^2	
Subscale								
Physical functioning	46.3 ± 21.9	45.3 ± 21.2	63.0 ± 20.9	75.8 ± 14.9		<0.001	0.451	2 vs. 3 (0.376) 3 vs. 4 (0.337) 1 vs. 2 (0.386)
Physical role functioning	43.0 ± 36.6	12.5 ± 23.8	57.0 ± 42.7	74.1 ± 30.3		<0.001	0.446	2 vs. 3 (0.500) 3 vs. 4 (0.221)
Bodily pain	31.7 ± 17.6	37.2 ± 14.7	57.3 ± 15.2	64.3 ± 16.3		<0.001	0.560	2 vs. 3 (0.562) 3 vs. 4 (0.212)
General health perception	57.4 ± 19.2	61.4 ± 18.9	68.2 ± 17.2	66.8 ± 15.9		0.007	0.134	2 vs. 3 (0.120)
Vitality	52.2 ± 18.3	50.9 ± 17.8	64.5 ± 18.1	65.8 ± 17.2		<0.001	0.267	2 vs. 3 (0.369)
Social role functioning	78.9 ± 27.6	71.1 ± 24.1	83.2 ± 24.9	86.3 ± 23.4		0.003	0.151	2 vs. 3 (0.226)
Emotional role functioning	78.1 ± 37.5	59.4 ± 44.6	78.3 ± 36.3	85.0 ± 29.6		0.008	0.126	1 vs. 2 (0.188) 2 vs. 3 (0.154)
Mental health	74.0 ± 15.9	78.4 ± 16.6	75.9 ± 23.9	77.5 ± 23.1		0.646	0.016	-
Total score								
physical health component summary score	31.4 ± 8.16	29.8 ± 7.22	40.5 ± 8.28	45.0 ± 6.36		<0.001	0.573	2 vs. 3 (0.569) 3 vs. 4 (0.365)
mental health component summary score	55.0 ± 11.4	53.5 ± 11.3	54.4 ± 11.1	53.6 ± 11.1		0.804	0.010	-

Values are given as mean ± standard deviation. Significance level: $p < 0.006$ or $\eta_p^2 \geq 0.10$. Significant differences and performance maxima marked in bold.

The smallest significant change was calculated for emotional role functioning ($\eta_p^2 = 0.126$). In contrast, bodily pain displayed the largest improvement ($\eta_p^2 = 0.560$), especially between exams 2 and 3 (37.2 ± 14.7 vs. 57.3 ± 15.2; $\eta_p^2 = 0.562$). The physical role functioning was the only subscale with significant improvements between all examinations. Similar to bodily pain, the largest change was observed between exams 2 and 3 (12.5 ± 23.8 vs. 57.0 ± 42.7; $\eta_p^2 = 0.500$). After a postoperative period of six weeks, the standard deviation was clearly higher than the mean (coefficient of variation: 190%). It was the only quality of life parameter with a coefficient of variation above 100% at any examination.

4. Discussion

The primary objective of this prospective, longitudinal (preoperative to six months postoperative) cohort study was to evaluate the effect of HTO and subsequent rehabilitation on load distribution postural stability and postural regulation. Regarding posturography, the cross-sectional comparison with asymptomatic matched individuals was also performed. Additionally, the parameters quality of life and pain perception were also investigated.

Our results supported hypothesis one indicating that the HTO leads to a strong weight relief of the injured side. Improvement of the mediolateral weight distribution needs at least a six-month postoperative period. After medial knee compartmental OA and HTO postural stability is strongly reduced (hypothesis two). The largest posturographic changes during the six-month investigation period were calculated for weight distribution ($\eta_p^2 = 0.152$). As expected, the mediolateral weight distribution (left-sided injury: $\eta_p^2 = 0.547$; right-sided injury: $\eta_p^2 = 0.163$) showed the largest improvements. Consistently, the largest differences (exam 1–4: 29–33%) and highest activity (hyperactivity/compensation) compared with the matched asymptomatic subjects (reference: median), were observed in cerebellar system after HTO (hypothesis three). A similar hyperactive pattern was found for the visual and nigrostriatal system during exam 2 (35%) and exam 3 (39%). At exam 4, these postural subsystems showed the smallest difference (14%) of all postural subsystems according to the median of the matched subjects.

The peripheral–vestibular system consistently showed the smallest differences (exam 1–4: 14–22%) compared to the matched subjects and lowest activity directly (exam 2: 16%) after HTO. In contrast to the postural stability and regulation, pain perception (main time effect: $\eta_p^2 = 0.438$) and the physical health component of quality of life $\eta_p^2 = 0.573$) were strongly improved following HTO and subsequent rehabilitation. In particular, the subscales bodily pain ($\eta_p^2 = 0.560$), physical functioning ($\eta_p^2 = 0.451$) and physical role functioning ($\eta_p^2 = 0.446$) showed the largest longitudinal improvements (hypothesis four).

4.1. Weight Distribution and Postural Stability

The comparability of our results with previous studies is limited because we used different assessments to measure postural stability. For example, Hunt et al. [14,36] used the single leg stand on a force platform to judge the balance of patients with OA (n = 49) prior to and 12 months following medial opening wedge HTO. In line with our longitudinal study design, they also found only small (d < 0.34) and not significant ($p > 0.05$) changes regarding center of pressure and standing balance following HTO. As in our study, these patients showed a reduction in pain as quantified by the WOMAC despite no changes in standing balance [14]. Hunt et al. [36] found that the amount of varus malalignment was inversely related to single-legged standing balance. Presumably, neuromuscular control is reduced in the presence of this malalignment. The authors discussed a reduced joint innervation or muscle reflexes as possible causes [37]. It seems, that asymptomatic subjects with varus alignment exhibit more changed postural control strategies than subjects with neutral alignment [38]. Kim et al. [39] also used the IBS and investigated 80 patients with primary OA, classified by the Kellgren–Lawrence score (mild vs. moderate to severe) and 40 age-matched controls. These authors detected a higher postural sway of the moderate to severe group compared to those of the mild or control groups.

4.2. Postural Regulation and Subsystems

Kim et al. [39] showed a larger amount of instability in their moderate-to-severe primary OA group than the mild or control groups except for the somatosensory and cerebellar systems. They deduced that moderate-to-severe patients with knee OA depend on their eyesight in order to compensate for their postural instability. The calculated values for all frequency bands were much higher comparable with this study and Bartels et al. [16].

Following ACL rupture and surgical reconstruction and consistent with our study, Bartels et al. [16] observed the largest reductions of postural subsystems for the somatosensory (consistently below the healthy median reference) and cerebellar systems. However, in contrast to Bartels et al. [16] we detected a hyperactivity in both systems (consistently above the healthy interquartile range; Figure 2C,D) and not a suppression, especially at six-months post-operation. Obviously, these types of lower limb surgeries would have completely different effects concerning postural subsystems. The change of somatosensory information, potentially caused by mechanoreceptor damage (e.g., HTO surgery), may subsequently lead to a reduction of postural stability and regulation [40]. Both investigations are examples and proofs for the neuroplasticity of biological systems and the model of selective compensatory optimization. For example, the relation between the somatosensory system and the spinocerebellum system, which is responsible for processing the afferent (somatosensory) information is very close. The relationship between the peripheral–vestibular system and the vestibulocerebellum system is comparable. In this context, the hyperactive effects are caused by reduced activity of other postural systems, in this case particularly the peripheral-vestibular system (consistently below the healthy percentile 75; Figure 2B). Brandt et al. [41] demonstrated that knee osteoarthritis (OA) causes changes not only in the tissues within the articular cavity, but also the ligaments, tendons, and periarticular tissues including the muscles. Furthermore, patients with knee OA have deficiencies in the number of sensory receptors and therefore their proprioception compared to similar age controls Barrett et al. [42].

At six-months post-HTO, postural regulation returned to an asymptomatic level for mediolateral weight distribution. The cross-sectional comparison to asymptomatic subjects at all examinations showed that OA and HTO led to hyperactivity of the cerebellar and somatosensory systems and postural instability. Obviously, the subsequent rehabilitation was not able to improve postural regulation and stability. This investigation provides further insight into the underlying mechanisms of postural regulation and in the understanding of the interaction of postural subsystems. Future research examining postural stability after one- and two-year postoperative periods will provide a subsequent midterm and long-term evaluation of surgery and rehabilitation. It is possible that improvements in postural stability and regulation need longer than six-months to occur. In relation to other studies [17,49], we wanted to establish a more holistic approach instead of the frequently used isolated orthopedic view (flexibility, strength, pain).

4.3. Clinical Outcomes

Previous research has shown the effectiveness of uni-compartmental arthrosis for joint-preservation. Floerkemeier et al. [43] described a multicenter study with a large patient population (n = 533). Of these patients, 80% were very satisfied with the result of the surgery, in relation to knee pain and function. Insall et al. [44] reported that over a 10-year period, until conversion to a prosthesis, HTO should be considered for more physically active patients and has better results with advanced implants. According to the Finnish National Hospital Discharge Register (NHDR), the survival rate for 3195 knee-related reconversion osteotomies was 89% over 5 years and 73% over 10 years [45]. Naudie et al. [46] reported slightly lower survival rates of 73% after 5 years, 51% after ten years, 39% after 15 years and 30% after 20 years.

4.4. Pain Situation and Quality of Life

Van der Woude et al. [6] compared the efficacy of knee joint distraction (n = 23) and HTO (n = 46). In line with our results, these authors found significant improvements for the HTO group in the VAS pain score ($p = 0.006$) and physical component of SF 36 ($p = 0.024$) one year after surgery. Bastard et al. [13] evaluated return to sports and quality of life after HTO in athletic patients less than 60 years of age. The patients had the same age (mean age: 55.6 years) as our patients (mean age: 55.3 years) and in line with our results, they observed a significant improvement ($p = 0.01$) in quality of life pre-operatively (65%) compared with one year postoperatively (73%). In this time interval, the SF-36 physical sub-score also increased significantly ($p = 0.02$) from 59 (55–63) to 67 (58–72). However, the level of quality of life was consistently higher than in our investigation (from 59 to 67 vs. 30 to 45). However, this comparison is only valid for the preoperative evaluation because the postoperative examination is (still) different (one-year vs. six-months). Bonnin et al. [7] reported a similar level of quality of life (SF-12 physical score: 53.6 ± 9.7) for a non-selected population of HTO patients (closing-wedge HTO: n = 88; opening-wedge HTO: n = 51) as in our study to exam 4 (45.0 ± 6.36). Ihle et al. [34] examined the health-related quality of life (assessment: SF-36) in patients (n = 120) after HTO. In line with our study, they also found significantly longitudinal (after 6, 12 and 18 months postoperatively) improvements in the physical score ($p < 0.001$) in contrast to small changes in the mental score of the SF-36 ($p = 0.360$). The amount of improvement (13.6 vs. 9.3) over the time (six months) in the physical score was much higher in our study compared those of Ihle et al. [34]. Saier et al. [47] also observed a significant increase in health related quality of life (SF-36) and decrease in pain (VAS; $p < 0.001$; $\eta_p^2 = 0.4$) among patients (n = 64) after open-wedge high tibial osteotomy across the same time period of six months. The improvements in the physical score ($p < 0.001$; $\eta_p^2 = 0.4$) of the SF-36 were also much higher than in the mental score ($p = 0.008$, $\eta_p^2 = 0.1$). Webster and Feller [48] reported an increase in the physical scores of patients (n = 414) with knee OA before surgery and at a minimum of 12 months following knee replacement (33.6 to 45.6). In contrast, the change regarding the mental score was clearly smaller (52.2 to 55.1). We hope that our future investigations (one year and two years postoperative) will provide further insight into the long-term outcomes after HTO and rehabilitation. In summary, the HTO and the subsequent rehabilitation led to a significant improvement of the physical component of the quality of life. However, the mental part of the quality of life remained unaffected.

4.5. Limitations

Our prospective cohort study has some limitations worth noting. First, we had a relatively small sample size (n = 32). Initially, we recruited 37 patients. In the interest of a homogeneous sample (only men to avoid sex effects), we decided to eliminate three women (exam 2: n = 34). Between exams 3 and 4, two additional patients dropped out of the study, because they did not want to continue (exam 4: n = 32).

Although our patients conducted a standardized rehabilitation program (Table A1), a limiting factor in this examination was that the investigators had no direct influence on the rehabilitation process. Therefore, we are not able to guarantee that each protocol was realized completely as recommended. In addition, there was no uniform standardized treatment 16 weeks after surgery as the patients were discharged from clinical surveillance. Comparable to the study design by Bartels et al. [16], the longitudinal comparison is limited due to the different temporal durations between the four examinations (e.g., six weeks, twelve weeks, six months). Consequently, the longest time interval (twelve weeks) from exam 3 to 4 was supposed to have the highest potential for changes.

In regards to the time periods of the postoperative examinations, there were small differences compared to the targeted time points: exam 1 (preoperative) occurred 6.38 ± 10.2 (0–40) days preoperatively, exam 2 (six weeks) occurred 41.8 ± 5.11 (33–53) days postoperatively, exam 3 (twelve weeks) occurred 88.3 ± 20.3 (74–193) days postoperatively, and exam 4 (six-months) occurred 182 ± 12.1 (137–203) days postoperatively.

Essentially, we were not able to guarantee a precise realization of the timeline. Preoperatively, 69% (n = 22) of the patients were examined between 0 and 5 prior to surgery. Based on a time interval of three days around the ideal time point, 66% (n = 21, exam 2), 44% (n = 14, exam 3) and 31% (n = 10, exam 4) of the patients were tested in this time window.

5. Conclusions and Clinical Implications

From a clinical perspective, the findings of this investigation indicate that HTO patients do not present with improvements in postural performance following surgery and rehabilitation. Therefore, similar to ACL surgery and rehabilitation [16], the rehabilitation program should implement unexpected disturbances in order to improve feedforward mechanisms. This could contribute to improvements in the somatosensory and cerebellar systems. For example, Bartels et al. [49] described and examined a rehabilitation concept using unexpected cues that cause a response time of less than 200 ms five-months after an ACL reconstruction. The study results identified the IBS as a scientific evaluation and a useful posturographic assessment in terms of HTO surgery and following rehabilitation. The center of pressure measurement using IBS allows for a functional distinction in postural stability of HTO patients and asymptomatic subjects. Based on these study results and our extensive experiences, the IBS might support the work of physicians and physical therapists and adjust rehabilitation demands in a more precise and evidence-based way.

The outcomes of this investigation indicate that patients with medial tibiofemoral osteoarthrosis have deficits in postural stability and regulation. HTO and rehabilitation is not able to generate substantial improvements in these parameters during the observed period of six months. Sole overload of the injured side foot decreased significantly over the six months after HTO. In contrast, pain perception and quality of life (physical component) significantly improved after HTO and rehabilitation.

Author Contributions: Conceptualization, R.S., K.B., T.B. and M.J.; methodology, R.S., K.B. and M.P.; formal analysis, K.-S.D., R.S. and K.G.L.; investigation, K.B., M.J. and R.S.; resources, T.B.; data curation, R.S.; writing—original draft preparation, R.S., M.J., K.B. and K.G.L.; writing—review and editing, R.S., K.G.L. and K.-S.D.; visualization, R.S.; supervision, M.P.; project administration, T.B., K.B. and R.S.; All authors have read and agreed to the published version of the manuscript.

Funding: This research received no external funding.

Acknowledgments: We are grateful to all the patients, who participated after HTO surgery and made this study possible.

Conflicts of Interest: The authors declare no conflict of interest.

Appendix A

Table A1. Phases (Ph) of rehabilitation after HTO.

Ph	Week	Goals and Content
1	1	• <u>Aim:</u> pain relief, no effusion, pain free Range of Motion (ROM) • Immediately: postoperative treatment with cryotherapy • Constant support with an orthopedic splint (Listra) • First day: removal of the drainage • Manual lymphatic drainage (2–3 times per week) • Partial weight bearing with crutches (20 kg) • Fourth day: change of bandages
2	2	• <u>Aim:</u> pain free full ROM, partial weight bearing, safe muscular stabilization of knee joint • Suture removal and change of bandages • Manual lymphatic drainage (2–3 times per week) • Partial weight bearing with crutches (20 kg) • Isometric exercises with special regard to knee extension ROM

Table A1. *Cont.*

Ph	Week	Goals and Content
3	3–10	• <u>Aim:</u> pain free full ROM, pain-adapted full weight bearing, safe muscular stabilization of knee joint • Fourth week: physical therapy (strength and endurance) • X-ray • Intense rehabilitation in clinic or institution if desired by patient
4	11–15	• <u>Aim:</u> recovery of full general function • X-ray if necessary
5	16st week and later	• <u>Aim:</u> Restoration of full working or sports ability • Patient receives instructions/recommendations for further independent training (without therapist) related to their specific sport or occupation • Patient should return to work or competitive sport after 4–6 months

References

1. Felson, D.T.; Naimark, A.; Anderson, J.; Kazis, L.; Castelli, W.; Meenan, R.F. The prevalence of knee osteoarthritis in the elderly. The Framingham osteoarthritis study. *Arthritis Rheum.* **1987**, *30*, 914–918. [CrossRef] [PubMed]
2. Kurtz, S.M.; Lau, E.; Ong, K.; Zhao, K.; Kelly, M.; Bozic, K.J. Future young patient demand for primary and revision joint replacement: National projections from 2010 to 2030. *Clin. Orthop. Relat. Res.* **2009**, *467*, 2606–2612. [CrossRef] [PubMed]
3. Lobenhoffer, P.; Agneskirchner, J.D. Improvements in surgical technique of valgus high tibial osteotomy. *Knee Surg. Sport. Traumatol. Arthrosc.* **2003**, *11*, 132–138. [CrossRef]
4. Lobenhofffer, P.; Agneskirchner, J.; Zoch, W. Open valgus alignment osteotomy of the proximal tibia with fixation by medial plate fixator. *Orthopade* **2004**, *33*, 153–160. [CrossRef]
5. Bode, G.; Schmal, H.; Pestka, J.M.; Ogon, P.; Südkamp, N.P.; Niemeyer, P. A non-randomized controlled clinical trial on autologous chondrocyte implantation (ACI) in cartilage defects of the medial femoral condyle with or without high tibial osteotomy in patients with varus deformity of less than 5°. *Arch. Orthop. Trauma Surg.* **2013**, *133*, 43–49. [CrossRef]
6. Van der Woude, J.A.D.; Wiegant, K.; van Heerwaarden, R.J.; Spruijt, S.; van Roermund, P.M.; Custers, R.J.H.; Mastberger, S.C.; Lafeber, F.P.J.G. Knee joint distraction compared with high tibial osteotomy: A randomized controlled trial. *Knee Surg. Sport. Traumatol. Arthrosc.* **2017**, *25*, 876–886. [CrossRef]
7. Bonnin, M.P.; Laurent, J.R.; Zadegan, F.; Badet, R.; Pooler Archbold, H.A.; Servien, E. Can patients really participate in sport after high tibial osteotomy? *Knee Surg. Sport. Traumatol. Arthrosc.* **2013**, *21*, 64–73. [CrossRef]
8. Spahn, G.; Klinger, H.M.; Harth, P.; Hofmann, G.O. Cartilage regeneration after high tibial osteotomy. Results of an arthroscopic study. *Z. Orthop. Unf.* **2012**, *150*, 272–279. [CrossRef]
9. Jung, W.H.; Takeuchi, R.; Chun, C.W.; Lee, J.S.; Ha, J.H.; Kim, J.H.; Jeong, J.H. Second-look arthroscopic assessment of cartilage regeneration after medial opening-wedge high tibial osteotomy. *Arthroscopy* **2014**, *30*, 72–79. [CrossRef]
10. Koh, Y.G.; Kwon, O.R.; Kim, Y.S.; Choi, Y.J. Comparative outcomes of open-wedge high tibial osteotomy with platelet-rich plasma alone or in combination with mesenchymal stem cell treatment: A prospective study. *Arthroscopy* **2014**, *30*, 1453–1460. [CrossRef]
11. Jung, W.H.; Takeuchi, R.; Chun, C.W.; Lee, J.S.; Jeong, J.H. Comparison of results of medial opening-wedge high tibial osteotomy with and without subchondral drilling. *Arthroscopy* **2015**, *31*, 673–679. [CrossRef] [PubMed]
12. Wiegant, K.; van Heerwaarden, R.J.; van der Woude, J.A.D.; Custers, R.J.H.; Emans, P.J.; Kuchuk, N.O.; Mastbergen, S.C.; Lafeber, F.P.J.G. Knee joint distraction as an alternative surgical procedure for patients with osteoarthritis considered for high tibial osteotomy or for a total knee prosthesis: Rationale and design of two randomized controlled trials. *Int. J. Orthop.* **2015**, *2*, 353–360. [CrossRef]
13. Bastard, C.; Mirouse, G.; Potage, D.; Silbert, H.; Roubineau, F.; Hernigou, C.H.; Flouzat-Lachaniette, C.H. Return to sports and quality of life after high tibial osteotomy in patients under 60 years of age. *Orthop. Traumatol. Surg. Res.* **2017**, *103*, 1189–1191. [CrossRef] [PubMed]

14. Hunt, M.A.; Birmingham, T.B.; Jones, I.C.; Vandervoort, A.A.; Giffin, J.R. Effect of tibial re-alignment surgery on single leg standing balance in patients with knee osteoarthritis. *Clin. Biomech.* **2009**, *24*, 693–696. [CrossRef]
15. Zhang, Z.; Lion, A.; Chary-Valckenaere, I.; Loeuille, D.; Rat, A.C.; Paysant, J.; Perrin, P.P. Diurnal variation on balance control in patients with symptomatic knee osteoarthritis. *Arch Gerontol. Geriatr.* **2015**, *61*, 109–114. [CrossRef] [PubMed]
16. Bartels, T.; Brehme, K.; Pyschik, M.; Pollak, R.; Schaffrath, N.; Schulze, S.; Delank, K.S.; Laudner, K.G.; Schwesig, R. Postural stability and regulation before and after anterior cruciate ligament reconstruction—A two-years longitudinal study. *Phys. Ther. Sport* **2019**, *38*, 49–58. [CrossRef]
17. Bartels, T.; Brehme, K.; Pyschik, M.; Schulze, S.; Delank, K.S.; Fieseler, G.; Laudner, K.G.; Hermassi, S.; Schwesig, R. Pre- and postoperative postural regulation following anterior cruciate ligament reconstruction. *J. Exerc. Rehab.* **2018**, *14*, 143–151. [CrossRef]
18. Miniaci, A.; Ballmer, F.T.; Ballmer, P.M.; Jakob, R.P. Proximal tibial osteotomy. A new fixation device. *Clin. Orthop. Relat. Res.* **1989**, *246*, 250–259.
19. Schwesig, R.; Fischer, D.; Kluttig, A. Are there changes in postural regulation across the lifespan? *Somatosens. Mot. Res.* **2013**, *30*, 167–174. [CrossRef]
20. Friedrich, M.; Grein, H.J.; Wicher, C.; Schuetze, J.; Müller, A.; Lauenroth, A.; Hottenrott, K.; Schwesig, R. Influence of pathologic and simulated visual dysfunctions on the postural system. *Exp. Brain Res.* **2008**, *186*, 305–314. [CrossRef]
21. Schwesig, R.; Becker, S.; Lauenroth, A.; Kluttig, A.; Leuchte, S.; Esperer, H.D. A novel posturographic method to differentiate sway patterns of patients with Parkinson's disease from patients with cerebellar ataxia. *Biomed. Tech.* **2009**, *54*, 347–356. [CrossRef] [PubMed]
22. Schwesig, R.; Goldich, Y.; Hahn, A.; Müller, A.; Kohen-Raz, R.; Kluttig, A.; Morad, Y. Postural control in subjects with visual impairment. *Eur. J. Ophthalmol.* **2011**, *21*, 303–309. [CrossRef] [PubMed]
23. Reinhardt, L.; Heilmann, F.; Teicher, M.; Wollny, R.; Lauenroth, A.; Delank, K.S.; Schwesig, R.; Wollny, R.; Kurz, E. Comparison of posturographic outcomes between two different devices. *J. Biomech.* **2019**, *86*, 218–224. [CrossRef] [PubMed]
24. Schwesig, R.; Becker, S.; Fischer, D. Intraobserver reliability of posturography in healthy subjects. *Somatosens. Mot. Res.* **2014**, *31*, 16–22. [CrossRef] [PubMed]
25. Schwesig, R.; Fischer, D.; Becker, S.; Lauenroth, A. Intraobserver reliability of posturography in patients with vestibular neuritis. *Somatosens. Mot. Res.* **2014**, *31*, 28–34. [CrossRef] [PubMed]
26. Schwesig, R.; Hollstein, L.; Plontke, S.K.; Delank, K.S.; Fieseler, G.; Rahne, T. Comparison of intraobserver single-task reliabilities of the Interactive Balance System (IBS) and Vertiguard in asymptomatic subjects. *Somatosens. Mot. Res.* **2017**, *34*, 9–14. [CrossRef]
27. Seiwerth, I.; Jonen, J.; Rahne, T.; Schwesig, R.; Lauenroth, A.; Hullar, T.; Plontke, S.K. Influence of hearing on vestibulospinal control in healthy subjects. *HNO* **2018**, *66*, 590–597. [CrossRef]
28. Seiwerth, I.; Jonen, J.; Rahne, T.; Lauenroth, A.; Hullar, T.; Plontke, S.; Schwesig, R. Postural regulation and stability with acoustic input in normal hearing subjects. *HNO* **2020**, *68*, 100–105. [CrossRef]
29. Rat, A.C.; Coste, J.; Pouchot, J.; Baumann, M.; Spitz, E.; Retel-Rude, N.; Le Quintrec, J.S.; Dumont-Fischer, D.; Guillemin, F. OAKHQOL: A new instrument to measure quality of life in knee and hip osteoarthritis. *J. Clin. Epidemiol.* **2005**, *58*, 47–55. [CrossRef]
30. Ware, J.E., Jr.; Sherbourne, C.D. The MOS 36-item short-form health survey (SF-36). Conceptual framework and item selection. *Med. Care* **1992**, *30*, 473–483. [CrossRef]
31. Bullinger, M. German translation and psychometric testing of the SF-36 Health Survey: Preliminary results from the IQOLA Project. International Quality of Life Assessment. *Soc. Sci. Med.* **1995**, *41*, 1359–1366. [CrossRef]
32. Mc Horney, C.A.; Ware, J.E., Jr.; Lu, J.F.; Sherbourne, C.D. The MOS 36-item Short-Form Health Survey (SF-36): III. Tests of data quality, scaling assumptions, and reliability across diverse patient groups. *Med. Care* **1994**, *32*, 40–66. [CrossRef] [PubMed]
33. Bullinger, M.; Alonso, J.; Apolone, G.; Leplege, A.; Sullivan, M.; Wood-Dauphinee, S. Translating health status questionnaires and evaluating their quality: The IQOLA Project approach. International Quality of Life Assessment. *J. Clin. Epidemiol.* **1998**, *51*, 913–923. [CrossRef]

34. Ihle, C.; Ateschrang, A.; Grünwald, L.; Stöckle, U.; Saier, T.; Schröter, S. Health-related quality of life and clinical outcomes following medial open wedge high tibial osteotomy: A prospective study. *BMC Musculoskelet. Disord.* **2016**, *17*, 215. [CrossRef] [PubMed]
35. Richardson, J.T.E. Eta squared and partial eta squared as measures of effect size in educational research. *Educ. Res. Rev.* **2011**, *6*, 135–147. [CrossRef]
36. Hunt, M.A.; McManus, F.J.; Hinman, R.S.; Bennell, K.L. Predictors of single-leg standing balance in individuals with medial knee osteoarthritis. *Arthritis Care Res.* **2010**, *62*, 496–500. [CrossRef] [PubMed]
37. Salo, P. The role of joint innervation in the pathogenesis of arthritis. *Can. J. Surg.* **1999**, *42*, 91–100. [PubMed]
38. Nyland, J.; Smith, S.; Beickman, K.; Armsey, T.; Caborn, D. Frontal plane knee angle affects dynamic postural control strategy during unilateral stance. *Med. Sci. Sport. Exerc.* **2001**, *34*, 1150–1157. [CrossRef]
39. Kim, H.S.; Yun, D.H.; Yoo, S.D.; Kim, D.H.; Jeong, J.S.; Yun, J.S.; Hwang, D.G.; Jung, P.K.; Choi, S.H. Balance control and knee osteoarthritis severity. *Ann. Rehabil. Med.* **2011**, *35*, 701–709. [CrossRef]
40. Lehmann, T.; Paschen, L.; Baumeister, J. Single-leg assessment of postural stability after anterior cruciate ligament injury: A systematic review and metaanalysis. *Sport. Med. Open* **2017**, *3*, 32. [CrossRef]
41. Brandt, K.D.; Dieppe, P.; Radin, E.L. Etiopathogenesis of osteoarthritis. *Rheum. Dis. Clin. N. Am.* **2008**, *34*, 531–539. [CrossRef] [PubMed]
42. Barrett, D.S.; Cobb, A.G.; Bentley, G. Joint proprioception in normal, osteoarthritic and replaced knees. *J. Bone Jt. Surg. Br.* **1991**, *73*, 53–56. [CrossRef]
43. Floerkemeier, S.; Staubli, A.E.; Schröter, S.; Goldhahn, S.; Lobenhoffer, P. Outcome after high tibial open-wedge osteotomy: A retrospective evaluation of 533 patients. *Knee Surg. Sport. Traumatol. Arthrosc.* **2013**, *21*, 170–180. [CrossRef] [PubMed]
44. Insall, J.N.; Joseph, D.M.; Msika, C. High tibial osteotomy for varus gonarthrosis. A long-term follow-up study. *J. Bone Jt. Surg. Am.* **1984**, *66*, 1040–1048. [CrossRef]
45. Niinimäki, T.T.; Eskelinen, A.; Mann, B.S.; Junnila, M.; Ohtonen, P.; Leppilahti, J. Survivorship of high tibial osteotomy in the treatment of osteoarthritis of the knee. *J. Bone Jt. Surg. Br.* **2012**, *94*, 1517–1521. [CrossRef]
46. Naudie, D.; Bourne, R.B.; Rorabeck, C.H.; Bourne, T.J. The Install award: Survivorship of the high tibial valgus osteotomy. *Clin. Orthop. Relat. Res.* **1999**, *367*, 18–27. [CrossRef]
47. Saier, T.; Minzlaff, P.; Feucht, M.J.; Lämmle, L.; Burghoff, M.; Ihle, C.; Imhoff, A.B.; Hinterwimmer, S. Health-related quality of life after open-wedge high tibial osteotomy. *Knee Surg. Sport. Traumatol. Arthrosc.* **2017**, *25*, 934–942. [CrossRef]
48. Webster, K.E.; Feller, J.A. Comparison of the short form-12 (SF-12) health status questionnaire with the SF-36 in patients with knee osteoarthritis who have replacement surgery. *Knee Surg. Sport. Traumatol. Arthrosc.* **2016**, *24*, 2620–2626. [CrossRef]
49. Bartels, T.; Proeger, S.; Brehme, K.; Pyschik, M.; Delank, K.S.; Schulze, S.; Schwesig, R.; Fieseler, G. The SpeedCourt system in rehabilitation after reconstruction surgery of the anterior cruciate ligament (ACL). *Arch. Orthop. Trauma Surg.* **2016**, *136*, 957–966. [CrossRef]

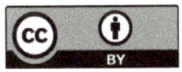

© 2020 by the authors. Licensee MDPI, Basel, Switzerland. This article is an open access article distributed under the terms and conditions of the Creative Commons Attribution (CC BY) license (http://creativecommons.org/licenses/by/4.0/).

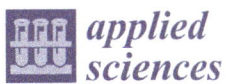

Article

Biomechanical Analysis of Allograft Spacer Failure as a Function of Cortical-Cancellous Ratio in Anterior Cervical Discectomy/Fusion: Allograft Spacer Alone Model

Ji-Won Kwon [1,2], Hwan-Mo Lee [1], Tae-Hyun Park [3], Sung Jae Lee [3], Young-Woo Kwon [3], Seong-Hwan Moon [1] and Byung Ho Lee [1,*]

1. Department of Orthopedic Surgery, Yonsei University College of Medicine, Seoul 03722, Korea; kwonjjanng@nhimc.or.kr (J.-W.K.); HWANLEE@yuhs.ac (H.-M.L.); SHMOON@yuhs.ac (S.-H.M.)
2. Department of Orthopedic Surgery, National Health Insurance Service Ilsan Hospital, Goyang 410719, Korea
3. Department of Biomedical Engineering, College of Biomedical Science & Engineering, Inje University, Gyeongnam 621749, Korea; thyun06@gmail.com (T.-H.P.); sjl@bme.inje.ac.kr (S.J.L.); voicians0908@gmail.com (Y.-W.K.)
* Correspondence: bhlee96@yuhs.ac; Tel.: +82-2-2228-2180

Received: 9 August 2020; Accepted: 7 September 2020; Published: 15 September 2020

Abstract: The design and ratio of the cortico-cancellous composition of allograft spacers are associated with graft-related problems, including subsidence and allograft spacer failure. Methods: The study analyzed stress distribution and risk of subsidence according to three types (cortical only, cortical cancellous, cortical lateral walls with a cancellous center bone) and three lengths (11, 12, 14 mm) of allograft spacers under the condition of hybrid motion control, including flexion, extension, axial rotation, and lateral bending,. A detailed finite element model of a previously validated, three-dimensional, intact C3–7 segment, with C5–6 segmental fusion using allograft spacers without fixation, was used in the present study. Findings: Among the three types of cervical allograft spacers evaluated, cortical lateral walls with a cancellous center bone exhibited the highest stress on the cortical bone of spacers, as well as the endplate around the posterior margin of the spacers. The likelihood of allograft spacer failure was highest for 14 mm spacers composed of cortical lateral walls with a cancellous center bone upon flexion (PVMS, 270.0 MPa; 250.2%) and extension (PVMS: 371.40 MPa, 344.2%). The likelihood of allograft spacer subsidence was also highest for the same spacers upon flexion (PVMS, 4.58 MPa; 28.1%) and extension (PVMS, 12.71 MPa; 78.0%). Conclusion: Cervical spacers with a smaller cortical component and of longer length can be risk factors for allograft spacer failure and subsidence, especially in flexion and extension. However, further study of additional fixation methods, such as anterior plates/screws and posterior screws, in an actual clinical setting is necessary.

Keywords: cervical spine surgery; allograft spacer; subsidence; finite element model

1. Introduction

The incidence of degenerative cervical spine diseases (DCSD) was varied from 1684 to 1767 per 100,000 population stratified according to disease codes in the Republic of Korea from 2012 to 2016 [1]. In the USA, the incidence of surgery for DCSD rose by almost 150% over the last three decades and stabilized at slightly over 70 operations/100,000 people [2]. The mean age at surgery was 53.3 years, and women underwent 44.4% of all cervical spine surgeries [2]. Anterior cervical discectomy and fusion (ACDF) is a standard treatment for DCSD [3,4]. Instead of using tricortical autologous bone grafts and titanium polyetheretherketone cages [3,5–8], cervical allograft spacers have been commonly utilized because of their absence of donor site morbidity and physical properties that are similar to those of the natural vertebral body [3,9–11]. A few studies have examined the biomechanical stability of allografts compared with autografts using cadaveric cervical spines; [10]. however, no study has examined allograft spacers and the risk of subsidence on endplates.

From a biomechanical point of view, the design and ratio of cortico-cancellous composition of allograft spacers have been shown to be associated with graft-related problems, including subsidence and allograft spacer failure, leading to breakage and dislodging in clinical settings [12,13]. The present study used finite element model (FEM) analysis to investigate the associations of different cortico-cancellous ratios of cervical allograft spacers with physical stress on the spacers and with subsidence risk on the endplate and vertebral body in involved spinal segments. All experiments were conducted under the condition of hybrid motion control, including flexion, extension, axial rotation, and lateral bending.

2. Materials and Methods

2.1. FEM of an Intact Cervical Spine

A previously validated, three-dimensional, intact model of a C3–7 segment from a 54-year-old male was used for the present study [14,15]. The geometrical data of the multi-segmental cervical model were reconstructed from computed tomography (CT) images. Axial CT scans were obtained with a slice thickness of 0.5 mm and a pixel width of 0.429 mm.

The material properties were selected from the published literature (Table 1). The detailed FEM included vertebral bodies, bony posterior elements, intervertebral discs, and six major groups of ligaments: anterior longitudinal, posterior longitudinal, ligament flavum, facet capsular, interspinous, and supraspinous. The origins and insertions of these ligaments were obtained from a morphological study. The spinal ligaments adopted the nonlinear load-displacement property for the physiological nonlinear behavior of the ligaments [14,16]. The vertebral body consisted of an outer shell of high strength cortical bone reinforced internally by cancellous bone and had an average thickness of 0.5 mm in both cancellous bone and endplates [17]. 3D hexahedral element (eight-node brick) were used as vertebral body-disc structures and posterior element of which material properties were assumed to be homogeneous and isotropic [18–21]. However, the structures of interface between implant and vertebral body were remeshed to 3D tetrahedron (four-node brick) for element refining at interest site. The region of interest between implants and the bone-implant interface was set up using different element sizes that could be distinguished from other parts (implant and periphery, element size = 0.5 mm; the others, 2 mm). Region of interest between implants and the bone-implant interface were set up using different element sizes that could be distinguished from other parts (implant and periphery, element size = 0.5 mm; the others, 2 mm) The mesh convergence in the present study was decided among varying element sizes ranging from 0.5 to 2.0 mm. With an element size of 0.5 mm, the peri-implant converged properly. Finally, a 0.5 mm element size was applied in our surgical model for the translation of experimental results. No unusual stress patterns were observed in this study for this setting.

The intervertebral disc was modeled as a fiber-reinforced structure surrounding the incompressible inviscid nucleus pulposus. The reinforcement structure annulus fibers were modeled by truss elements with modified tension-only properties, with an orientation of about 25° [19,22]. The facet joint was oriented at 45° from the horizontal plane, where the initial surface gaps between each facet region was assumed to be 0.5 mm based upon CT imaging. The facet joint was oriented at 45° from the horizontal plane, where initial surface gaps between each facet region are assumed to be 0.5 mm based upon CT imaging. The interaction of facet joints worked toward increasing the contact force with the narrowing initial gap distance between the upper and lower facet surfaces [22]. The segmental angular measures used to create the lordotic curve for the model were as follows: C3–4, 4.35°; C4–5, 1.87°; and C5–6, 3.94° [23]. For this study, the general-purpose FEA package ABAQUS (Abaqus 2017, Dassault Systèmes

Simulia Corp., Providence, RI, USA.)- the non-linear geometry parameter (NLGEON=ON) in ABAQUS step module was used.

Table 1. Peak stress levels of motion in the motion model.

Component Name	Young's Modulus (MPa)	Poisson's Ratio	Ref.
Cortical bone	12,000	0.3	[22]
Cancellous bone	100	0.29	[18]
Posterior element	3.500	0.29	[16]
End plate	500	0.4	[19]
Annulus matrix	4.2	0.45	[19]
Annulus Fibers	500	Cross-sectional Area 0.1 (mm^2)	[20]
Nucleus pulposus	1.0	0.499 (Incompressible)	[19]

2.2. Allograft Spacer Model

The geometries of a cortical cervical spacer (cortical only: CO; DCI Donor Services Tissue Bank, Nashville, TN, USA), a cortical cancellous cervical spacer (cortical cancellous: CC; DCI Donor Services), and a Cornerstone^{TM} ASR (cortical lateral walls with a cancellous center bone: CLC; Medtronic Sofamor Danek, Memphis, TN, USA) were constructed based on measuring the allograft spacer using SolidWorks CAD drawings (Solidworks 2013, Dassault systemes Solidworks Corporation, Waltham, MA, USA) (Figure 1, Table 2) and imported into Abaqus (Abaqus 2017, Dassault Systèmes Simulia Corp., Providence, RI, USA) for meshing. The size of three different allograft spacers was meshed 0.5 mm. And then, the interface behavior, such as CC and CLC, between cortical bone and cancellous bone of the allograft spacer was accomplished through a "tie" contact condition.

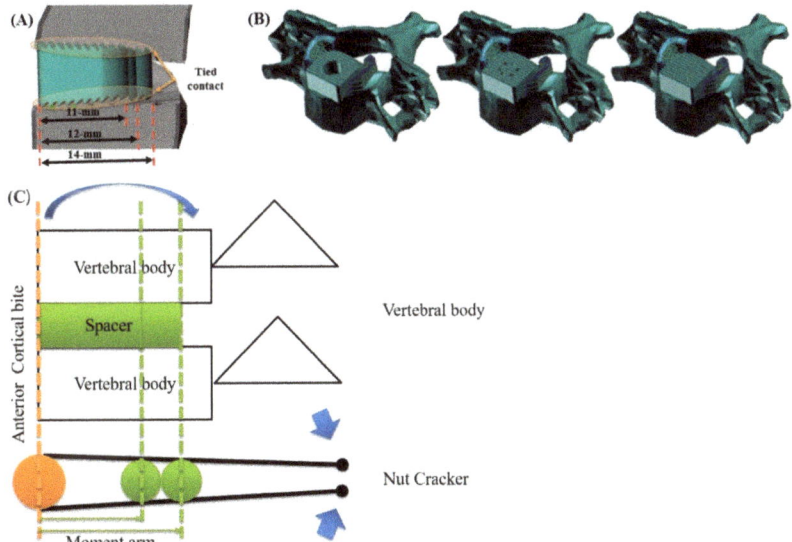

Figure 1. Design of allograft spacers. Length and position of allograft spacers. (A) Anterior cortical bite positioning of allograft spacers (B) Types of allograft spacers: CO, cortical only; CC, cortico-cancellous; CLC, cortical lateral walls with a cancellous center bone, in that order. (C) Schema of the nutcracker mechanism upon flexion and extension in anterior cortical bite positioning of allograft spacers.

Table 2. Cortical-cancellous bone ratio of allospacers.

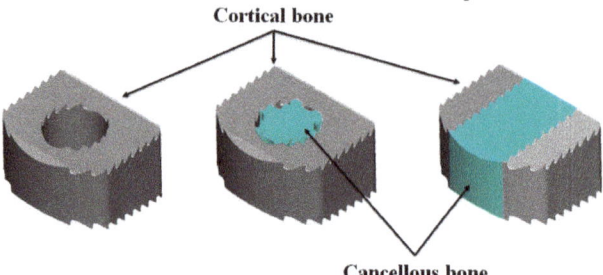

	Cortical only		Cortico-Cancellous		Cortical lateral Walls with a Cancellous Center Bone	
	Cortical	Cancellous	Cortical	Cancellous	Cortical	Cancellous
11 mm	1	0	1	0.32	0.46	0.54
12 mm	1	0	1	0.28	0.47	0.53
14 mm	1	0	1	0.23	0.47	0.53

Then, each meshed spacer model was inserted into the C5–6 disc without plate fixation in the previously constructed, intact cervical FEM. The spacers used for modeling were 11, 12, or 14 mm in length, had 6° of lordotic angle, and were 7 mm in height, which best fit the vertebral anatomy at the C5–6 level of the cervical model used in this study. The material properties of the allograft spacers (cortical bone, elastic modulus (E) = 18,200 MPa, Poisson's ratio (v) = 0.38; cancellous bone, E = 389 MPa, (v) = 0.3) were measured on a donor femur according to previous research [24,25]. The devices were designed to be implanted via an anterior surgical approach, as recommended by the manufacturer. By simulating this surgical procedure [26], the anterior longitudinal ligament, the superior and inferior endplates, and the anterior and posterior parts of the annulus fibrosus were excised. Then, the spacers were positioned at the anterior margin of the vertebral body (Figures 1 and 2). Because our model aimed to simulate biomechanical behavior after bony fusion, specific corresponding constraint conditions were set up, especially at the bone-implant interface. In this study, interface behavior was accomplished through a "tie" contact condition, which enabled the allograft spacer and vertebrae to be bonded together permanently with full constraint.

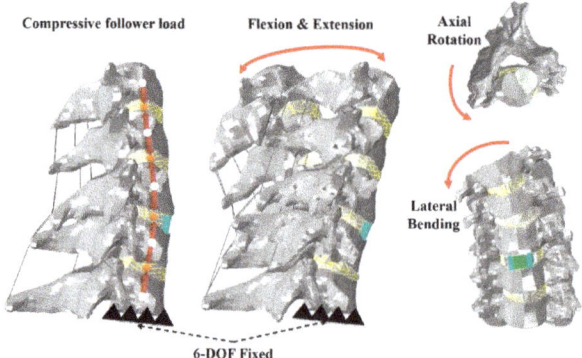

Figure 2. Finite element model of allograft spacers with hybrid motion control.

2.3. Loading and Boundary Conditions

The inferior endplate of the most caudal vertebra (C7) was fixed in all degrees of freedom, while loads were applied to the superior endplate of the most cephalic vertebral vertebra (C3).

The follower load allows each individual vertebra to be loaded in nearly pure compression. In the present FEM, the intervertebral body was connected at approximately the center of rotation of vertebral bodies C3 through C7 [27]. In loading control, pure moments of 1.0 Nm were generated by a force coupled to flexion, extension, lateral bending, or axial rotation of the cervical spine.

A compressive follower load of 73.6 N was considered to approximate the head weight and local muscle stabilization during daily activity (Figure 2) [14]. A hybrid protocol was used to predict range of motion (ROM) at the surgical site and adjacent levels [28].

3. Results

3.1. Range of Motion

The validated ROM of our intact FEM model was within the acceptable range, compared with cadaver studies [29,30] Upon flexion, the ROM at C4–5 was increased in all spacer models, compared with that in the intact model. The ROM of C5–6 (fused segment) was significantly decreased in all spacer models (Figure 3). Upon extension, when compared with the intact model, the ROM at the C4–5 and C6–7 segments was increased in all spacer models. The ROM of C5–6 was significantly decreased in all spacer models. In axial rotation and lateral bending, when compared with the intact model, the ROM at the C4–5 and C6–7 segments was increased in all spacer models. The ROM of C5–6 was significantly decreased in all spacer models.

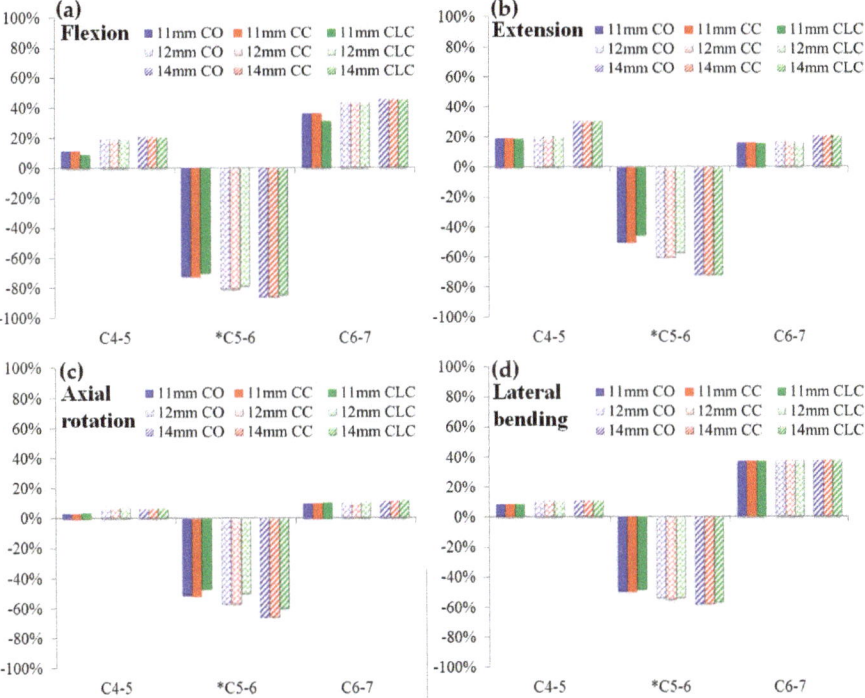

Figure 3. Effects of different cervical allograft spacers on the range of motion, compared with that in an intact model: (a) flexion (b) extension (c) axial rotation (d) lateral bending. * indicates fused cervical segment with allograft spacers. CO, cortical only; CC, cortico-cancellous; CLC, cortical lateral walls with a cancellous center bone.

3.2. Stress Analysis of Cervical Spacers with Different Cortico-Cancellous Ratios

In flexion and extension, von Mises stress increased as the length of spacers increased for all types of allograft spacers. The CLC spacer demonstrated the highest stress among the three types of spacers. In counterclockwise axial rotation, von Mises stress decreased as the lengths of spacers increased. In right lateral bending, von Mises stress decreased as the lengths of the CO and CC spacers increased. However, among CLC spacers, PVMS increased as the length of the spacer increased. Stress on the anterior cortical portion increased as the length of spacers increased. The CLC spacers demonstrated the highest stress on the anterior cortical portion among the three types of spacers in the study. (Figure 4). The likelihood of allograft spacer failure was calculated on the basis of the yield strength of the femoral cortical bone (107.9 MPa). The allograft failure risk was calculated using the following formula [31]:

$$\text{Failure risk} = \frac{\text{Stress on the cortial portion of allograft spacer}}{\text{Yield strength of Femoral cortical bone } (107.9 MPa)} \times 100. \qquad (1)$$

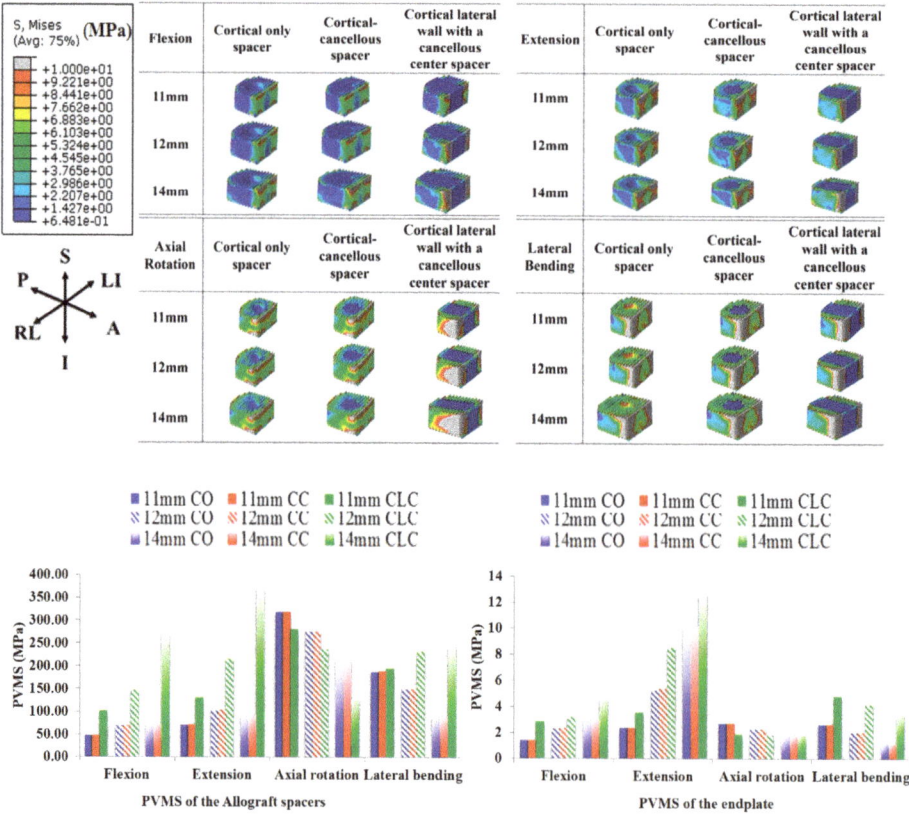

Figure 4. Peak von Mises stress (PVMS) on the allograft spacers and endplates under hybrid motion.

In flexion motion, the risk of allograft spacer failure was lowest for the 11 mm CO spacer (PVMS, 48.04 MPa; 44. 5%) and highest for the 14 mm CLC spacer (PVMS, 270.0 MPa; 250.2%). In extension, the risk of allograft spacer failure was highest for the 14 mm CLC spacer (PVMS: 371.40 MPa, 344.2%) and lowest for the 11 mm CO spacer (PVMS: 71.05 MPa; 65.8%). In axial rotation, the risk of allograft spacer failure was highest for the 11 mm CC spacer (PVMS: 317.20 MPa, 294.0%) and lowest for the 14 mm CLC spacer (PVMS: 128.30 MPa, 118.9%). In lateral bending, the risk of allograft spacer failure was highest for 14 mm CLC spacers (PVMS: 244.20 MPa, 226.3%) and lowest for 14 mm CO spacers (PVMS: 150.20 MPa, 139.2%) (Figure 4).

3.3. Stress Analysis of Endplates of Involved Lower Cervical Segments

In flexion, von Mises stress increased as the lengths of spacers increased, especially at the endplates around the posterior wall of the allograft spacers, and was most prominent in the CLC spacers. In extension, von Mises stress increased as the lengths of spacers increased, especially around the posterior margin of each spacer. In both counterclockwise axial rotation and right lateral bending, von Mises stress decreased as the lengths of the spacers increased. In lateral bending, von Mises stress was higher with CLC spacers than with other spacers. The likelihood of allograft spacer subsidence was calculated on the basis of the yield strength of the cancellous bone of the C6 vertebral body (16.3 MPa). The subsidence risk was calculated using the following formula [31]:

$$\text{Subsidence risk} = \frac{\text{Stress on the cortial portion of allograft spacer}}{\text{Yield strength of vertebral body}(16.3 \text{ MPa})} \times 100. \quad (2)$$

In flexion motion, the risk of allograft spacer subsidence was lowest for 11 mm CO and CC spacers (PVMS, 1.41 MPa; 8.7%) and highest for the 14 mm CLC spacer (PVMS, 4.58 MPa; 28.1%). The subsidence risk was highest for the 14 mm CLC spacer (PVMS: 12.71 MPa, 78.0%) in extension, 11 mm CO and CC spacers (PVMS: 2.71 MPa, 16.6%) in axial rotation, and the 11 mm CLC spacers (PVMS 4.81 MPa, 29.5%) in lateral bending. Subsidence risk was lowest for the 11 mm CO and CC spacers (PVMS: 2.39 MPa, 14.7%) in extension, the 14 mm CO spacer (PVMS: 1.76 MPa, 10.8%) in axial rotation, and the 14 mm CO and CC spacers (PVMS: 1.13 MPa, 6.9%) in lateral bending.

4. Discussion

Graft failure with subsidence and breakage leading to non-union are major concerns in ACDF surgery and have been shown to be associated with the use an autologous bone substitute, stand-alone cages, allospacers, reinforcement with anterior plates and screws, and posterior fixation, as well as age and other factors [13,15,32–35]. However, no study has analyzed associations of biomechanical stress with cervical spacer design, length, and the ratio of cortical and cancellous portions of the spacers. It is expected that the cortical and cancellous portions play a different role once they are fused after insertion [10]. The cortical portion usually supports the endplates until the cancellous portion can form a firm union of bone. It could be postulated that a larger cortical component could result in breakage of allograft spacers or more subsidence into the vertebral body through the endplates if they fail to be fused properly postoperatively because of the different properties of E and v of the allograft-cortical bone and the cancellous portions of the recipient vertebral body [36]. Cortical breakage or subsidence could then result in a decrease of disc height and lead to foraminal restenosis [37]. It is commonly accepted that greater stress on the endplate and spacers and less contact with the surface of the cancellous portion could lead to an increased risk of subsidence and delayed fusion [10]. In one clinical study, CO-type allospacers, which have a smaller cancellous fusion bed, exhibited more breakage and displacement with disc height loss causing fixation instability, compared with other spacers [13]. In our study, the smaller cortical portion conversely led to an increased subsidence risk and a relatively higher risk of allograft spacer failure despite the wider fusion bed of cancellous bone, especially upon flexion and extension.

We analyzed the results of predicted FE study using von Mises stress. The reasons are as follows: Generally, stress has direction, but von Mises stress is scalar and not a vector. Therefore, it is easy to analyze stresses in various directions, such as principal stress, at complex loading on the human body. Additionally, the von Mises is a theoretical measure of stress used to estimate yield failure criteria and is also popular in fatigue strength calculations. While significant differences in von Mises stress on different types of spacers and endplates were noted (Figure 4), the results did not fall in line with our initial hypothesis that longer spacers could supply a wider surface area of stress distribution and result in less von Mises stress on allograft spacers and endplates. The longer spacers showed a higher level of concentrated stresses on the posterior wall of the allograft spacers and in the contacted endplate area in flexion and extension. This could be explained by the nutcracker mechanism with anterior cortical-bite positioning of allograft spacers (Figure 1), wherein the longer spacer exerts greater compression force at the posterior margin of the allograft spacer and contacting endplate, as well as greater posterior shear force from the superior anterior corner to the inferior posterior corner of the allograft spacer. This could lead to allograft spacer failure or graft subsidence, even though it is known that posterior endplates are stronger than the anterior component [38]

The ROM in all motion modes was easily understandable because of the decreased ROM in the fused segment of C5–6 and increased ROM in the adjacent C4-5 and C6–7 segments. The longer spacers produced greater stress on the endplate and posterior complex of the vertebral body in flexion and extension. Along with higher preloading on the distal cervical segment, this increased stress could play a role in increased subsidence and result in a decreased ROM relative to the intact segment of C6–7. This needs to be clarified in further research.

This study had a few limitations. This study was designed only for allograft spacers and vertebral bodies without additional fixation methods, such as anterior plates and screws, lateral mass screws, or pedicle screws [15,31]. However, using our basic stress analyses on allograft spacers and endplate-vertebral bodies for spacer composition and length, a series of biomechanical studies will be performed with variable fixation methods, spacer sizes, and cervical sagittal alignments. Also, the ROM of the intact model was compared with that previously reported by Ivancic and Panjabi et al [29,30]. This approach confirmed that the kinematics of the developed FEM reflect real soft tissue functions. However, in our study, we calculated the distribution of stress on endplates, which is a different context for the use of this FEM. Therefore, this study could lack sufficient evidence in support of the validation of this FEM. Nevertheless, in many biomechanical studies, ROM was utilized to validate and verify models, as well as to predict stress and forces reflective of real-world settings [39–46]. Considering the relative comparisons between the design and lengths of the allograft spacers, the results in the present study could be helpful to understanding the biomechanical differences between allospacers.

This study could help to decide the best combination of surgical approach and type of allograft spacer depending on a patient's conditions. As a potential ethnic anthropometric limitation, the FEM model was designed for the average Korean, middle-aged male, and Caucasian individuals tend to have larger profiles than Koreans [47,48]. Additional analysis on post-menopausal women with weaker bone quality is ongoing and will provide a better understanding of biomechanical properties in that clinical settings.

5. Conclusions

Smaller cortical portions and longer cervical spacers could be risk factors for allograft spacer failure and subsidence, especially in flexion and extension, in an allograft spacer only model. However, further study in combination with additional fixation methods, such as anterior plates/screws and posterior screws, in an actual clinical setting is necessary.

Author Contributions: Conceptualization, B.H.L., J.-W.K., T.-H.P., S.J.L., Y.-W.K., S.-H.M., H.-M.L.; Methodology, B.H.L., J.-W.K., T.-H.P., S.J.L., Y.-W.K., S.-H.M., H.-M.L.; Software, B.H.L., J.-W.K., T.-H.P., S.J.L., Y.-W.K., S.-H.M., H.-M.L.; Validation, B.H.L., J.-W.K., T.-H.P., S.J.L., Y.-W.K., S.-H.M., H.-M.L.; Formal Analysis, B.H.L., T.-H.P., S.J.L.; Investigation, B.H.L., T.-H.P., S.J.L.; Resources, B.H.L., T.-H.P., S.J.L.; Data Curation, B.H.L., T.-H.P., S.J.L.; Writing—Original Draft Preparation, B.H.L.; Writing—Review & Editing, B.H.L.; Visualization, B.H.L., T.-H.P., S.J.L.; Supervision, B.H.L., J.-W.K., T.-H.P., S.J.L., Y.-W.K., S.-H.M., H.-M.L.; Project Administration, B.H.L., T.-H.P., S.J.L.; Funding Acquisition, none. All authors have read and agreed to the published version of the manuscript.

Funding: This research was funded by NRF-2017R1C1B5017402.

Conflicts of Interest: The authors declare no conflict of interest.

References

1. Lee, C.-H.; Chung, C.-K.; Kim, C.H.; Kwon, J.-W. Health Care Burden of Spinal Diseases in the Republic of Korea: Analysis of a Nationwide Database From 2012 Through 2016. *Neurospine* **2018**, *15*, 66–76. [CrossRef] [PubMed]
2. Kotkansalo, A.; Leinonen, V.; Korajoki, M.; Salmenkivi, J.; Korhonen, K.; Malmivaara, A. Surgery for degenerative cervical spine disease in Finland, 1999–2015. *Acta Neurochir.* **2019**, *161*, 2147–2159. [CrossRef] [PubMed]
3. Yang, J.J.; Yu, C.H.; Chang, B.-S.; Yeom, J.S.; Lee, J.H.; Lee, C.-K. Subsidence and Nonunion after Anterior Cervical Interbody Fusion Using a Stand-Alone Polyetheretherketone (PEEK) Cage. *Clin. Orthop. Surg.* **2011**, *3*, 16–23. [CrossRef] [PubMed]
4. Pandita, N.; Gupta, S.; Raina, P.; Srivastava, A.; Hakak, A.Y.; Singh, O.; Darokhan, M.A.-U.-D.; Butt, M.F. Neurological Recovery Pattern in Cervical Spondylotic Myelopathy after Anterior Surgery: A Prospective Study with Literature Review. *Asian Spine J.* **2019**, *13*, 423–431. [CrossRef]
5. Viswanathan, V.K.; Manoharan, S.R. To Plate or Not to Plate after a Single- or Two-Level Anterior Cervical Discectomy: Fusion with Cage-Plate Construct or Stand-Alone Cage. *Asian Spine J.* **2017**, *11*, 1–3. [CrossRef]
6. Schmieder, K.; Wolzik-Grossmann, M.; Pechlivanis, I.; Engelhardt, M.; Scholz, M.; Harders, A. Subsidence of the Wing titanium cage after anterior cervical interbody fusion: 2-year follow-up study. *J. Neurosurg. Spine* **2006**, *4*, 447–453. [CrossRef]
7. Čabraja, M.; Oezdemir, S.; Koeppen, D.; Kroppenstedt, S. Anterior cervical discectomy and fusion: Comparison of titanium and polyetheretherketone cages. *BMC Musculoskelet. Disord.* **2012**, *13*, 172. [CrossRef]
8. Chen, Y.; Wang, X.; Lu, X.; Yang, L.; Yang, H.; Yuan, W.; Chen, D. Comparison of titanium and polyetheretherketone (PEEK) cages in the surgical treatment of multilevel cervical spondylotic myelopathy: A prospective, randomized, control study with over 7-year follow-up. *Eur. Spine J.* **2013**, *22*, 1539–1546. [CrossRef]
9. Chau, A.M.T.; Mobbs, R.J. Bone graft substitutes in anterior cervical discectomy and fusion. *Eur. Spine J.* **2009**, *18*, 449–464. [CrossRef]
10. Ryu, S.I.; Lim, J.T.; Kim, S.M.; Paterno, J.; Willenberg, R.; Kim, D.H. Comparison of the biomechanical stability of dense cancellous allograft with tricortical iliac autograft and fibular allograft for cervical interbody fusion. *Eur. Spine J.* **2006**, *15*, 1339–1345. [CrossRef]
11. Lee, J.C.; Jang, H.-D.; Ahn, J.; Choi, S.-W.; Kang, D.; Shin, B.-J. Comparison of Cortical Ring Allograft and Plate Fixation with Autologous Iliac Bone Graft for Anterior Cervical Discectomy and Fusion. *Asian Spine J.* **2019**, *13*, 258–264. [CrossRef] [PubMed]
12. Ordway, N.R.; Rim, B.C.; Tan, R.; Hickman, R.; Fayyazi, A.H. Anterior cervical interbody constructs: Effect of a repetitive compressive force on the endplate. *J. Orthop. Res.* **2011**, *30*, 587–592. [CrossRef] [PubMed]
13. Park, K.J.; Kim, D.H.; Park, K.D.; Park, J.H.; Yoo, N.K.; Cho, K.H.; Kim, S.H. Clinical Outcomes and Finite Element Method Results of Anterior Cervical Discectomy and Fusion Using H-Beam Shaped Allospacer: A Comparison with Rim-Shaped Allospacer. *Nerve* **2019**, *5*, 49–54. [CrossRef]
14. Jung, T.-G.; Woo, S.-H.; Park, K.-M.; Jang, J.-W.; Han, D.-W.; Lee, S.J. Biomechanical behavior of two different cervical total disc replacement designs in relation of concavity of articular surfaces: ProDisc-C® vs. Prestige-LP®. *Int. J. Precis. Eng. Manuf.* **2013**, *14*, 819–824. [CrossRef]
15. Kwon, J.-W.; Bang, S.H.; Park, T.H.; Lee, S.-J.; Lee, H.-M.; Lee, S.-B.; Lee, B.H.; Moon, S.-H. Biomechanical comparison of cervical discectomy/fusion model using allograft spacers between anterior and posterior fixation methods (lateral mass and pedicle screw). *Clin. Biomech.* **2020**, *73*, 226–233. [CrossRef]
16. Galbusera, F.; Bellini, C.M.; Raimondi, M.T.; Fornari, M.; Assietti, R. Cervical spine biomechanics following implantation of a disc prosthesis. *Med. Eng. Phys.* **2008**, *30*, 1127–1133. [CrossRef]
17. Ritzel, H.; Amling, M.; Pösl, M.; Hahn, M.; Delling, G. The Thickness of Human Vertebral Cortical Bone and its Changes in Aging and Osteoporosis: A Histomorphometric Analysis of the Complete Spinal Column from Thirty-Seven Autopsy Specimens. *J. Bone Miner. Res.* **1997**, *12*, 89–95. [CrossRef]
18. Zhang, Q.H.; Teo, E.C.; Ng, H.W.; Lee, V.S.; Lee, P.V.S. Finite element analysis of moment-rotation relationships for human cervical spine. *J. Biomech.* **2006**, *39*, 189–193. [CrossRef]

19. Ha, S.K. Finite element modeling of multi-level cervical spinal segments (C3–C6) and biomechanical analysis of an elastomer-type prosthetic disc. *Med. Eng. Phys.* **2006**, *28*, 534–541. [CrossRef]
20. Kim, J.-D.; Kim, N.-S.; Hong, C.-S.; Oh, C.-Y. Design optimization of a xenogeneic bone plate and screws using the Taguchi and finite element methods. *Int. J. Precis. Eng. Manuf.* **2011**, *12*, 1119–1124. [CrossRef]
21. Whyne, C.M.; Hu, S.S.; Klisch, S.; Lotz, J.C. Effect of the Pedicle and Posterior Arch on Vertebral Body Strength Predictions in Finite Element Modeling. *Spine* **1998**, *23*, 899–907. [CrossRef] [PubMed]
22. Faizan, A.; Goel, V.K.; Garfin, S.R.; Bono, C.M.; Serhan, H.; Biyani, A.; Elgafy, H.; Krishna, M.; Friesem, T. Do design variations in the artificial disc influence cervical spine biomechanics? A finite element investigation. *Eur. Spine J.* **2009**, *21*, 653–662.
23. Harrison, D.E.; Harrison, D.D.; Cailliet, R.; Troyanovich, S.J.; Janik, T.J.; Holland, B. Cobb Method or Harrison Posterior Tangent Method: Which to choose for lateral cervical radiographic analysis. *Spine* **2000**, *25*, 2072–2078. [CrossRef] [PubMed]
24. Shi, D.; Wang, F.; Wang, N.; Li, X.; Wang, Q. 3-D finite element analysis of the influence of synovial condition in sacroiliac joint on the load transmission in human pelvic system. *Med. Eng. Phys.* **2014**, *36*, 745–753. [CrossRef]
25. Black, J.; Hastings, G. *Handbook of Biomaterial Properties*; Springer: Berlin/Heidelberg, Germany, 1998.
26. Smith, G.W.; Robinson, R.A. The Treatment of Certain Cervical-Spine Disorders by Anterior Removal of the Intervertebral Disc and Interbody Fusion. *J. Bone Jt. Surg.* **1958**, *40*, 607–624. [CrossRef]
27. Sis, H.L.; Mannen, E.M.; Wong, B.M.; Cadel, E.S.; Bouxsein, M.L.; Anderson, D.E.; Friis, E.A. Effect of follower load on motion and stiffness of the human thoracic spine with intact rib cage. *J. Biomech.* **2016**, *49*, 3252–3259. [CrossRef]
28. Panjabi, M.M. Hybrid multidirectional test method to evaluate spinal adjacent-level effects. *Clin. Biomech.* **2007**, *22*, 257–265. [CrossRef]
29. Panjabi, M.M.; Crisco, J.J.; Vasavada, A.; Oda, T.; Cholewicki, J.; Nibu, K.; Shin, E. Mechanical Properties of the Human Cervical Spine as Shown by Three-Dimensional Load–Displacement Curves. *Spine* **2001**, *26*, 2692–2700. [CrossRef]
30. Ivancic, P.C. Biomechanics of Sports-Induced Axial-Compression Injuries of the Neck. *J. Athl. Train.* **2012**, *47*, 489–497. [CrossRef]
31. Kwon, J.-W.; Bang, S.-H.; Kwon, Y.-W.; Cho, J.-Y.; Park, T.-H.; Lee, S.-J.; Lee, H.-M.; Moon, S.-H.; Lee, B.-H. Biomechanical comparison of the angle of inserted screws and the length of anterior cervical plate systems with allograft spacers. *Clin. Biomech.* **2020**, *76*, 105021. [CrossRef]
32. Kao, T.H.; Wu, C.H.; Chou, Y.C.; Chen, H.T.; Chen, W.H.; Tsou, H.K. Risk factors for subsidence in anterior cervical fusion with stand-alone polyetheretherketone (PEEK) cages: A review of 82 cases and 182 levels. *Arch. Orthop. Trauma Surg.* **2014**, *134*, 1343–1351. [CrossRef] [PubMed]
33. Goel, V.K.; Faizan, A.; Palepu, V.; Bhattacharya, S. Parameters that effect spine biomechanics following cervical disc replacement. *Eur. Spine J.* **2012**, *21*, 688–699. [CrossRef] [PubMed]
34. Lee, Y.S.; Kim, Y.B.; Park, S.W. Risk factors for postoperative subsidence of single-level anterior cervical discectomy and fusion: The significance of the preoperative cervical alignment. *Spine (Phila Pa 1976)* **2014**, *39*, 1280–1287. [CrossRef] [PubMed]
35. De Leo–Vargas, R.A.; Muñoz–Romero, I.; Mondragón–Soto, M.G.; Martínez–Anda, J.J. Locking Stand-Alone Cage Constructs for the Treatment of Cervical Spine Degenerative Disease. *Asian Spine J.* **2019**, *13*, 630. [CrossRef]
36. Roberts, T.T.; Rosenbaum, A.J. Bone grafts, bone substitutes and orthobiologics: The bridge between basic science and clinical advancements in fracture healing. *Organogenesis* **2012**, *8*, 114–124. [CrossRef]
37. Karikari, I.O.; Jain, D.; Owens, T.R.; Gottfried, O.; Hodges, T.R.; Nimjee, S.M.; Bagley, C.A. Impact of subsidence on clinical outcomes and radiographic fusion rates in anterior cervical discectomy and fusion: A systematic review. *J. Spinal Disord. Tech.* **2014**, *27*, 1–10. [CrossRef]
38. Cheng, C.C.; Ordway, N.R.; Zhang, X.; Lu, Y.M.; Fang, H.; Fayyazi, A.H. Loss of cervical endplate integrity following minimal surface preparation. *Spine (Phila Pa 1976)* **2007**, *32*, 1852–1855. [CrossRef]
39. Chiang, M.-F.; Teng, J.-M.; Huang, C.-H.; Cheng, C.-K.; Chen, C.-S.; Chang, T.-K.; Chao, S.-H. Finite element analysis of cage subsidence in cervicalinterbody fusion. *J. Med. Biol. Eng.* **2004**, *24*, 201–208.

40. Liu, N.; Lu, T.; Wang, Y.; Sun, Z.; Li, J.; He, X. Effects of new cage profiles on the improvement in biomechanical performance of multilevel anterior cervical Corpectomy and fusion: A finite element analysis. *World Neurosurg.* **2019**, *129*, e87–e96. [CrossRef]
41. Zhang, Y.; Zhou, J.; Guo, X.; Cai, Z.; Liu, H.; Xue, Y. Biomechanical Effect of Different Graft Heights on Adjacent Segment and Graft Segment Following C4/C5 Anterior Cervical Discectomy and Fusion: A Finite Element Analysis. *Med. Sci. Monit. Int. Med J. Exp. Clin. Res.* **2019**, *25*, 4169. [CrossRef]
42. Wang, J.; Qian, Z.; Ren, L. Biomechanical Comparison of Optimal Shapes for the Cervical Intervertebral Fusion Cage for C5–C6 Cervical Fusion Using the Anterior Cervical Plate and Cage (ACPC) Fixation System: A Finite Element Analysis. *Med. Sci. Monit. Int. Med. J. Exp. Clin. Res.* **2019**, *25*, 8379. [CrossRef]
43. Lee, J.H.; Park, W.M.; Kim, Y.H.; Jahng, T.-A. A biomechanical analysis of an artificial disc with a shock-absorbing core property by using whole-cervical spine finite element analysis. *Spine* **2016**, *41*, E893–E901. [CrossRef]
44. Lee, S.-H.; Im, Y.-J.; Kim, K.-T.; Kim, Y.-H.; Park, W.-M.; Kim, K. Comparison of cervical spine biomechanics after fixed-and mobile-core artificial disc replacement: A finite element analysis. *Spine* **2011**, *36*, 700–708. [CrossRef] [PubMed]
45. Lin, C.-Y.; Chuang, S.-Y.; Chiang, C.-J.; Tsuang, Y.-H.; Chen, W.-P. Finite element analysis of cervical spine with different constrained types of total disc replacement. *J. Mech. Med. Biol.* **2014**, *14*, 1450038. [CrossRef]
46. Kim, Y.H.; Khuyagbaatar, B.; Kim, K. Recent advances in finite element modeling of the human cervical spine. *J. Mech. Sci. Technol.* **2018**, *32*, 1–10. [CrossRef]
47. Kim, M.K.; Kwak, D.S.; Park, C.K.; Park, S.H.; Oh, S.M.; Lee, S.W.; Han, S.H. Quantitative anatomy of the endplate of the middle and lower cervical vertebrae in Koreans. *Spine (Phila Pa 1976)* **2007**, *32*, E376–E381. [CrossRef] [PubMed]
48. Yao, Q.; Yin, P.; Khan, K.; Tsai, T.Y.; Li, J.S.; Hai, Y.; Tang, P.; Li, G. Differences of the Morphology of Subaxial Cervical Spine Endplates between Chinese and White Men and Women. *Biomed. Res. Int.* **2018**, *2018*, 2854175. [CrossRef] [PubMed]

© 2020 by the authors. Licensee MDPI, Basel, Switzerland. This article is an open access article distributed under the terms and conditions of the Creative Commons Attribution (CC BY) license (http://creativecommons.org/licenses/by/4.0/).

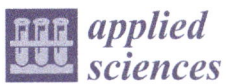

Article

Fixation Stability and Stiffness of Two Implant Systems for Proximal Femoral Varization Osteotomy

Kerstin Radtke [1], Fabian Goede [1], Michael Schwarze [2], Peter Paes [1], Max Ettinger [1] and Bastian Welke [2,*]

[1] Department of Orthopaedic Surgery, Hannover Medical School, Anna-von-Borries Straße 1-7, 30625 Hannover, Germany; kerstin.radtke@diakovere.de (K.R.); fabian.goede@diakovere.de (F.G.); peter.paes@diakovere.de (P.P.); max.ettinger@diakovere.de (M.E.)
[2] Laboratory for Biomechanics and Biomaterials, Department of Orthopaedic Surgery, Hannover Medical School, Anna-von-Borries Straße 1-7, 30625 Hannover, Germany; schwarze.michael@mh-hannover.de
* Correspondence: welke.bastian@mh-hannover.de; Tel.: +49-511-5354-652; Fax: +49-511-5354-875

Received: 24 June 2020; Accepted: 24 July 2020; Published: 25 August 2020

Abstract: Proximal femoral varization osteotomy is a well-established surgical procedure in children with severe hip problems. This study aimed to evaluate the fixation stability and stiffness of two new implant systems. A biomechanical testing model was created with a total of 12 synthetic femora. Proximal femoral varization osteotomy was performed in every femur, and the synthetic femora were fixed with two different implant systems (PediLoc Locking Proximal Femur Plate System versus PediLoc Locking Cannulated Blade Plate System; OrthoPediatrics, Warsaw, IN, USA). The average torsional stiffness of the locking plate group was higher than for the cannulated blade plate group. Differences in internal and external rotations were seen between the two groups, but they were not significant. Using the tested implants in severe osteoporotic bones might show other results. Therefore, it might be helpful to use the locking plate system in osteoporotic bones and in cases of revision operations where stability is of critical focus.

Keywords: proximal femoral varization osteotomy; blade plate; screw side plate

1. Introduction

Proximal femoral varization osteotomy is a well-established surgical procedure in children with different hip problems, such as developmental dysplasia of the hip (DDH), containment in Perthes disease, and hip dislocation or subluxation in severe cerebral palsy (CP) [1–9]. In the literature, older implant systems had higher complication rates and longer time to bone union [8].

To simplify the procedure and to stabilize the fixation, new blade plate systems were developed [9]. Given the low complication rates and postoperative mobilization under full weight bearing, fixed-angle blade plates became the most used implant over time [2,4–6].

Clinical studies with the new implant systems comparing blade plate and screw-side plate show generally good results [2,10–12]. Jain et al. described a rate of implant-related fractures of 2.5% in all patients, and they found no significant difference between the blade plate and screw-side plate [11]. Trainee surgeons had preference for cannulated blade plate when learning proximal femoral osteotomy, analyzing cannulated blade plate versus fixed angled blade plate. The fixed angled blade plate group had a higher prevalence of technical errors. However, radiological results were similar regarding migration and neck shaft angle [12]. In contrast, little is known about the biomechanical stability of the new implant systems used in proximal femoral varization osteotomy [1–3].

Synthetic bones are often used as a substitute for human tissue in biomechanical in vitro investigations. In certain applications, they show good agreement in terms of macroscopic mechanical properties and anatomy [13]. A further advantage is their standardization and the associated low variance.

This study aimed to evaluate fixation stability and stiffness of two new implant systems (PediLoc Locking Proximal Femur Plate System versus PediLoc Locking Cannulated Blade Plate System) using a synthetic bone model.

2. Materials and Methods

2.1. Specimens

A total of 12 synthetic femora with medium-sized and left-side geometry (#3403, 4th generation, Sawbone, Pacific Research Laboratories Inc., Vashon, WA, USA) bones were used for the study. The specimens were divided into two groups of patients using PediLoc Locking Proximal Femur Plate System (F-PL group) and PediLoc Locking Cannulated Blade Plate System (G-CBP group).

On every femur, proximal femoral varization osteotomy was performed by a surgeon and in accordance to the user manual. The closing was 10° from the medial side: five femora were fixed with a PediLoc Locking Proximal Femur Plate (size 90° × 3.5-mm plate, 12-mm offset, 3 holes, OrthoPediatrics, Warsaw, IN, USA) and seven with a PediLoc Locking Cannulated Blade Plate System (size 90° − 50 × 10 × 3, OrthoPediatrics, Warsaw, IN, USA). The proximal end of the prepared specimens was embedded into a metal shell using cold-curing three-component resin (Rencast FC52/53 Isocyanate, FC53 Polyol, Füller DT 082, gössl&pfaff GmbH, Karlskron/Braulach, Germany).

2.2. Mechanical Testing

Biomechanical investigations were carried out on a servohydraulic material testing machine (MTS MiniBionix I, Model 858, Eden Prairie, MN, USA) and a custom-made experimental setup. Two different loading scenarios were selected. First, the torsional stiffness of all specimens was investigated without harming them. After axial torsion, the so-called Hayes fall investigations were carried out. The experimental setup allowed measuring the force applied to fracture the proximal femur or damage the implant, and was based on the Hayes fall [14,15].

2.3. Axial Torsion

The synthetic femora were mounted between two universal joints to apply a purely torsional load (Figure 1). The distal part of the specimens was fixed to the lower cardan joint. The load was applied to the specimen via the second cardan joint at the top. The specimens were axially loaded with a static force (compression) of 100 N. First, a cyclic internal rotation was performed by introducing a torsional moment of 0 to 3 Nm into the proximal end of the specimens. After 100 cycles of internal rotation, an external rotation with 100 cycles was performed with the same load. The specimens were not harmed during the torsional test. Time, cycles, angle, torque, and force were recorded with a sampling rate of 1 kHz.

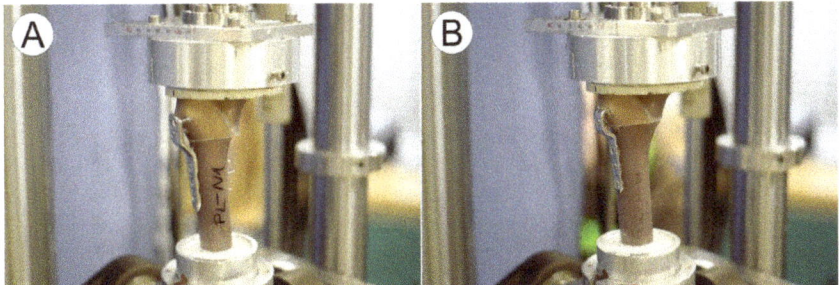

Figure 1. Test setup for axial torsion on the material test machine with mounted synthetic femora specimen: (**A**) F-PL with PediLoc Locking Proximal Femur Plate and (**B**) G-CBP with PediLoc Locking Cannulated Blade Plate System.

2.4. Proximal Femoral Strength

The proximal strength of the osteotomized synthetic femora was determined using a custom-made setup designed to simulate a sideways fall onto the greater trochanter region [14,15]. The distal embedding was free to rotate around the mediolateral axis. The specimens were positioned in the assembly with 15° internal rotation and 10° adduction (Figure 2). Proximally, the trochanter lay on a 6-mm thick rubber mat. The table under the rubber mat can be moved in the proximal-distal direction. The force and torque sensors of the material testing machine were located below the table. The force was applied directly to the femoral head via a sliding plate that permitted translational movements in the frontal plane of the femur. A position-controlled test protocol was used. First, a preload of 20 N was applied. The actuator then moved downward at a traversing speed of 0.5 mm/s. The abort criterion was manual after the failure of the sample. The transversal position, force, and time were recorded at 1 kHz.

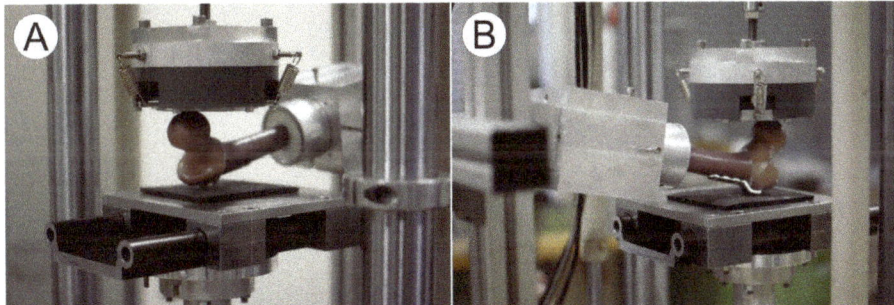

Figure 2. Test setup for the determination of the proximal femoral strength on the material test machine with mounted synthetic femora specimen. (**A**) Experimental setup to determine the proximal femoral strength based on the Hayes fall. The force is applied on the femoral head via a sliding plate that permits translational movements. The greater trochanter lies on a 6-mm thick rubber mat. The table under the rubber mat can be moved in the proximal–distal direction. (**B**) In the left part of the picture, the aluminum shell with the distal embedding is shown. The embedding can be rotated about the mediolateral axis. The specimens are positioned with internal rotation of 15° and an adduction of 10°.

2.5. Statistics

Due to the small sample size of the groups, the statistics were carried out with a Mann–Whitney U test for unrelated samples using R software (R version 3.5.1, The R Foundation for Statistical Computing, Vienna, Austria). A significance level of $\alpha = 0.05$ was applied.

3. Results

3.1. Axial Torsion

All synthetic femora could be tested for axial torsion without causing damage. The average torsional stiffness of the F-PL group was 4.26 ± 2.38 Nm/deg for internal rotation and 4.28 ± 1.40 Nm/deg for external rotation (Figure 3A). For the G-CBP group, the average torsional stiffness was 2.63 ± 1.23 Nm/deg for internal rotation and 2.85 ± 1.61 Nm/deg for external rotation (Figure 3B). The differences for internal and external rotations were not significant between the two groups.

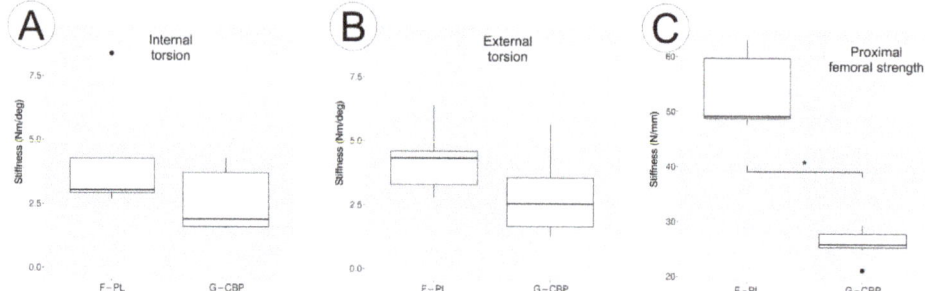

Figure 3. Box plots of the torsional stiffness for (**A**) internal, (**B**) external rotations, and (**C**) proximal femoral strength for both subgroups.

3.2. Proximal Femoral Strength

All specimens of both groups showed plastic deformation of the osteosynthesis plates at the end of the tests. The bone screws did not tear out, and the synthetic bones were not fractured.

The mean stiffness of the F-PL group was 53.9 ± 6.4 N/mm and that of the G-CBP group was 26.1 ± 2.7 N/mm (Figure 3C). This difference was also significant ($p = 0.018$). The mean force for the F-PL group and G-CBP group where implant failure occurred was 554 ± 71 N and 399 ± 33 N, respectively (Figure 4). This difference was significant ($p = 0.003$).

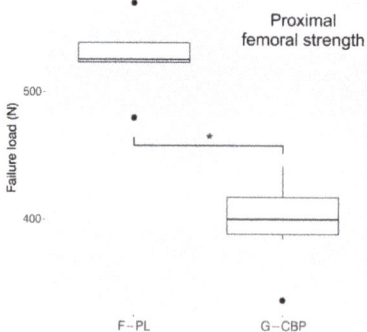

Figure 4. Box plots of the load to failure of the proximal femora for both tested groups.

4. Discussion

In this biomechanical comparative study, we investigated the torsional stiffness for internal and external rotations and the proximal strength of the osteotomized synthetic femora for two implant systems (PL and CBP). The average torsional stiffness of the F-PL group was higher than that for the G-CBP group. Differences in internal and external rotations were found between the two both groups.

However, this difference was not significant (Figure 3A,B). Moreover, the F-PL system has proximal locking screws to ensure that bending moments were further reduced during loading.

The proximal femoral strength of the osteotomized synthetic femora was tested with a setup to simulate a sideways fall onto the great trochanteric region. All specimens (both groups) showed plastic deformation of the implants at the end of the testing. No fractured synthetic bones or torn screws were seen in any group. The mean force where implant failure occurred was significantly higher in the F-PL group than in the G-CBP group. That the F-PL plate has a significantly higher rigidity and load to failure can be due to its construction. With 19 mm, the F-PL is 8 mm wider in the proximal and highly stressed gap area than the G-CBP. Both plates have approximately the same 3-mm thickness. This results in a higher moment of inertia of the F-PL, which is reflected in the results of the proximal strength. That there were no significant differences in torsion can be due to the fact that the G-CBP has a cannulated blade plate.

A recent study has shown that the design of the blade plate is relevant for stability [16]. After the addition of a proximal screw, the pullout strength increased even if the axial loading properties of the blade plate did not increase [16]. Considering these and our results, we suspect that design modifications might influence biomechanical results, and we hypothesize that adding a screw to the blade plate will not necessarily lead to better results. Further investigation might be helpful.

The fourth-generation synthetic femoral sawbones were used for testing. In a previous study, these femoral sawbones showed generally good agreement in terms of mean anatomy and macroscopic mechanical properties [13]. They are standardized and have low variance because of their biomechanical behavior. As regards testing, we expect comparable good results in vivo, as previously described [4,9]. However, most varization operations are performed in growing children [8,11,12]. The diversity of the growing skeleton cannot be represented by the sawbones used. Due to ethical consideration, we would disclaim interventional clinical trials analyzing stability with pediatric patients. Further studies, for example, on failed implants after osteotomy of the femur (in vivo) might help us better understand the stability and stiffness of the implants used.

A typical indication for the operation is coxa valga and excessive anteversion in spastic CP [2,3,12]. In severe cases, the hip is subluxated or luxated, and additive soft tissue operation is necessary [3]. Younger patients are often between 4 and 8 years [3]. The synthetic femora used cannot be representative for this pathologic anatomic situation. Furthermore, these patients have osteoporotic bone and reduced state of health, causing problems during treatment. This has to be investigated further in vivo.

In this study, comparable results were described in both groups. Using the tested implants in severe osteoporotic bones might show other results. Torn screws or fractured bones might occur. Concerning our results, we decided to use the F-PL in osteoporotic bones and in cases of revision operations. However, further biomechanical and in vivo tests in osteoporotic bones are necessary.

One further limitation of the study is the simplification of the loads that actually affect the musculoskeletal system. No combined load scenarios were applied, which do not fully correspond to reality, but facilitates the interpretation and comprehensibility of the results. However, the simulation of a sideways fall on the greater trochanter region is a frequently used method to examine the load capacity in the area of the osteotomy gap [14,15].

The results of this study showed that it is not possible to make a statement about possible intra- and postoperative complications. Blood loss, operation time, delayed union, implant loosening, and wound infections are typical parameters that should be evaluated in further comparative in vivo studies. Radiographic analyses of changes in containment should also be evaluated. In regard to existing studies, we expect comparable good results for these parameters [9,11,12].

Implant-related fractures along the two different implant systems (blade plate versus screw side plate) have been evaluated [11]. A previous study showed that no observed significant differences [11] may support our results on stiffness and stability. Therefore, differences in the design of the plates do not necessarily lead to significant differences in stability, even if we must await further studies with our two implant systems in vivo before making a definitive statement.

The correlation between surgeon experience and operative results is well explored [12]. All osteotomies in this study were performed by a well-experienced senior surgeon to prevent learning curve effects.

In a study analyzing CBP versus fixed angled blade plate, trainee surgeons were found to have preference for CBP when learning proximal femoral osteotomy [11]. In the present study, we decided to use the CBP for our trainee surgeons in their first year. Severe cases, such as osteoporotic bones and the use of PL, are reserved to senior surgeons in our department.

In conclusion, the average torsional stiffness of the locking plate group was higher than for the cannulated blade plate group. Differences in internal and external rotations were seen between the two groups, but they were not significant. Using the tested implants in severe osteoporotic bones might show other results. Therefore, it might be helpful to use the locking plate system in osteoporotic bones and in cases of revision operations where stability is of critical focus.

Author Contributions: Conceptualization, K.R. and F.G.; methodology, K.R., F.G., B.W., and M.E.; software, M.S. and B.W.; validation M.S. and B.W.; operation/implantation, F.G. and P.P.; biomechanical testing, M.S. and B.W.; data curation, B.W. and M.S.; writing—original draft preparation, K.R., B.W., and M.S.; writing—review and editing, K.R., B.W., and M.S.; visualization, B.W. and M.S.; supervision, B.W.; funding acquisition, F.G. All authors have read and agreed to the published version of the manuscript.

Funding: This research received no external funding.

Acknowledgments: We thank Robert Martin from OrthoPediatrics (now NuVasive Germany GmbH, Bremen, Germany) for supporting our study with the used implants and sawbones. We acknowledge support by the German Research Foundation (DFG) and the Open Access Publication Fund of Hannover Medical School (MHH).

Conflicts of Interest: All authors declare that we received implants and sawbones from Robert Martin, OrthoPediatrics, Warsaw, IN, USA, for this study. The sponsors had no role in the design, execution, interpretation, or writing of the study.

References

1. Thielemann, F.; Schneider, A. Long-term management results of Pemberton's ilium osteotomy in combination with inter-trochanter derotation-varisation osteotomy in hip dysplasia of childhood. *Z Orthop. Ihre Grenzgeb.* **2003**, *141*, 459–464. [CrossRef] [PubMed]
2. Rutz, E.; Brunner, R. The pediatric LCP hip plate for fixation of proximal femoral osteotomy in cerebral palsy and severe osteoporosis. *J. Pediatr. Orthop.* **2010**, *30*, 726–731. [CrossRef] [PubMed]
3. Eilert, R.E.; MacEwen, D. Varus derotational osteotomy of the femur in cerebral palsy. *Clin. Orthop. Relat. Res.* **1977**, *125*, 168–172. [CrossRef]
4. Zhou, L.; Camp, M. Cannulated, locking blade plates for proximal femoral osteotomy in children and adolescents. *J. Child. Orthop.* **2015**, *9*, 121–127. [CrossRef] [PubMed]
5. Beauchesne, R.; Miller, F. Proximal femoral osteotomy using the AO fixed-angle blade plate. *J. Pediatr. Orthop.* **1992**, *12*, 735–740. [CrossRef] [PubMed]
6. Hau, R.; Dickens, D.R.V. Which implant for proximal femoral osteotomy in children? A comparison of the AO (ASIF) 90° fixed-angle blade plate and the Richards intermediate hip screw. *J. Pediatr. Orthop.* **2000**, *20*, 336–343. [CrossRef] [PubMed]
7. Maranho, D.A.; Pagnano, R.G. Tension band wiring for proximal femoral varus osteotomy fixation in children. *Medicine* **2014**, *93*, e61. [CrossRef] [PubMed]
8. Canale, S.T.; Holand, R.W. Coventry screw fixation of osteotomies about the pediatric hip. *J. Pediatr. Orthop.* **1983**, *3*, 592–600. [CrossRef] [PubMed]
9. Grant, A.D.; Lehman, W.B. Cannulated blade plate for proximal femoral varus osteotomy. *Clin. Orthop. Relat. Res.* **1990**, *259*, 111–113. [CrossRef]
10. Heiner, A.D.; Brown, T.D. Structural properties of a new design of composite replicate femurs and tibia. *J. Biomech.* **2001**, *34*, 773–781. [CrossRef]
11. Jain, A.; Thompson, J.M. Implant-related fractures in children with proximal femoral osteotomy: Blade plate versus screw-side plate construct. *J. Pediatr. Orthop.* **2016**, *36*, e1–e5. [CrossRef] [PubMed]
12. Zhou, L.; Camp, M. Proximal femoral osteotomy in children with cerebral palsy: The perspective of the trainee. *J. Child. Orthop.* **2017**, *11*, 6–14. [CrossRef] [PubMed]

13. Gardner, M.P.; Chong, A.C.M. Mechanical evaluation of large-size fourth-generation composite femur and tibia models. *Ann. Biomed. Eng.* **2010**, *38*, 613–620. [CrossRef] [PubMed]
14. Beckmann, J.; Ferguson, S.J. Femoroplasty-augmentation of the proximal femur with a composite bone cement-feasibility, biomechanical properties and osteosynthesis potential. *Med. Eng. Phys.* **2007**, *29*, 755–764. [CrossRef] [PubMed]
15. Cheng, X.G.; Lowet, G. Assessment of the strength of proximal femur in vitro: Relationship to femoral bone mineral density and femoral geometry. *Bone* **1997**, *20*, 213–218. [CrossRef]
16. Ruzbarsky, J.J.; Swarup, I. Biomechanical comparison of two pediatric blade plate designs in proximal femoral osteotomies. *HSS J.* **2020**, *16*, 81–85. [CrossRef] [PubMed]

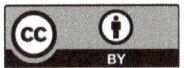

© 2020 by the authors. Licensee MDPI, Basel, Switzerland. This article is an open access article distributed under the terms and conditions of the Creative Commons Attribution (CC BY) license (http://creativecommons.org/licenses/by/4.0/).

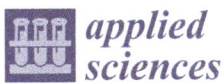

Article

Intra- and Interobserver Reliability Comparison of Clinical Gait Analysis Data between Two Gait Laboratories

René Schwesig [1,*], Regina Wegener [2], Christof Hurschler [3], Kevin Laudner [4] and Frank Seehaus [5]

1. Department of Orthopaedic and Trauma Surgery, Martin-Luther-University Halle-Wittenberg, Ernst-Grube-Str. 40, 06120 Halle, Germany
2. Private Practice for Neurology Dr. Wegener, Lienaustr. 2, 23730 Neustadt, Holstein, Germany; reginawegener@gmx.net
3. Laboratory for Biomechanics and Biomaterials, Hannover Medical School, Anna-von-Borries-Str. 1-7, 30625 Hannover, Germany; hurschler.christof@mh-hannover.de
4. Department of Health Sciences, University of Colorado, Colorado Springs, CO 80918, USA; klaudner@uccs.edu
5. Department of Orthopaedic Surgery, Friedrich-Alexander-University Erlangen-Nürnberg, Rathsberger Str. 57, 91054 Erlangen, Germany; frank.seehaus@fau.de
* Correspondence: rene.schwesig@uk-halle.de; Tel.: +49-345-557-1317; Fax: +49-345-557-4899

Received: 7 July 2020; Accepted: 22 July 2020; Published: 23 July 2020

Featured Application: Clinical gait analysis (CGA) is an in vivo method used to measure the movement behavior/gait patterns of patients before and after an orthopedic treatment. It monitors joint kinematics and kinetics under dynamic conditions within the musculoskeletal system. This study contributes to a better understanding of the comparability and significance of motion analysis data recorded in different gait laboratories using different technical qualities.

Abstract: Comparing clinical gait analysis (CGA) data between clinical centers is critical in the treatment and rehabilitation progress. However, CGA protocols and system configurations, as well as choice of marker sets and individual variability during marker attachment, may affect the comparability of data. The aim of this study was to evaluate reliability of CGA data collected between two gait analysis laboratories. Three healthy subjects underwent a standardized CGA protocol at two separate centers. Kinematic data were captured using the same motion capturing systems (two systems, same manufacturer, but different analysis software and camera configurations). The CGA data were analyzed by the same two observers for both centers. Interobserver reliability was calculated using single measure intraclass correlation coefficients (ICC). Intraobserver as well as between-laboratory intraobserver reliability were assessed using an average measure ICC. Interobserver reliability for all joints (ICC_{total} = 0.79) was found to be significantly lower ($p < 0.001$) than intraobserver reliability (ICC_{total} = 0.93), but significantly higher ($p < 0.001$) than between-laboratory intraobserver reliability (ICC_{total} = 0.55). Data comparison between both centers revealed significant differences for 39% of investigated parameters. Different hardware and software configurations impact CGA data and influence between-laboratory comparisons. Furthermore, lower intra- and interobserver reliability were found for ankle kinematics in comparison to the hip and knee, particularly for interobserver reliability.

Keywords: motion analysis; kinematics, repeatability; lower extremity; optical infrared camera motion capturing system

1. Introduction

Three-dimensional clinical gait analysis (CGA) is an important diagnostic tool within the field of movement disorders [1]. Optical marker tracking systems are considered the gold standard for this type of assessment [2,3]. However, discrepancies in CGA data across multiple analyses can be caused by differences in marker sets [4], observer error [5], marker placement [6] and patient variability [7]. Despite applied standardized protocols (e.g., marker-set, measurement pipeline), incompatibilities and discrepancies within CGA data of the same patient cohorts collected by different institutions are often observed, and have caused reservations concerning the applicability of CGA among multicenter studies [3,4,8]. Ferrari et al. [4] compared the trunk, pelvis and lower limb kinematics of five separate measurement protocols (different marker sets), using a single data pool of subjects. These authors reported good correlations between kinematic variables in the sagittal plane (flexion/extension), but poorer correlations for out-of-sagittal-plane rotations, such as knee abduction/adduction. They also reported good correlations among protocols with similar biomechanical models [4]. Ferrari et al. [4] concluded that the comparison of different measurement protocols results in higher data variability when compared to interobserver and interlaboratory comparisons for most gait characteristics. Obviously, model conventions and definitions are crucial for data comparison. Gorton et al. [8] identified the marker placement procedure of examiners as the largest source of error. The use of a standardized protocol for marker placement decreased data variability by up to 20%. Based on clinical experience, the authors of the current study hypothesized that significant discrepancies would exist between CGA data sets collected using different hardware and software infrastructures or configurations.

Due to the observed limitations in the reproducibility of CGA data, efforts have focused on the reduction of measurement error, with the aim of producing data with the highest possible degree of reproducibility. To improve our understanding of the accuracy and reproducibility of CGA data, cross-laboratory studies must be performed using a single cohort of subjects. Previous research has reported on the repeatability of motion capture data using separate trials, sessions and observers under various conditions for a specific CGA setup or laboratory [5–7,9,10]. However, reports for multi-center repeatability are limited and have focused on differences in hardware configurations, marker placement, as well as between trials and days of measurement [3,8,11]. Unfortunately, a validation using the same motion capturing technology, but different hardware and software infrastructure/configurations (e.g., capturing software, camera type), among a single cohort of subjects is lacking.

It is critical for clinicians and researchers to have reliable examination tools to accurately and objectively assess the functional status of a joint [12–16]. A high level of intraobserver reliability is imperative to accurately evaluate the longitudinal effects of the rehabilitation process and to identify differences between subjects [17,18]. A central research question is whether the findings of clinical gait analyses conducted by multiple laboratories are consistent and reliable enough for making clinical decisions—or is the dependence on observers, repeat measurements or measurement and analysis protocols too large?

The specific aims of this study were to evaluate the intra- and interobserver reliability and the equivalence of CGA data between two gait analysis laboratories (between-laboratory intraobserver reliability) using the same motion capturing technology, but different hardware and software infrastructure/configurations among a single cohort of subjects. The following two hypotheses were specifically investigated:

1) Intraobserver reliability of CGA data for the lower extremity obtained for the same cohort of subjects and captured at one laboratory will be good-to-excellent, whereas interobserver reliability will be fair-to-good.
2) CGA data for the lower extremity obtained for the same cohort of subjects, captured at two separate laboratories by the same observers, using different hardware and software systems, will be equivalent.

2. Materials and Methods

2.1. Subjects

A standardized measurement protocol was performed repeatedly on three adult subjects (one female, two males) who were asymptomatic at the time of testing and did not display any movement disorders. This cohort had a mean (±SD) age of 33.3 (±4.0) years, mean body weight of 77.3 (±16.3) kg, mean body height of 176.7 (±9.1) cm, and a mean body mass index of 24.3 (±2.9) kg·m^{-2} (Table A1). The study was approved by the ethical committee of Martin-Luther-University Halle-Wittenberg (approval number: 217/08.03.10/10). Written consent from study participants was obtained prior to data collection.

2.2. Measurement Set-Up

Gait analyses were performed in two gait laboratories (Figure 1). Both laboratories used an optical infrared camera-based motion capturing system provided by one manufacturer (Vicon Motion System Ltd., Oxford, UK).

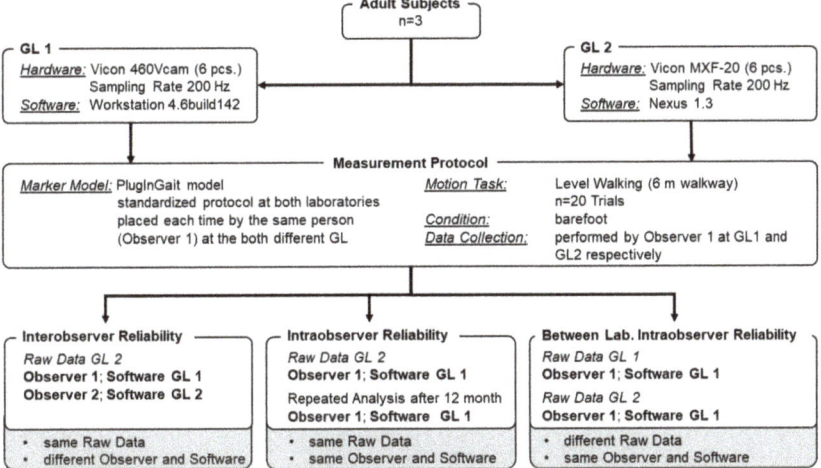

Figure 1. Data processing chart—clinical gait analysis (CGA) data collected on three healthy test-subjects (n = 20 barefoot trials per person). The data were captured using the same measurement protocols in both the first (GL1) and the second laboratories (GL2). Three reliability tests were performed with the datasets from GL1 and GL2. Interobserver reliability was tested for two observers using the CGA data collected at GL2. Observer 1 used the data processing software from GL 1 (Workstation 4.6), which was different to that of Observer 2 (GL2: Nexus 1.3). To assess intraobserver reliability, the same data set was analyzed a second time by observer 1 after a time interval of 12 months, using the CGA data collected at GL2 and the software from GL1. To test between-laboratory intraobserver reliability, the CGA data collected at both sites (GL1 and GL2) were analyzed by Observer 1 using software from GL1.

The first laboratory (GL1) was equipped with a six-camera system (460 Vcam cameras, Workstation 4.6 build 142 software). The second laboratory (GL2) used a six-camera system (MXF-20 cameras, Nexus 1.3 software). These systems thus differed in their respective configurations, both in terms of analysis software (Workstation vs. Nexus) and camera type (Vcam vs. MXF). Both laboratories applied the same sampling rate (200 Hz) and the same reflective markers (14 mm diameter). Capture space represented the full dimensions (length, width and height) of the motion capture room for GL1 (7 m, 4 m and 3 m) and for GL2 (15.5 m, 8.8 m and 4.8 m). Capture volume was defined as the area within the capture space, for which motion capturing cameras were able to capture the motion task of each subject. The GL1 capture volume was 6 m, 2 m and 2 m. The capture volume for GL2 was 10.0 m, 8.5 m and 2.9 m. Captured marker data were processed and trajectories were labeled using the PlugInGait model under a standardized protocol at both laboratories. All kinematic data were Woltring filtered using a mean squared error setting of 10. These gait data were reduced to 100% of one gait cycle using gait cycle event detection, based on the available force plates (threshold: 20 N). All subsequent measurement conditions were consistent at both laboratories.

2.3. Measurement Protocol

Calibration of the optical infrared camera-based motion capturing systems at both laboratories were performed according to the manufacturer's guidelines. This calibration process consisted of two main steps: (*i*) a static calibration to calculate the origin of the capture volume and define the 3D workspace orientation (x, y, z directions) and (*ii*) a dynamic calibration to calculate the relative position and orientation of each camera within the capture volume. Calibration quality was checked according to the manufacturer's guidelines.

The PlugInGait marker setup for the lower extremity (kinematic model V 2.3) was used in both laboratories, based on the work of Kadaba et al. [19]. Markers were attached to each subject by the same experienced staff member (Observer 1) at both gait analysis laboratories, according to a standardized protocol for anthropometric measurements, landmark identification and marker mounting.

Each of the three subjects performed 20 barefoot gait trials with a self-selected walking speed resulting in a total of 60 CGA trials per gait laboratory. Individual gait speed was controlled and standardized between data collection sessions. The same two staff members (Observer 1 and Observer 2) performed data processing and analysis at both laboratories, using a standardized protocol for data processing, labeling and gait event detection. For each reliability analysis variation, the observer started with the original raw data in their data processing routine. These raw data were labeled, gait events were detected and possible gaps of reconstructed marker trajectories were filled. The kinematic parameters were extracted using the same template and again used a standardized workflow for both observers. Kinematic data used for reliability analysis, which consisted of specific movement parameters in the sagittal and frontal plane for the hip, knee and ankle. Parameters were selected according to the specifications of Benedetti et al. [20] (Figure 2).

Data from the right leg of each subject were used for the analyses of reliability. Three different measures of reliability were performed (Figure 1):

- Interobserver Reliability: The reliability of the two observers, using the same data set, was assessed using separate analysis software (Observer 1: GL1 (Workstation); Observer 2: GL2 (Nexus)).
- Intraobserver Reliability: The reliability of the same data set among the same observer was tested. This assessment was performed with a time interval of 12 months between analyses using the same software (Workstation). The CGA data for this assessment were collected at the GL2 site.
- Between-Laboratory Intraobserver Reliability: To compare the effect of laboratory environment and instrumentation while excluding observer-dependent influences, CGA data collected at both laboratories were analyzed by a single observer using the same analysis software.

The following reliability variables were assessed. ICC_{mean} was the average of all parameters for hip, knee and ankle. ICC_{total} (Equation (1)) was the average of hip ICC_{mean}, knee ICC_{mean} and ankle ICC_{mean} for all three types of reliability (intraobserver, interobserver, between-laboratory intraobserver).

$$ICC_{total} = hip\ ICC_{mean} + knee\ ICC_{mean} + ankle\ ICC_{mean} / 3 \qquad (1)$$

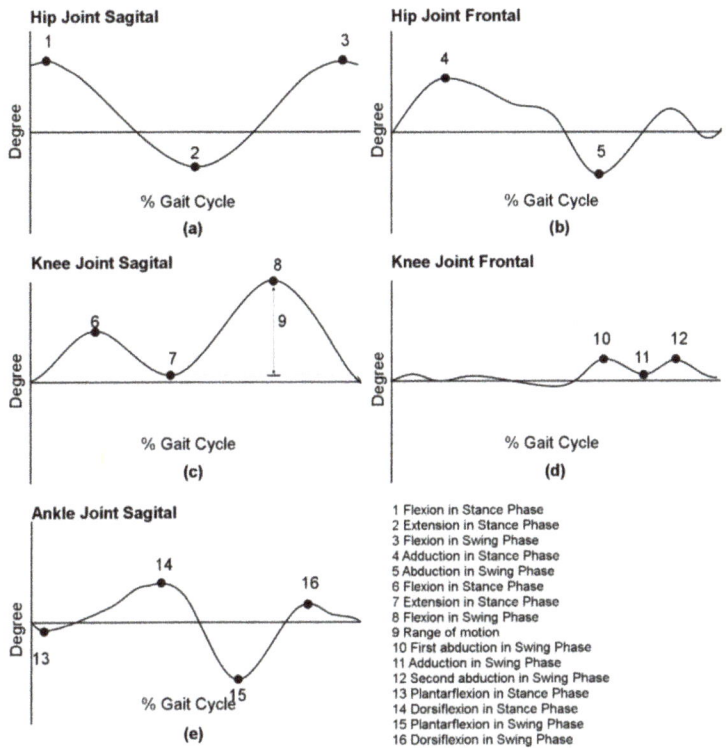

Figure 2. Parameters extracted (No. 1 to 16) out of processed kinematic data for sagittal (**a**) and frontal (**b**) plane of the hip joint, for sagittal (**c**) and frontal (**d**) plane of the knee joint, as well as data for sagittal (**e**) plane of the ankle joint.

2.4. Statistics

Descriptive statistics (mean, standard deviation) were based on 20 barefoot trials and were calculated for 31 kinematic parameters in the sagittal and frontal plane for the hip, knee and ankle joints. Reliability analyses were divided into five parts:

1. For interobserver reliability, a single measure intraclass correlation coefficient (ICC) was calculated. The number of measures (k) was 60 (n = 20 barefoot trials from three subjects).
2. For intraobserver reliability, an average measure ICC was calculated. The number of measures (k) was 60.
3. To assess between-laboratory intraobserver reliability, an average measure ICC was calculated and again referenced to the same ICC value classification [21]. The ICC indicated excellent reliability if the value was above 0.75, fair-to-good reliability between 0.40 and 0.75 and poor reliability when less than 0.40. A two-way mixed-effects model (definition: absolute agreement) was used for all calculations. For all ICC values, 95% confidence intervals were reported.
4. To estimate experimental errors of a joint angle, the standard error was calculated (for intra- ($\sigma^{repeated}$), inter- ($\sigma^{observer}$) and between-laboratory intraobserver reliability ($\sigma^{sess(lab)}$)) as described by Schwartz et al. [10], as well as the magnitude of the interobserver error and its ratio to intra-subject error r (Equations (2)–(4)).

$$r = \sigma^{repeated}/\sigma^{trial} \qquad (2)$$

$$r = \sigma^{observer}/\sigma^{trial} \tag{3}$$

$$r = \sigma^{sesss(lab)}/\sigma^{trial} \tag{4}$$

5. A scatter-plot technique suggested by Bland and Altman [22] was used to assess interchangeability (equivalence) of CGA data between laboratories. Calculated differences for joint angles were plotted against their average value for each subject. The interchangeability of CGA data was tested by a bounding criterion defined as the mean ± two standard deviations of the measured differences (approximately 95% of all measured values).

6. To evaluate the variability within and between subjects, the standard error of measurement (SEM) was calculated in conjunction with the ICCs, using the following equation from Portney and Watkins [23]:

$$SEM = SD \times \sqrt{(1 - ICC)} \tag{5}$$

ICC values may be influenced by inter-subject variability of scores, because a large ICC may be reported despite poor trial-to-trial consistency if the inter-subject variability is too high [23,24]. However, the SEM is not affected by inter-subject variability [24].

7. Mean differences for multicenter comparisons were tested using variance analysis. A one-factor, univariate general linear model (GLM; dependent variable: hip flexion during stance; independent variable: CGA center; covariate: walking speed) was performed. Prior to inference statistical analyses, all variables were tested for normal distribution (Kolmogorov–Smirnov test). To estimate practical relevance and to quantify the differences between GL1 and GL2, effect sizes (partial eta squared, η_p^2 [25,26]) were calculated for the main effects (η_p^2) and the mean differences divided by the pooled standard deviations (d). To evaluate effect sizes, d or η_p^2 were classified, with $d \geq 0.2$, $d \geq 0.5$, $d \geq 0.8$ or $\eta_p^2 \geq 0.01$, $\eta_p^2 \geq 0.06$, $\eta_p^2 \geq 0.14$ indicating small, medium or large effects, respectively [27]. Level of significance was adjusted to $p \leq 0.002$ (0.05/31 = 0.002) for multiple tests by means of a Bonferroni correction.

All statistical analyses were performed using SPSS version 25.0 for Windows (SPSS Inc., IBM, Armonk, NY, USA).

3. Results

Because of the controlled and standardized CGA data collection, walking speed and stride length parameters did not differ between laboratory measurement sessions (walking speed: 1.40 ± 0.06 m·s^{-1} vs. 1.40 ± 0.04 m·s^{-1}; stride length: 1.38 ± 0.09 m vs. 1.40 ± 0.10 m).

3.1. Interobserver Reliability

All interobserver reliability variables fulfilled the assumption of normality. Interobserver reliability at one laboratory (GL2), showed excellent reliability for 71% of the parameters observed (22/31). Based on the lower limit of the 95% CI, 58% (18/31) displayed an ICC value of at least 0.75. Nineteen percent (6/31) of the parameters showed fair-to-good reliability, whereas 10% (3/31) were poor (Table 1).

Table 1. Single site inter- and intraobserver intraclass correlation coefficient (ICC) values and results of repeated single observer analysis at both laboratories (between-laboratory intraobserver values) of an ICC greater than 0.75 were considered excellent and marked in bold.

Parameter	Intraobserver			Interobserver			Between-Laboratory Intraobserver		
	ICC	95% CI lower	95% CI upper	ICC	95% CI lower	95% CI upper	ICC	95% CI lower	95% CI upper
Hip (degree)									
Flexion ST	**1.00**	1.00	1.00	**0.97**	0.95	0.98	0.60	0.10	0.80
Extension ST	**1.00**	1.00	1.00	**0.76**	0.63	0.85	0.72	0.54	0.83
Flexion SW	**1.00**	1.00	1.00	**0.99**	0.97	0.99	0.71	0	0.89
Adduction ST	**1.00**	1.00	1.00	**0.98**	0.97	0.99	**0.88**	0.55	0.95
Abduction SW	**1.00**	1.00	1.00	**0.93**	0.89	0.96	0.59	0.06	0.80
Hip (% gait cycle)									
Flexion ST	**1.00**	0.99	1.00	**0.96**	0.92	0.97	**0.90**	0.83	0.94
Extension ST	**0.92**	0.77	0.97	**0.81**	0.64	0.90	0.46	0.00	0.71
Flexion SW	**0.83**	0.72	0.90	0.71	0.56	0.81	0.31	0.00	0.57
Adduction ST	**1.00**	1.00	1.00	**0.95**	0.92	0.97	**0.78**	0.63	0.87
Abduction SW	**0.99**	0.98	0.99	**0.94**	0.90	0.97	0.53	0.23	0.72
Knee (degree)									
Flexion ST	**1.00**	1.00	1.00	**0.91**	0.86	0.95	0.57	0.08	0.78
Extension ST	**1.00**	1.00	1.00	**1.00**	0.99	1.00	0.74	0.56	0.84
Flexion SW	**1.00**	1.00	1.00	0.47	0.25	0.65	**0.82**	0.70	0.89
Range of motion	**1.00**	1.00	1.00	0.40	0.17	0.59	0.46	0.10	0.68
First abduction SW	**1.00**	1.00	1.00	**0.99**	0.98	0.99	0.00	0.00	0.35
Adduction SW	**1.00**	1.00	1.00	**0.97**	0.94	0.98	0.41	0.00	0.67
Second abduction SW	**1.00**	1.00	1.00	**0.97**	0.95	0.96	0.41	0.00	0.67
Knee (% gait cycle)									
Flexion ST	**0.99**	0.98	0.99	**0.88**	0.81	0.93	**0.81**	0.18	0.93
Extension ST	**0.98**	0.97	0.99	**0.94**	0.83	0.97	0.21	0.00	0.53
Flexion SW	**0.89**	0.66	0.95	**0.84**	0.75	0.90	0.13	0.00	0.42
First abduction SW	**0.97**	0.93	0.98	**0.84**	0.74	0.90	0.48	0.12	0.69
Adduction SW	**0.98**	0.92	0.99	0.72	0.55	0.83	0.19	0.00	0.52
Second abduction SW	**0.98**	0.81	1.00	**0.91**	0.85	0.95	**0.75**	0.55	0.86
Ankle (degree)									
Plantarflexion ST	0.23	0.00	0.51	0.11	0	0.314	0.33	0.00	0.60
Dorsiflexion ST	0.61	0.28	0.78	0.47	0.02	0.721	0.74	0.57	0.85
Plantarflexion SW	**0.98**	0.94	0.99	**0.93**	0.79	0.968	**0.86**	0.62	0.94
Dorsiflexion SW	**0.82**	0.63	0.90	0.72	0.25	0.875	**0.83**	0.65	0.91
Ankle (% gait cycle)									
Plantarflexion ST	**0.98**	0.96	0.99	**0.82**	0.69	0.90	**0.77**	0.07	0.92
Dorsiflexion ST	**0.95**	0.92	0.97	0.22	0.00	0.44	0.36	0.00	0.62
Plantarflexion SW	**0.92**	0.82	0.96	**0.84**	0.75	0.90	0.27	0.00	0.55
Dorsiflexion SW	**0.95**	0.92	0.97	0.50	0.26	0.68	0.45	0.06	0.68
ICC ≥ 0.75 (%)	94% (29/31)			71% (22/31)			29% (9/31)		

Remarks: ST = stance phase; SW = swing phase.

The highest ICC value was observed for knee extension in the stance phase (ICC = 0.97, excellent reliability). In contrast, dorsiflexion during the stance phase showed poor reliability (ICC = 0.22) (Table 1). After averaging all parameters for interobserver reliability, an ICC_{total} = 0.79 (95% CI: 0.67–0.86) was observed (Table 2).

For interobserver reliability, the largest standard error was observed for hip adduction (% gait cycle) during stance phase, as well as for ankle dorsiflexion (% gait cycle) during swing phase, with each presenting with a standard error of $\sigma^{observer}$ = 4.4% (Table 3). Plantarflexion during the stance phase had the worst detected angle ($\sigma^{observer}$ = 3.8°). The largest ratio of interobserver to intrasubject error was observed for knee abduction angle in the stance phase ($\sigma^{observer}$ = 2.4°, r = 3.2; Table 3).

Table 2. Calculated mean ICC values (ICC_{mean} = mean of all parameters for hip, knee and ankle) and 95% confidence intervals (95% CI) for the ankle, knee and hip, as well as total mean ICC values (ICC_{total} = ICC_{mean} hip + ICC_{mean} knee + ICC_{mean} ankle). Values for ICC above 0.75 were considered excellent and marked in bold.

Joint	Intraobserver (95% CI)	Interobserver (95% CI)	Between-Laboratory Intraobserver (95% CI)
Hip ∅ ICC_{mean}	0.97 (0.95–0.99)	0.90 (0.84–0.94)	0.65 (0.27–0.81)
Knee ∅ ICC_{mean}	0.98 (0.94–0.99)	0.83 (0.74–0.89)	0.46 (0.05–0.68)
Ankle ∅ ICC_{mean}	0.81 (0.66–0.88)	0.58 (0.33–0.73)	0.58 (0.21–0.76)
∅ ICC_{total}	0.93 (0.87–0.96)	0.79 (0.67–0.86)	0.56 (0.16–0.74)
Analysis of Variance (ICC_{total})	\multicolumn{3}{l}{Comparison of all three types of reliability: $p < 0.001$; $\eta_p^2 = 0.533$ Intraobserver vs. Interobserver: $p < 0.001$; $\eta_p^2 = 0.399$ Intraobserver vs. Between-laboratory intraobserver: $p < 0.001$; $\eta_p^2 = 0.676$ Interobserver vs. Between-laboratory intraobserver: $p < 0.001$; $\eta_p^2 = 0.374$}		

Remarks: ICC_{mean} = mean of all parameters for hip, knee and ankle; ICC_{total} = ICC_{mean} hip + ICC_{mean} knee + ICC_{mean} ankle divided by 3 (for all three types of reliability).

Table 3. Standard errors for intra- ($\sigma^{repeated}$), inter- ($\sigma^{observer}$) and between-laboratory intraobserver ($\sigma^{sess(lab)}$) reliability. The inter-trial error is represented by r (r = $\sigma^{repeated}$ / σ^{trial}; r = $\sigma^{observer}$ / σ^{trial}; r = $\sigma^{sess(lab)}$ / σ^{trial}). Kinematic parameters for ankle-, knee- and hip-joints are presented by peak values (amplitude) and associated time point during the gait cycle.

		Parameter	Intraobserver $\sigma^{observer}$	r	Interobserver $\sigma^{repeated}$	r	Between-Laboratory Intraobserver $\sigma^{sess(lab)}$	r
Joint Angles (degree)	Hip	Flexion ST	1.2	1.0	1.3	1.0	1.6	1.4
		Extension ST	0.8	1.0	0.9	1.0	1.6	1.7
		Flexion SW	0.7	1.0	0.9	1.0	1.2	1.5
		Adduction ST	1.0	1.0	1.2	1.0	1.5	1.6
		Abduction SW	0.7	1.0	0.9	1.2	1.3	1.4
	Knee	Flexion ST	2.1	1.0	2.4	1.0	2.3	1.2
		Extension ST	1.3	1.0	1.9	1.3	1.7	1.4
		Flexion SW	1.1	1.0	1.8	1.4	1.6	1.5
		Range of motion	1.6	1.0	1.8	1.0	1.7	1.1
		First abduction SW	0.8	1.0	2.4	3.2	4.2	5.1
		Adduction SW	1.0	1.0	1.5	1.6	3.4	3.7
		Second abduction SW	0.7	1.0	1.3	1.6	3.2	3.8
	Ankle	Plantarflexion ST	1.6	1.4	1.5	1.5	1.6	1.4
		Dorsiflexion ST	1.7	1.3	1.5	1.3	1.4	1.1
		Plantarflexion SW	2.5	1.1	3.8	1.7	3.6	1.5
		Dorsiflexion SW	1.5	1.5	1.6	1.4	1.3	1.4
Time at % Gait Cycle	Hip	Flexion ST	1.4	1.0	1.9	1.2	1.3	1.2
		Extension ST	0.8	1.0	0.9	1.2	1.2	1.2
		Flexion SW	2.9	1.0	3.2	1.0	4.2	1.1
		Adduction ST	3.8	1.0	4.4	1.0	5.4	1.0
		Abduction SW	1.5	1.0	2.5	1.5	5.0	1.0
	Knee	Flexion ST	0.8	1.0	1.1	1.1	1.0	1.2
		Extension ST	1.4	1.0	1.7	1.1	1.4	1.1
		Flexion SW	0.9	1.0	1.0	1.1	0.9	1.2
		First abduction SW	2.7	1.0	3.0	1.0	2.1	1.0
		Adduction SW	2.0	1.0	3.1	1.0	2.4	0.9
		Second abduction SW	1.7	1.0	3.0	1.2	2.3	0.9
	Ankle	Plantarflexion ST	1.0	1.0	1.3	1.4	1.1	1.3
		Dorsiflexion ST	1.0	1.0	1.2	1.2	1.2	1.0
		Plantarflexion SW	0.9	1.0	1.0	1.1	1.1	1.3
		Dorsiflexion SW	4.2	1.0	4.4	1.1	4.8	1.1
		Analysis of Variance	\multicolumn{6}{l}{Intraobserver vs. Interobserver: $p < 0.001$; $\eta_p^2 = 0.498$ Intraobserver vs. Between-Laboratory Intraobserver: $p = 0.001$; $\eta_p^2 = 0.325$ Interobserver vs. Between-Laboratory Intraobserver: $p = 0.083$; $\eta_p^2 = 0.097$}					

Remarks: ST = stance phase; SW = swing phase.

3.2. Intraobserver Reliability

All intraobserver reliability variables fulfilled the assumption of normality. Intraobserver reliability (ICC$_{total}$ = 0.93) was significantly ($p < 0.001$, $\eta_p^2 = 0.399$) higher than interobserver reliability (ICC$_{total}$ = 0.79). When considering the total intraobserver ICC, excellent values were observed for 94% (29/31) of parameters, 3% (1/31) were fair to good and 3% (1/31) were poor (Table 1). Based on the lower limit of the 95% CI, 87% (27/31) of the parameters showed an ICC value of at least 0.75 (excellent reliability). For intraobserver reliability, the calculated standard errors ($\sigma^{repeated}$) and SEM were smaller than those for interobserver reliability ($\sigma^{repeated}$) (Table 3, Tabel A2); however, these values were not compared statistically. The highest error for intraobserver reliability existed for ankle dorsiflexion during the swing phase (% gait cycle) ($\sigma^{repeated} = 4.2\%$), as well as plantarflexion during the swing phase (mean $\sigma^{observer} = 2.5°$).

Intraobserver reliability across laboratories (between-laboratory intraobserver) was excellent in 29% (9/31) of all parameters, fair to good for 48% (15/31), and poor for 26% (8/31) (Table 1). The highest ICC (0.90) was observed for hip flexion during the stance phase (% gait cycle). The worst ICC (0) was calculated for knee abduction angle in the swing phase.

3.3. Between-Laboratory Intraobserver Reliability

All between-laboratory intraobserver reliability variables fulfilled the assumption of normality. Between-laboratory intraobserver reliability for the entire lower limb (hip, knee, ankle) was poor (ICC$_{total}$ = 0.56, Table 2). Excellent ICC values were only calculated for 29% (9/31) of parameters (Table 1). Considering the lower limit of the 95% CI, no parameter reached an ICC level of 0.75. Calculated standard errors between-laboratory intraobserver reliability ($\sigma^{sess(lab)}$) were larger than those for interobserver and intraobserver reliability (Table 3). The largest standard errors were the same as those found for interobserver reliability, which included hip adduction (% gait cycle) at the stance phase with a mean $\sigma^{sess(lab)} = 5.4\%$, and for ankle dorsiflexion (% gait cycle) at the stance phase with a mean $\sigma^{sess(lab)} = 4.8\%$. The largest ratio was again observed for knee abduction in the swing phase ($\sigma^{sess(lab)} = 4.2°$, $r = 5.1$) whereas its smallest inter-trial error was 0.8°.

3.4. Variance Analysis

When comparing the between-site CGA data from GL1 and GL2, the general linear model revealed significant differences (adjusted significance level: $p \leq 0.002$) for 39% of all parameters (12/31) (Table 4). Only three parameters (hip abduction swing phase (degree), hip extension stance phase (% gait cycle), knee flexion swing phase (% gait cycle)) fulfilled all three statistical criteria ($p \leq 0.002$ and $\eta_p^2 \geq 0.14$ and $d \geq 0.80$).

Table 4. Single observer comparison between laboratories (means, standard deviations, general linear model (GLM), standard error of measurement (SEM)). Significance level was set at 0.002. Large effect sizes (d ≥ 0.8; η_p^2 ≥ 0.14) marked in bold.

Parameter	GL1		GL2		Analysis of Variance			d	SEM
	Mean	SD	Mean	SD	F	p	η_p^2		
Hip (degree)									
Flexion ST	36.5	2.79	38.1	1.68	2.44	0.121	0.02	0.72	1.41
Extension ST	−7.19	2.00	−6.57	3.67	20.0	**<0.001**	**0.15**	0.22	1.50
Flexion SW	35.9	2.34	37.6	1.58	0.03	0.855	0.00	**0.87**	1.06
Adduction ST	5.04	3.94	6.71	3.72	3.32	0.071	0.03	0.44	1.33
Abduction SW	−8.44	2.12	−7.02	1.37	141	**<0.001**	**0.55**	**0.81**	1.12
Hip (% gait cycle)									
Flexion ST	3.00	3.65	3.45	3.17	79.2	**<0.001**	**0.40**	0.13	1.08
Extension ST	52.0	1.64	50.7	1.10	35.2	**<0.001**	**0.32**	**0.95**	1.01
Flexion SW	88.7	5.32	86.6	3.94	0.13	0.721	0.00	0.45	3.85
Adduction ST	27.1	10.4	25.2	8.15	25.7	**<0.001**	**0.18**	0.21	4.35
Abduction SW	67.2	8.23	65.4	3.20	0.67	0.416	0.01	0.32	3.92
Knee (degree)									
Flexion ST	24.7	3.30	27.1	3.02	1.62	0.206	0.01	0.76	2.07
Extension ST	7.25	3.81	7.96	2.35	40.4	**<0.001**	**0.26**	0.23	1.57
Flexion SW	67.9	4.49	68.3	2.36	16.0	**<0.001**	0.12	0.12	1.45
Range of motion	60.7	1.72	60.4	2.27	3.35	0.070	0.03	0.15	1.47
First abduction SW	6.33	6.77	8.62	4.06	1.90	0.171	0.02	0.42	5.42
Adduction SW	−0.07	7.73	0.46	2.48	9.26	0.003	0.08	0.10	3.92
Second abduction SW	4.96	7.33	5.83	1.60	0.00	0.960	0.00	0.20	3.43
Knee (% gait cycle)									
Flexion ST	12.9	1.70	11.8	1.82	12.1	**0.001**	0.09	0.63	0.77
Extension ST	39.1	1.49	38.7	1.72	0.09	0.769	0.00	0.25	1.43
Flexion SW	72.9	0.78	72.0	1.03	19.2	**<0.001**	**0.14**	**1.00**	0.84
First abduction SW	64.5	1.80	64.5	3.01	0.11	0.740	0.00	0	1.73
Adduction SW	75.1	2.21	76.2	2.24	0.80	0.374	0.01	0.49	2.00
Second abduction SW	85.3	3.52	85.7	3.37	4.45	0.035	0.04	0.12	1.72
Ankle (degree)									
Plantarflexion ST	0.06	2.79	1.34	1.11	39.1	**<0.001**	**0.25**	0.66	1.60
Dorsiflexion ST	18.0	2.66	17.5	2.00	3.06	0.083	0.03	0.22	1.19
Plantarflexion SW	−11.3	10.7	−7.68	6.69	110	**<0.001**	**0.49**	0.42	3.25
Dorsiflexion SW	8.69	2.96	9.76	2.77	9.06	0.003	0.07	0.37	1.18
Ankle (% gait cycle)									
Plantarflexion ST	6.43	1.83	5.22	1.65	12.7	**0.001**	0.10	0.70	0.84
Dorsiflexion ST	47.3	1.48	46.9	1.27	0.01	0.940	0.00	0.29	1.10
Plantarflexion SW	64.4	1.02	63.1	1.21	3.66	0.058	0.03	**1.17**	0.95
Dorsiflexion SW	91.4	5.37	87.7	5.37	0.20	0.656	0.00	0.69	3.98

Remarks: ST = stance phase; SW = swing phase; GL1 = laboratory 1; GL2 = laboratory 2.

3.5. Scatter-Plot Technique Suggested by Bland and Altman [22]

The Bland and Altman [22] scatter-plot technique revealed that the largest (worst) bounding criterion was for frontal plane knee angle (−2.3 ± 16.1°) (Figure 3d). The hip joint angles (Figure 3a,b), as well as the sagittal plane angles of the knee joint (Figure 3c,d), had the lowest bounding range. Ankle angles in general had a small bounding range (Figure 3e,f), with the exception of the maximum plantarflexion angle during the swing phase (−3.6 ± 10.7°).

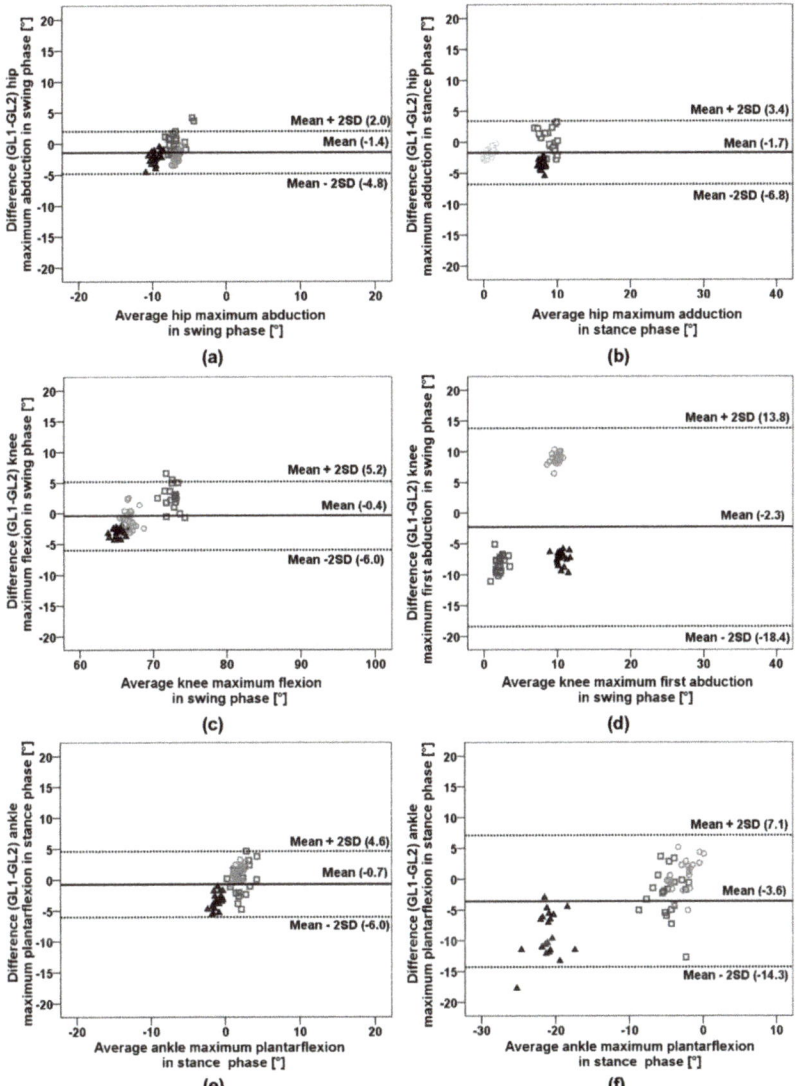

Figure 3. Bland and Altman plots presenting the computed differences between the clinical gait analysis data from the first laboratory (GL1) and the second laboratory (GL2) for (**a**,**b**) hip joint, (**c**,**d**) knee joint and (**e**,**f**) ankle joint. Each data point (test subject 1 = circle, test subject 2 = triangle, test subject 3 = square) represents the computed difference between CGA data of GL1 and GL2 (ordinate) which was plotted vs. the mean difference (abscissa) respectively, from the same healthy test subjects. The solid horizontal line represents the mean of all the differences plotted, and the two dashed lines represent the mean ± 2 SD (standard deviation) agreement interval, as defined by Bland and Altman [22].

3.6. Joint-Related Reliability

Inter- and intraobserver reliability for the ankle was in the fair-to-good and excellent ranges, in contrast to the knee and hip, which showed excellent reliability only (Table 2, Table A2). The within-site interobserver reliability for the ankle was ICC_{mean} = 0.58 (95% CI: 0.33–0.73) compared with $ICC_{mean} = 0.81$ (95% CI: 0.66–0.88) for intraobserver reliability. This was much lower than the reliability for the knee (interobserver $ICC_{mean} = 0.83$ (95% CI: 0.74–0.89), intraobserver $ICC_{mean} = 0.98$ (95% CI: 0.94–0.99)) and hip (interobserver $ICC_{mean} = 0.90$ (95% CI: 0.84–0.94), intraobserver $ICC_{mean} = 0.97$ (95% CI: 0.95–0.99)) (Table 2).

Between-laboratory intraobserver reliability showed fair-to-good reliability for all joints. Within this reliability level, small differences were found for the knee ($ICC_{mean} = 0.46$ (95% CI: 0.05–0.68)) in comparison to the ankle (between-laboratory intraobserver $ICC_{mean} = 0.58$) and hip (between-laboratory intraobserver $ICC_{mean} = 0.65$ (95% CI: 0.27–0.81)).

Based on the ICC_{total}, significant differences were calculated between all three types of reliability ($p < 0.001$) (Table 2).

4. Discussion

The ability to exchange and compare clinical gait analysis data between laboratories is a valuable tool to improve the monitoring of clinical treatments and rehabilitation progressions for patients with musculoskeletal disease. Gait analysis data was thus compared in three ways in the present study. First, to determine interobserver reliability; second, to determine intraobserver reliability; and finally, to determine between-laboratory intraobserver reliability of CGA data between two gait laboratories.

In support of our first hypothesis, the total mean reliability was excellent for interobserver ($ICC_{total} = 0.79$, 95% CI: 0.67–0.86) and intraobserver reliability ($ICC_{total} = 0.93$, 95% CI: 0.87–0.96) (Table 2). For a single laboratory, we found fair-to-good or poor interobserver reliability, which suggests an observer influence dependent on subjective observer variability and the different software used for analysis (Workstation vs. Nexus) (Table 1). These results support those of previous work by Schwartz et al. [10] (Table 3). We found excellent intraobserver reliability for one observer processing the data using the same software (excluding observer and software error). Nonetheless, ICC values for inter- and intraobserver reliability still fall under the excellent classification for a majority of the parameters observed (interobserver: 71% parameters; intraobserver: 94% parameters).

The ankle displayed fair-to-good and excellent interobserver reliability, whereas the knee and hip showed excellent reliability only (Table 2). This outcome is in general agreement with the systematic review of McGinley et al. [3], who reported excellent intra- and interobserver reliability for the parameters of the hip and knee joints in the sagittal-plane, and a lower reliability for the ankle joint. However, the observed differences within ankle kinematics may in part be attributed to technical improvements in the applied software (Nexus, version 1.3 vs. Workstation, version 4.6 build 142). However, future research is needed to investigate this possibility.

For total mean reliability, we observed fair-to-good between-laboratory intraobserver reliability ($ICC_{total} = 0.56$, 95% CI: 0.16–0.74) and excellent inter- ($ICC_{total} = 0.79$, 95% CI: 0.67–0.86) and intraobserver reliability ($ICC_{total} = 0.93$, 95% CI: 0.87–0.96). Only 26% of the between-laboratory intraobserver parameters revealed excellent ICC values, whereas the remaining 74% fell within the fair-to-good and poor ranges. Significant differences ($p \leq 0.002$) were found in 39% of the compared parameters (Table 4). This fair-to-good and poor reliability may be caused by differences in the measurement system hardware configurations and by slight differences in marker placement between data collection sessions. Both laboratories employed electro-optical motion capturing from the same manufacturer, but use a different hardware configuration (capturing software, camera type).

According to our second hypothesis, we believed that CGA data could be accurately collected between two gait laboratories, making such data interchangeable. An acceptance of this hypothesis could be affirmed for 61% of the parameters, with significant differences ($p \leq 0.002$) in the remaining 39% (Table 4). Between-laboratory intraobserver reliability of CGA data captured at two different gait analysis laboratories had total ICC values at the fair-to-good level, which was lower than the excellent inter- and intraobserver reliability values (Table 2). In general, differences were found at each joint (ankle, knee, hip) for angle as well as for time-dependent (% gait cycle) analysis. The Bland–Altman plots indicated a detectable amount of variation for specific parameters, such as the knee in the frontal plane (Figure 3d), when compared between laboratories. These plots also showed a small data distribution for each individual observer, when compared between laboratories and the largest (worst) bounding criteria for frontal plane knee angle (2.3 ± 16.1°) (Figure 3d).

The standard errors for between-laboratory intraobserver analysis (maximum abduction at stance phase $\sigma^{sess(lab)}$ = 4.2, maximum adduction at swing phase $\sigma^{sess(lab)}$ = 3.4, maximum second abduction swing phase $\sigma^{sess(lab)}$ = 3.2) supports the low between-laboratory intraobserver reliability found for the knee (ICC_{mean} = 0.46, Table 2). These values are twice as large as for inter- (maximum first abduction stance phase $\sigma^{observer}$ = 2.4; maximum adduction/abduction swing phase $\sigma^{observer}$ = 1.5; maximum second abduction swing phase $\sigma^{observer}$ = 1.3) and intraobserver reliability (maximum first abduction stance phase $\sigma^{repeated}$ = 0.8; maximum adduction/abduction swing phase $\sigma^{repeated}$ = 1.0; maximum second abduction swing phase $\sigma^{repeated}$ = 0.7). The lower between-laboratory intraobserver reliability and significant differences observed indicate an influence of the applied motion capturing camera technology on the captured CGA data between testing sites. In contrast to our measure of intra- and interobserver variability in the between-laboratory comparison, the effect of different hardware (cameras, lenses, Analog-to-digital (A/D) converter, etc.), as well as marker removal and replacement between data sets can also contribute to lower reliability. The reduction in reliability suggests that the detection of tracked markers may be affected by the different camera resolutions investigated (Vcam with 0.3 million pixels, 659 x 439 black/white pixel sensor resolution vs. MXF with 2 million pixels, 1600 x 1280 grayscale pixel sensor resolution). We believe the effect of the measurement protocol and observer dependence are probably small in comparison to available technical requirements, existing in the different generations of cameras (i.e., sensor technology) because the ICC values of the one-site interobserver reliability were much higher, falling well within the excellent classification. These findings were somewhat different than those reported by Bucknall et al. [11], who observed apparent differences during motion data captured simultaneously using three camera systems (612, MX-13 and MX-F40).

Results of this study support the findings of Gorton et al. [8] and Bucknall et al. [11], which showed a dependence of CGA data quality on system resources, as well as applying standardized measurement protocols. The fact that CGA data quality could be affected by different camera types, even ones from the same manufacturer, is problematic, not only in the context of multicenter investigations, but it could also be a problem when comparing CGA data within institutions that have recently updated their laboratory equipment. Based on these findings when multicenter investigations are considered, it is important that both laboratories use the same or comparable camera equipment and software.

A limitation of this investigation was the sample size (n = 3). Each subject performed 20 barefoot gait trials using a self-selected walking speed. Subjects had no gait pathologies, resulting in similar gait patterns. This approach included the risk of correlated observations. On the other hand, it was not feasible to conduct our investigation with actual patients (with gait pathologies) and a powered sample, due to time restrictions in subject preparation (e.g., time required for marker application) and transportation limitations between testing sites.

5. Conclusions

The results of this study showed higher intraobserver reliability than interobserver reliability for CGA data conducted in a single gait analysis laboratory. There was weaker intra- and interobserver reliability ankle kinematics when compared to the hip and knee. Inter- or intraobserver reliability for data collected at a single laboratory was much stronger compared to data collected between laboratories. The outcomes of this study indicate that CGA results are probably influenced by testing conditions, such as laboratory equipment and software (capturing software and camera type). Peer-reviewed literature has reported an effect on the repeatability of motion capture data using separate trials, sessions and observers, etc. [5–7,9,10], and for multicenter repeatability focused on different applied hardware configurations, marker placement, as well as between trials and days of measurement [3,8,11]. The results of the current study support these previous investigations, and suggest that when multicenter investigations are considered, it is important that both laboratories use the same or comparable camera equipment and software. The reduced between-laboratory intraobserver reliability implies that comparisons of CGA data between centers with varying measurement equipment are generally not recommended.

Author Contributions: Conceptualization, R.S., F.S., C.H. and R.W.; methodology, R.W., R.S., F.S. and C.H.; formal analysis, R.W., R.S. and F.S.; investigation, R.W., R.S. and F.S.; resources, C.H.; data curation, R.S.; writing—original draft preparation, R.W., R.S. and F.S.; writing—review and editing, R.S., F.S., C.H., K.L. and R.W.; visualization, F.S.; supervision, C.H.; project administration, R.S. and F.S.; All authors have read and agreed to the published version of the manuscript.

Funding: This research received no external funding.

Acknowledgments: The authors wish to thank Gavin D. Olender for his assistance during preparing this manuscript. We would although like to thank Martin Scott-Löhrer from prophysics AG (Zürich, Switzerland) for his assistance and support. We thank Siegfried Leuchte and Henning Windhagen for the supervision and support of this project. This manuscript is dedicated to Siegfried Leuchte, who passed away unexpectedly at the end of 2018. We honor him as a committed and insightful Professor and keep him in honorable memory. This research was made possible out of research cooperation between members of the Musculoskeletal Biomechanics Network (www.msb-net.org) of the DGOOC (German Association of Orthopedics and Orthopedic Surgery).

Conflicts of Interest: The authors declare no conflict of interest.

Appendix A

Table A1. Anthropometric data for each individual test subject.

	Age [years]	Body Weight [kg]	Body Height [cm]	Body Mass Index [kg·m^{-2}]
Subject 1	29	59	167	21
Subject 2	37	83	178	26
Subject 3	34	90	185	26
Mean	33.3	77.3	177	24.3
SD	4.04	16.3	9.07	2.89

Table A2. Descriptive statistics (mean ± standard deviation) and SEM values reported for intra- and interobserver reliability to describe the variability within and between subjects.

Parameter	Intraobserver			Interobserver		
	Exam 1	Exam 2	SEM	Observer 1	Observer 2	SEM
Hip (degree)						
Flexion ST	38.2 ± 1.73	38.1 ± 1.68	0	38.1 ± 1.68	38.1 ± 1.69	0.29
Extension ST	−6.58 ± 3.68	−6.57 ± 3.67	0	−6.57 ± 3.67	−6.24 ± 4.49	2.00
Flexion SW	37.6 ± 1.62	37.6 ± 1.58	0	37.6 ± 1.58	37.7 ± 1.61	0.16
Adduction ST	6.69 ± 3.71	6.71 ± 3.72	0	6.71 ± 3.72	6.53 ± 3.74	0.53
Abduction SW	−7.01 ± 1.38	−7.02 ± 1.37	0	−7.02 ± 1.37	−6.96 ± 1.45	0.37
Hip (% gait cycle)						
Flexion ST	3.55 ± 3.19	3.45 ± 3.17	0	3.45 ± 3.17	3.73 ± 3.38	0.66
Extension ST	51.0 ± 1.17	50.7 ± 1.10	0.32	50.7 ± 1.10	51.0 ± 1.13	0.49
Flexion SW	86.6 ± 3.05	86.6 ± 3.94	1.44	86.6 ± 3.94	86.2 ± 3.26	1.94
Adduction ST	25.2 ± 8.38	25.2 ± 8.15	0	25.2 ± 8.15	24.8 ± 7.81	1.78
Abduction SW	65.7 ± 3.39	65.4 ± 3.20	0.33	65.4 ± 3.20	65.1 ± 3.53	0.82
Knee (degree)						
Flexion ST	27.2 ± 3.03	27.1 ± 3.02	0	27.1 ± 3.02	27.1 ± 3.16	0.93
Extension ST	7.91 ± 2.39	7.96 ± 2.35	0	7.96 ± 2.35	7.86 ± 2.44	0
Flexion SW	68.3 ± 2.33	68.3 ± 2.36	0	68.3 ± 2.36	67.7 ± 4.58	2.53
Range of motion	60.4 ± 2.27	60.4 ± 2.27	0	60.4 ± 2.27	59.9 ± 4.48	2.61
First abduction SW	8.61 ± 4.03	8.62 ± 4.06	0	8.62 ± 4.06	8.44 ± 3.81	0.39
Adduction SW	0.44 ± 2.41	0.39 ± 2.45	0	0.39 ± 2.45	0.60 ± 2.33	0.41
Second abduction SW	5.79 ± 1.58	5.86 ± 1.60	0	5.86 ± 1.60	5.75 ± 1.47	0.27
Knee (% gait cycle)						
Flexion ST	11.9 ± 1.88	11.8 ± 1.82	0.19	11.8 ± 1.82	11.9 ± 1.69	0.61
Extension ST	38.8 ± 1.75	38.7 ± 1.72	0.25	38.7 ± 1.72	38.4 ± 1.89	0.44
Flexion SW	72.4 ± 0.97	72.0 ± 1.03	0.33	72.0 ± 1.03	71.9 ± 1.09	0.42
First abduction SW	65.0 ± 3.22	64.5 ± 3.01	0.54	64.5 ± 3.01	64.8 ± 2.96	1.19
Adduction SW	76.6 ± 2.20	76.1 ± 2.23	0.31	76.1 ± 2.23	75.5 ± 3.11	1.41
Second abduction SW	86.4 ± 3.31	85.8 ± 3.30	0.47	85.8 ± 3.30	85.8 ± 3.78	1.06
Ankle (degree)						
Plantarflexion ST	0.37 ± 1.32	1.34 ± 1.11	1.07	1.34 ± 1.11	−0.17 ± 1.24	1.11
Dorsiflexion ST	16.6 ± 1.11	17.5 ± 2.00	0.97	17.5 ± 2.00	16.0 ± 1.68	1.34
Plantarflexion SW	−8.66 ± 6.08	−7.68 ± 6.69	0.90	−7.68 ± 6.69	−9.01 ± 5.64	1.63
Dorsiflexion SW	8.92 ± 1.56	9.76 ± 2.77	0.92	9.76 ± 2.77	8.45 ± 2.25	1.33
Ankle (% gait cycle)						
Plantarflexion ST	5.35 ± 1.49	5.22 ± 1.65	0.22	5.22 ± 1.65	5.57 ± 1.31	0.42
Dorsiflexion ST	47.0 ± 1.41	46.9 ± 1.27	0.30	46.9 ± 1.27	45.7 ± 4.46	2.53
Plantarflexion SW	63.4 ± 1.12	63.1 ± 1.21	0.33	63.1 ± 1.21	62.9 ± 1.04	0.45
Dorsiflexion SW	87.6 ± 5.16	87.7 ± 5.37	1.18	87.7 ± 5.37	85.7 ± 3.81	3.25

Remarks: ST = stance phase; SW = swing phase; Exam = examination.

References

1. Sander, K.; Rosenbaum, D.; Bohm, H.; Layher, F.; Lindner, T.; Wegener, R.; Wolf, S.I.; Seehaus, F. Instrumented gait and movement analysis of musculoskeletal diseases. *Orthopade* **2012**, *41*, 802–819. [CrossRef] [PubMed]
2. Baker, R. Gait analysis methods in rehabilitation. *J. Neuroeng. Rehabil.* **2006**, *3*, 4. [CrossRef] [PubMed]
3. McGinley, J.L.; Baker, R.; Wolfe, R.; Morris, M.E. The reliability of three-dimensional kinematic gait measurements: A systematic review. *Gait Posture* **2009**, *29*, 360–369. [CrossRef] [PubMed]
4. Ferrari, A.; Benedetti, M.G.; Pavan, E.; Frigo, C.; Bettinelli, D.; Rabuffetti, M.; Crenna, P.; Leardini, A. Quantitative comparison of five current protocols in gait analysis. *Gait Posture* **2008**, *28*, 207–216. [CrossRef] [PubMed]
5. Noonan, K.J.; Halliday, S.; Browne, R.; O'Brien, S.; Kayes, K.; Feinberg, J.R. Interobserver variability of gait analysis in patients with cerebral palsy. *J. Pediatr. Orthop.* **2003**, *23*, 279–287. [CrossRef]

6. Kadaba, M.P.; Ramakrishnan, H.K.; Wootten, M.E.; Gainey, J.; Gorton, G.; Cochran, G.V. Repeatability of kinematic, kinetic, and electromyographic data in normal adult gait. *J. Orthop. Res.* **1989**, *7*, 849–860. [CrossRef]
7. Steinwender, G.; Saraph, V.; Scheiber, S.; Zwick, E.B.; Uitz, C.; Hackl, K. Intrasubject repeatability of gait analysis data in normal and spastic children. *Clin. Biomech.* **2000**, *15*, 134–139. [CrossRef]
8. Gorton, G.E., 3rd; Hebert, D.A.; Gannotti, M.E. Assessment of the kinematic variability among 12 motion analysis laboratories. *Gait Posture* **2009**, *29*, 398–402. [CrossRef]
9. Growney, E.; Meglan, D.; Johnson, M.; Cahalan, T.; An, K.-N. Repeated measures of adult normal walking using a video tracking system. *Gait Posture* **1997**, *6*, 147–162. [CrossRef]
10. Schwartz, M.H.; Trost, J.P.; Wervey, R.A. Measurement and management of errors in quantitative gait data. *Gait Posture* **2004**, *20*, 196–203. [CrossRef]
11. Bucknall, V.; Gibbs, S.; Arnold, G.P. Comparison of the kinematic data from three different Vicon systems. Gait Posture. *Gait Posture* **2008**, *28*, S33–S34. [CrossRef]
12. Kolber, M.J.; Beekhuizen, K.; Cheng, M.S.; Fiebert, I.M. The reliability of hand-held dynamometry in measuring isometric strength of the shoulder internal and external rotator musculature using a stabilization device. *Physiother. Theory Pract.* **2007**, *23*, 119–124. [CrossRef] [PubMed]
13. Kolber, M.J.; Hanney, W.J. The reliability and concurrent validity of shoulder mobility measurements using a digital inclinometer and goniometer: A technical report. *Int. J. Sports Phys. Ther.* **2012**, *7*, 306–313.
14. Cools, A.M.; De Wilde, L.; Van Tongel, A.; Ceyssens, C.; Ryckewaert, R.; Cambier, D.C. Measuring shoulder external and internal rotation strength and range of motion: Comprehensive intrarater and interrater reliability study of several testing protocols. *J. Shoulder Elbow Surg.* **2014**, *23*, 1454–1461. [CrossRef] [PubMed]
15. Mullaney, M.J.; McHugh, M.P.; Johnson, C.P.; Tyler, T.F. Reliability of shoulder range of motion comparing a goniometer to a digital level. *Physiother. Theory Pract.* **2010**, *26*, 327–333. [CrossRef] [PubMed]
16. Muir, S.W.; Corea, C.L.; Beaupre, L. Evaluating change in clinical status: Reliability and measures of agreement for the assessment of glenohumeral range of motion. *N. Am. J. Sports Phys. Ther.* **2010**, *5*, 98–110.
17. May, S.; Littlewood, C.; Bishop, A. Reliability of procedures used in the physical examination of non-specific low back pain: A systematic review. *Aust. J. Physiother.* **2006**, *52*, 91–102. [CrossRef]
18. Wilhelmsen, K.; Strand, L.I.; Nordahl, S.H.G.; Eide, G.E.; Ljunggren, A.E. Psychometric properties of the Vertigo symptom scale: Short form. *BMC Ear Nose Throat Disord.* **2008**, *8*, 2. [CrossRef]
19. Kadaba, M.P.; Ramakrishnan, H.K.; Wootten, M.E. Measurement of lower extremity kinematics during level walking. *J. Orthop. Res.* **1990**, *8*, 383–392. [CrossRef]
20. Benedetti, M.G.; Catani, F.; Leardini, A.; Pignotti, E.; Giannini, S. Data management in gait analysis for clinical applications. *Clin. Biomech.* **1998**, *13*, 204–215. [CrossRef]
21. Shrout, P.E.; Fleiss, J.L. Intraclass correlations: Uses in assessing rater reliability. *Psychol. Bull.* **1979**, *86*, 420–428. [CrossRef] [PubMed]
22. Bland, J.M.; Altman, D.G. Statistical methods for assessing agreement between two methods of clinical measurement. *Lancet* **1986**, *1*, 307–310. [CrossRef]
23. Portney, L.G.; Watkins, M.P. *Foundations of Clinical Research: Applications to Practice*, 3rd ed.; Pearson Prentice Hall: Upper Saddle River, NJ, USA, 2009.
24. Weir, J.P. Quantifying Test-Retest Reliability Using the Intraclass Correlation Coefficient and the SEM. *J. Strength Cond. Res.* **2005**, *19*. [CrossRef]
25. Richardson, J.T.E. Eta squared and partial eta squared as measures of effect size in educational research. *Edu. Res. Rev.* **2011**, *6*, 135–147. [CrossRef]
26. Hartmann, A.; Herzog, T.; Drinkmann, A. Psychotherapy of bulimia nervosa: What is effective? A meta-analysis. *J. Psychosom. Res.* **1992**, *36*, 159–167. [CrossRef]
27. Cohen, J. *Statistical Power Analysis for the Behavioural Sciences*, 2nd ed.; Lawrence Erlbaum: Hillsdale, NJ, USA, 1998.

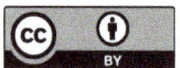

© 2020 by the authors. Licensee MDPI, Basel, Switzerland. This article is an open access article distributed under the terms and conditions of the Creative Commons Attribution (CC BY) license (http://creativecommons.org/licenses/by/4.0/).

MDPI
St. Alban-Anlage 66
4052 Basel
Switzerland
Tel. +41 61 683 77 34
Fax +41 61 302 89 18
www.mdpi.com

Applied Sciences Editorial Office
E-mail: applsci@mdpi.com
www.mdpi.com/journal/applsci

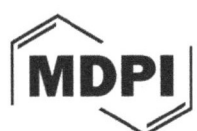

www.ingramcontent.com/pod-product-compliance
Lightning Source LLC
LaVergne TN
LVHW070453100526
838202LV00014B/1716